PHYSIOLOGY
OF
SPORTS AND EXERCISE

PHYSIOLOGY OF SPORTS AND EXERCISE

Dr Pralay Majumdar MSc, PhD
Physiologist
Sports Authority of India

New Central Book Agency (P) Ltd
LONDON
HYDERABAD ERNAKULAM BHUBANESWAR
DELHI KOLKATA PUNE

REGD OFFICE

8/1 Chintamoni Das Lane, Kolkata 700 009, India
email: ncbapvtltd@eth.net

OVERSEAS

NCBA (UK) Ltd, 149 Park Avenue North, Northampton, NN3 2HY, UK

EXPORT

NCBA Exports Pvt. Ltd, 212 Shahpur Jat, New Delhi 110 049
email: ncbaexp@ncbapvtltd.com

BRANCHES

208B Peacock Lane, Shahpur Jat
New Delhi 110 049
email: ncbadel@ncbapvtltd.com

Shop Nos. 3 & 4, Vinayak Towers
681/B Budhwar Peth, Appa Balwant Chowk
Pune 411 002
email: ncbapune@ncbapvtltd.com

House No. 3-1-315, 1st Floor
Nimboliadda, Kachiguda, **Hyderabad** 500 027
email: ncbahydb@ncbapvtltd.com

GSS Shopping Complex, 1st Floor
Opposite College Post Office, Convent Road
Ernakulam 682 035
email: ncbaernk@ncbapvtltd.com

Shop No. 15, Bharati Towers, Ground Floor
Forest Park, **Bhubaneswar** 751 001
email: ncbabub@ncbapvtltd.com

PHYSIOLOGY OF SPORTS AND EXERCISE

First Published: October 2002
Reprinted: February 2005
Reprinted: July 2011

PUBLISHER AND TYPESETTER
New Central Book Agency (P) Ltd
8/1 Chintamoni Das Lane, Kolkata 700 009

PRINTER
New Central Book Agency (P) Ltd
Web-Offset Division, Dhulagarh, Sankrail, Howrah

COVER DESIGNER
Ankit, Kolkata

COVER PRINTER
Biswanath Studio, Kolkata

PROOF CHECKING
Subas Maita, Suchismita Sengupta

PROJECT TEAM
Sukumar Patra, Prabir Ghosh, Prabhat Jas and Ananta Bhowmik

ISBN: 81-7381-426-7

Price: ₹ 235.00

PREFACE

Modern competitive sports training rely on the principles of Exercise Physiology. In the recent decades interest in this subject has increased to a great extent in India, both among academicians and professionals. Information in this field of speciality is proliferating at the international level with publication of books by several authors at a time. However, these books could not meet the demand of the Indian situation because of reasons like cost-effectiveness of foreign publications and availability of a limited number of international books in the Indian market.

In undertaking the preparation and development of **PHYSIOLOGY OF SPORTS AND EXERCISE** the author wanted to provide some background on why he decided to take on the challenge of writing a text book of this magnitude. **In India, Exercise Physiology is being taught at various levels of academic courses that include M. Sc. in Physiology, B. P. Ed., M. P. Ed. and the courses offered by Sports Authority of India (SAI) viz. Diploma in Sports Coaching (NIS Diploma), Master in Sports coaching (MS) and Diploma in Sports Medicine (DSM). A comprehensive text book of Exercise Physiology (by Indian author) with recent information is not available at present,** although a few books were written by Indian authors too. They primarily deal with Physiology as a basic subject and are devoid of information about the physiological changes related to exercise.

This endeavor by the author was taken up to fill the void and present a book containing material of both academic and professional interest. The author experienced the need as an academic professional that **careful integration of information from both text book and recent research is important to present the timely and logical progression of both knowledge and data.** In improving on the structure and organization of material, **it is important that the content be as current as possible, while simultaneously addressing the increasingly diverse needs for the Exercise Physiology student.**

In the past, texts had divided content biased on systems, physiology and have presented specific examples of how exercise affects physiology. However, **students may still be struggling to simply understand the basic concepts.** Acute and chorionic adaptation to exercise may be dispersed throughout the text, further leaving their importance under-emphasized and vague. Consistently confusion and frustration can be the result. Rather, adaptation of exercise during acute and chronic time frame provides a knowledge base that is a logical extension of pure physiology as well as a logical format in which to present research findings. **So, in this treatise, application of exercise physiology to exercise testing of various population are also addressed since these represent areas for growth as well as for future direction, for the field of Exercise Physiology.**

The concepts in these texts are presented in a simple and a straight-forward style.

Illustration and examples have been frequently used to clarify the subject more and are further explained as a concept. All topics in Exercise Physiology addressed within this text are presented in a contemporary fashion supported by uptodate references.

The text contains sixteen chapters. Special emphasis has been laid in **Chapter 1 about the physiological development in India**. In **Chapter 2**, the author **deals with the cellular function and the homeostatic control which help the students to have a deeper understanding about the unique and complex cellular function**. In **Chapter 3**, which **deals with the cardiovascular system,** more stress has been given on the cardiovascular adaptation to methodical training and the monitoring of heart rate to identify training load. In **Chapter 4, the respiratory system**, emphasis has been laid on the mechanics and mechanism of breathing and the exchange of gases (oxygen & carbon dioxide) across the membrane. **Chapter 5**, which **deals with the muscular system** more inputs have been given on the neuromuscular control, the mechanism of muscular contraction and the fiber type and athletic success. **Chapter 6 denotes the energy system** where the emphasis has been laid for measuring energy use during exercise and the predominant energy released in various games and sports activities. **Chapter 7 deals with fatigue and exhaustion** which entails about the factors limiting all-out anerobic performance and the aerobic activities. **Chapter 8 deals with growth and development** where emphasis has been given about the physiological implication of training the young athlete. **Chapter 9**, which **primarily deals with woman and sports performance,** gives the information about the physiological differences of male and female and physiological adaptation to exercise and training between the population. **Chapter 10 deals with thermoregulation of exercise** where more information is given about the physiological adjustments during heat and cold acclimatization and the effects of age, sex and obesity. **Chapter 11 entails the altitude and performance** where information are available about the altitude training and its benefits. **Chapter 12 deals with the hormonal regulation of exercise** where special reference has been given about the endocrine response to exercise. In **Chapter 13**, which **deals with food nutrition and sports performance**, the emphasis is laid about carbohydrate and its usage during exercise and nutrition for improved sports performance. In **Chapter 14**, which **deals with the training for performance**, the principal focus is physiological and metabolic adaptation to aerobic training and the neuromuscular adaptation to strength training. **Various information about overtraining, detraining and retraining are also updated. Chapter 15 deals with the references** and **Chapter 16 deals with the scientific contributions of the author**.

Again, I wish to express my deepest appreciation to all the persons who have helped in the preparation of this book. I am particularly grateful to Shir M. P. Ganesh, Executive Director, SAI, Southern Center, Bangalore, for constant inspiration. I extend my gratitude to all my colleagues in the Dept. of Exercise Physiology and my students who are the driving force for this effort.

Bangalore, India
September 2002

Dr. P. Majumdar

CONTENTS

CONTENTS

CONTENTS

CONTENTS

CONTENTS

CONTENTS

CONTENTS

CONTENTS

CONTENTS

CONTENTS

1

INTRODUCTORY NOTE

Exercise physiology has evolved from its parent discipline, Physiology. It is concerned with the study of how the body adapts physiologically to the acute stress of exercise, or physical activity, and the chronic state of physical training. Exercise physiology is a relative newcomer to the world of science. Exercise physiology can be defined as the study of how exercise alters the structure and function of human body.

Organized research to specifically learn more about how the body functions during exercise has a history of chemistry and nutrition (**Lusk, 1928**). At the same time the ability of the body to combust foodstuffs during exercise was researched (**Lusk, 1928**) and allowed calculations of efficiency, the energy expended during exercise, and the principles of using energy expenditure as a measure of exercise intensity.

The first text book published on exercise physiology was by Fernand La Grange entitled 'Physiology of Bodily Exercise' in 1889 (**La Grange, 1889**). That was an initial attempt to explain the body's response to exercise which was earlier limited to many of rambling theory and little fact. During the late 1800s many theories were proposed to explain the source of energy for muscle contraction. Because the energy demands for muscle action is high, this tissue served as an ideal model to expose the mysteries of cellular metabolism. In 1921 A. V. Hill was awarded the Nobel prize for his finding on energy metabolism.

A surprising large volume of research was also being conducted using exercise during the first three decades of the twentieth century. **Hill, 1923,** of Great Britain, studied oxygen consumption during exercise. Rubner and Voit (**in Lusk, 1928**) extended the theoretic findings of Lavoisier with human research of indirect calorimetry in differing nutritional, environmental and exercise conditions. Hill and Meyerhoff published extensive findings of carbohydrate catabolism and the production of lactic acid in skeletal muscles. Three physiologists, A. V. Hill, August Krogh and Otto Meyerhoff, received the Noble prize for work related to muscular exercise. At that time Biochemistry was in its infancy, which gradually established itself by pioneering scientific effort of such Nobel laureates as Albert Szent Gorgyi, Otto Meyerhoff, August Krogh and Hans Krebs, who were actively studying how living cells generate energy. Although much of Hill's research was conducted with isolated frog muscle, he also conducted some physiological studies on distance runners. Such studies were possible through the technical contributions of J. S. Haldane, who developed the method and equipment needed to measure oxygen during exercise. J. S. Haldane did some of the original work on the role of CO_2 in the control of breathing. Haldane also developed the respiratory gas analyzer that bears his name. C. G. Douglas did pioneering work with Haldane in role of O_2 and lactic acid in control of breathing during exercise; including some work conducted at various altitudes. A contemporary of Douglus, who did the classic work on how O_2 binds to hemoglobin was Christian Bohr's dissociation curve due to the addition of CO_2 bears his name (Bohr effect). It was in Bohr's lab that Krogh got his start on a carrier studying respiration and exercise in humans (**Fenn W. O. and Rahn H., 1964**) The other investigators provided the basic frame-work of our understanding of whole body energy production, which became the focus of considerable research during the middle of the 20th century.

In the United States an organized effort investigating the effects of exercise on the human body began after the formation of the Harvard Fatigue Lab in 1927. The Harvard Fatigue Laboratory (HFL) became the Mecca of exercise physiology in the late 1920s until its closure in 1947. HFL was founded by the biochemist L. J. Henderson and directed by David Bruce Dill. D. B. Dill was the research director of the lab, he remained in this position until the laboratory closed in 1947. Throughout his life Dr. Dill was intrigued by the physiology and adaptability of many animals who survived in extreme environmental conditions, but he is best remembered for his research on human responses to exercise, heat, high altitude and other environmental factors. Dr. Dill always served as one of the human 'guinea pigs' in these studies. During the Harvard Fatigue Laboratory's 20 years of existence, he and his co-workers produced 330 scientific papers along with a classic book Life Heat and Altitude (**Dill 1938**). Research from HFL was conducted in the area of environmental physiology (altitude, dry and moist heat), skeletal muscle metabolism during exercise, the effect of aging on metabolism at rest and during exercise, blood transport and acid base balance and nutrition (**Buskirk, 1992**).

After the Harvard Fatigue Laboratory closed its doors in 1947, Dr. Dill began a second career as Dy. Director of Medical Research for the Army Chemical Corps, a position he held until his retirement from the post in 1961. Dr. Dill was then 70 years old, an age he considered too young for retirement, so he moved his exercise research to Indiana University, where he served as a senior physiologist until 1966. In 1967 he obtained funding to establish the Desert Research Lab at the University of Nevada at Las Vegas. Dr. Dill used this lab as a base for his studies on human tolerance to exercise in the desert and at high altitude. He continued his research and writing until his final retirement at age 93, the same year he produced his last publication, a book entitled 'The Hot Life of Man and Beast' (**Dill, 1985**).

In the earlier years the HFL focused primarily on general problems of exercise, nutrition and health. For example, studies on exercise and aging were first conducted in 1939 by Sid Robinson, a student in the HFL. Based on his studies of subjects aged 6-91 years, Robinson described the effects of aging on maximum heart rate (HR) and Oxygen (O_2) uptake. But with the onset of World War II (1939-45), the HFL took a different direction used for military research. HFL trained most of those who became world leaders in exercise physiology through the 1950s and 1960s. Most contemporary exercise physiologists can trace their roots back to the HFL.

THE SCANDINAVIAN INFLUENCE

Early contact between D. B. Dill and August Krogh, a Danish Nobel prize winner, led to the coming of 3 exceptional Danish physiologists to the HFL in 1930s. Krogh encouraged Erik-Hohw Christensen, Erling Asmussen and Marius Nielsen to spend time at Harvard, studying exercise in the heat and at high altitude. After returning to Scandinavia, each man established a separate line of research. Asmussen and Nielsen became professors at the University of Copenhagen. Asmussen studied the mechanical properties of muscle and Nielsen studied body temperature control. Both remained active at the University of Copenhagen's August Krogh Institute until their retirements. In 1941, Hohw Christensen moved to Stockholm to become the first physiology professor at the college of physical education at Gymnastic-Och Idrottshog-skolan (GIH). In the late 1930s he joined with Ole Hansen to conduct and publish a series of five important studies of carbohydrate and fat metabolism during exercise.

Hohw Christensen introduced Olof Astrand to the field of exercise physiology. Astrand who — conducted numerous studies related to physical fitness and endurance capacity during the 1950s and 1960s — became the Director of GIH after Christensen retired in 1960. Astrand and Christensen were also the mentors of Bengt Saltin, one of today's leading contributors to our understanding of muscle metabolism during exercise. Beyond their work at Gymnastic-Och-Idrottshog-skolan both Christensen and Astrand interacted with physiologists at the Karolinska Institute in Stockholm who studied clinical application of exercise. It is hard to single out the most exceptional contributions from this institute, but Bergstrom's reintroduction of the biopsy needle (1960) to sample muscle tissue was a pivotal point to conduct histological and biochemical studies on human muscle before, during and after exercise. Other invasive studies of blood circulation have subsequently been conducted by physiologists at GIH and at the Karolinska Institute.

At about the time Bergstrom reintroduced the needle biopsy procedure, a new breed of exercise physiologists were well trained as biochemistry emerged. In Stockholm, Bengt Saltin realized the value of this procedure for studying muscle structure and biochemistry. He first collaborated with Bergstrom in the late 1960s to study the effect of diet on muscle endurance and muscle nutrition (**Bergstrom, 1962**). About the same time Reggie Edgerton (University of California, LA) and Phil Gollnick (Washington State University) was using rats to study the characteristics of muscle fiber and their responses to training. Saltin combined his knowledge of the biopsy procedure with Gollnick's biochemical talents. These researchers were responsible for many early studies on human muscle fibre characteristics and use during exercise. Although many biochemists have used exercise to study metabolism, few have had more impact on the current direction of human exercise physiology than Bergstrom, Saltin and Gollnick. As the HFL had been the Mecca of exercise physiology between 1927 and 1947, the Scandinavian Labs have been equally noteworthy since many leading investigations during the past 20 years were collaborations between American and Scandinavian exercise physiologists.

EXERCISE PHYSIOLOGY IN INDIA

Emergence of exercise physiology in India is a relatively new development. Teaching in physiology as a basic science was started in the year 1913 at Calcutta University. The focus was mostly on clinical aspects until 1950. Preliminary studies were initiated at Presidency College, Kolkata, under the leadership of Prof. S. N. Banerjee. The research was carried out on energy metabolism, measurement of body surface area and the changes in blood chemistry (**Sen, 1954; Banerjee and Sen, 1955; Sen, 1955; Banerjee and Sen, 1958; Sen & Banerjee, 1958**). During the 1960s a number of scientists started research on work physiology which includes environmental stress (**Maitra et al, 1968; Sen et al, 1964; Malhotra et al, 1966; Mathur, 1969**), industrial load & efficiency of the worker (**Sen et al, 1965; Sen et al, 1966**), respiratory physiology, metabolic changes (**Maitra et al, 1966; Maitra et al, 1967; Das et al, 1968**), and biochemical changes related to exercise stress (**Banerjee et al, 1969**).

Probably the first ever work on sports in India was by **D. N. Mathur (1969)** on interval training changes on blood sugar. Seventh decade had marked for growth of the work physiology in many directions. The scientists of Defence Institute of

Physiology and Allied Sciences contributed significantly in the area of environmental physiology, nutrition and sports (**Malhotra, 1966; Nair et al, 1971a,b; Brahmachari et al, 1972a,b; Sengupta et al, 1972; Malhotra et al, 1971, 1973; Bhardwaj et, al 1973**).

Specialized work on sports physiology was also carried out at Calcutta University in the beginning of the 1970s but the projects undertaken by the scientists were mostly academic rather than applied research (**Banerjee et al, 1974; Chatterjee et al, 1978**). Holding of Asian Games at New Delhi in 1982 gave a boost to this field of specialization and research work was started in a large scale all over the country. Leadership was taken by the then National Institute of Sports, Patiala. International Scientific Congress of Sports Sciences was held at Patiala in this year and scientists from all over the country took part in the discussion (**Proc. International Congress of Sports Sciences, 1982**). The scientists of NIS embraced a variety of topics directly related to the sports performance which broadly include studies on sports population, physiological variables influencing training load and recovery; physiological changes at altitude etc. (**Sodhi, 1980a, 1980b, 1983; Malhotra et al, 1982; Khanna et al, 1983; Malhotra et al, 1983; Malhotra and Khanna, 1984; Khanna et al, 1983, 1985, 1986,a,b. Ghosh et al, 1984; Ghosh et al, 1985a,b,c,d,e,f; Ghosh et al, 1986,a,b,c,d,e; Ghosh et al, 1987; Ghosh et al, 1988**). Further extensive studies were completed after the development of sports sciences in four regional centers of Sports Authority of India in the year 1990s (**Dey et al, 1991; Ghosh et al, 1990; Ghosh et al, 1991,a,b; Ghosh et al, 1993; Ghosh et al, 1995; Goswami et al, 1995; Gupta et al, 1996; Khanna et al, 1991; 1992a,b,c; 1993a,b; 1995a,b,c; 1996a,b,c,d; 1998; Majumdar, 1994, 1997, 1998.**)

EXERCISE PHYSIOLOGY AND OTHER FIELDS

Physiology has always been the basis for Clinical Medicine. In the same manner, exercise physiology has provided essential knowledge for many other areas, such as physical education, physical fitness and health promotion. Although physical educators such as Dudley Sargent, J. H. McCurdy, and others studied the effect of physical training on strength and endurance, Peter Karpovich, a Russian immigrant who had been briefly associated with HFL, must be credited with introducing physiology to physical education in USA. Karpovich established his own research faculty and taught physiology at Springfield College (Massachusetts) from 1927 until his death in 1968. Although he made numerous contributions to physical education and exercise physiology research, he is best remembered for the outstanding students he advised. Another Springfield faculty member, Swimming Coach T. K. Cureton created an exercise physiology lab at the University of Illinois in 1941. He continued his research and taught many of today's leaders in physical fitness and exercise physiology until his retirement in 1971. Physical fitness programs developed by Cureton and his students and Kenneth Cooper's 1968 book 'Aerobics' established a physiological rationale for using exercise to promote a healthy lifestyle (**Cooper, 1968**). A major area of interest for exercise physiologist as the body's acute responses to individual bout of exercise. Few selected physiological variables can be monitored during exercise in the field, but some can be assessed accurately without disrupting performance. For example radiotelemetry and miniature tape recorders can be used to monitor during activity :

- — Heart activity (HR & ECG).
- — Respiration rate.
- — Skin and deep body temp.
- — Muscle activity (Electromyogram).
- — O_2 consumption (**Cosmed K2** system).

Athletes have served as subjects in exercise physiology studies since the early days at HFL. Most often, these athletes were used to assess the upper limits of human strength and endurance and ascertain the characteristics needed for record setting performances. Some attempts have been made to use the technology and knowledge derived from exercise physiology to predict performance, to prescribe training or to identify athlete's exceptional potential.

Most often participants must be evaluated in the laboratory where they can be studied more thoroughly and under tightly controlled condition. Conditions under which research participants are monitored, both at rest and during exercise, must be carefully controlled. Environmental factors, such as temperature, humidity, altitude and noise, can affect the magnitude of response of all basic physiological systems. Similarly, diurnal and menstrual cycles must be controlled for.

Table 1 : Variations in HR response to running at 14 Kph on a treadmill with environmental alterations

Environmental factor	Heart rate (bpm) Rest	Exercise
Temperature (50% humidity)		
21 °C (70 °F)	60	165
35 °C (95 °F)	70	190
Humidity (21C)		
50%	60	165
90%	65	175
Noise level (21C, 50% Humidity)		
Low	60	165
High	70	165
Food intake		
Small meal 3hrs before exercise	60	165
Large meal 30 min before exercise	70	175

Table 2 : An Example of Diurnal Variation in HR at Rest and During Exercise

Condition	2 AM	6 AM	10 AM	2 PM	6 PM	10 PM
	Heart rate (beats per minute)					
Resting	65	69	73	74	72	69
Light Exercise	100	103	109	109	105	104
Moderate Exercise	130	131	138	139	135	134
Maximal Exercise	179	179	183	184	181	181
Recovery 3 min.	118	122	129	128	128	125

(Data from **Railly and Brooks, 1990**)

Research in exercise physiology has undergone several transitions identified as "the beginning", "the era of sports and athletics" and "the era of Medical Awakening". Nutrition and muscle metabolism are good examples of topics in which research progressed from resting conditions to the conditions that provides the greatest challenge to homeostasis in each example : Exercise. This early research soon provided adequate knowledge from which scientists could begin to ask and the answer applied questions that concerned exercise (**Chapman and Mitchell, 1965**).

Table 3 : Development of research and interest areas involving exercise

Historical Category	Important research topic	Dates
Beginning	Nutrient needs that accompany exercise Body's cardiorespiratory responses to exercise. Potential causes of muscle fatigue during exercise. Body's response to exercise in hot and cold environments. Regulating of chemical reaction in skeletal muscle and fever.	1960
Era of sports and athletics	Influence of diet and exercise on muscle carbohydrate stores. Muscle metabolic demands of different exercise intensities. Motor unit and muscle fibre type determinants of exercise performance. Effects of training on cardio-vascular and muscle function. Effects of training on exercise performance Effects of exercise performed in different environment.	1960-1980
Era of Medical awakening	Effects of exercise training on health and quality of life. Effects exercise training on cholesterol Effects of exercise training on heart function in diseased population. Effects of exercise training on disease prevention and rehabilitation. Role of exercise in health promotion.	1970
Present Status of Exercise Research and Knowledge	Role of exercise in supplying body functions in microgravity	1990-Present

Exercise as on independent risk factor for heart disease. Benefit of exercise for special populations disabled, elderly, children, pregnant women, etc., Molecular adaptations of skeletal muscle to exercise. Regulation of blood flow through skeletal muscle during exercise. During the 1960s and 1970s research findings were presented that indicated the potential for exercise to aid not only to athlete but also the average citizen had fewer signs of degenerative diseases and arguably had a higher quality of life. Indirect research evidence linked these differences to the adaptation of the body to continued exercise stress.

The vocalization of the medical doctors who are hooked on exercise, such as George Sheehan, Kenneth Cooper, assisted the recognition of the important health benefits of exercise by the medical community. In conjunction with the known deteriorating fitness of Western societies children with those of the United States being a notable example, and the increasing incidence of and the mortality from coronary artery disease, the role of exercise in health maintenance and disease prevention was given increased attention. Today exercise is used as a therapy during rehabilitation from injury and illness and as a preventive strategy to combat atherosclerotic cardiovascular disease. The medical interest in exercise physiology is developing a separate discipline, clinical exercise physiology and textbooks are being written to satisfy this need.

The recent history of exercise physiology is best categorised into the divisions of pure research and applied research. Pure research uses exercise to understand physiology whereas applied research uses physiology to further understand exercises. Despite the overwhelming medical interest in exercise physiology, applied research remains an important, if not primary, component of the discipline. The quest for fostering optimal athletic performance remains driving force for this research. However, today the focus of the research is not just on elite athletes but also the increasing population of individuals now participating in regular physical activity.

In the last 50 years, tremendous achievements have been possible in both pure and applied research because of the application of techniques to new conditions. During the late 1960s the application of the needlè biopsy of percutaneous muscle to research of muscle biochemistry stimulated a wealth of research. Today, the use of stable isotopes to study cellular metabolism in humans during rest exercise and post exercise conditions has contributed to the further understanding of substrates used during exercise. Similarly, non-invasive techniques such as magnetic resonance (MR), imaging and MR spectroscopy are providing insight into the function and adaptability of skeletal muscle metabolism to different exercise intensities.

INSTRUMENT USED IN EXERCISE PHYSIOLOGY

An ergometer is a device that allows the amount and rate of physical work to be measured under standardize conditions. For many years the cycle ergometer was the primary testing devise in use.

Cycle ergometers are generally based on one of four types of resistance: (a) Mechanical friction (Power output depends on pedal rate). (b) Electrical resistance (electrical resistance device) resistance is provided by an electrical conductor that moves through a magnetic or electromagnetic field. The strength of magnetic field determines the resistance to pedaling. The resistance increases automatically as the pedal rate increases, to provide a constant power output. (c) Air resistance cycle ergometer, the fly wheel of a standard mechanically braked ergometer is replaced by a free wheel that contains a series of fan blades arranged like

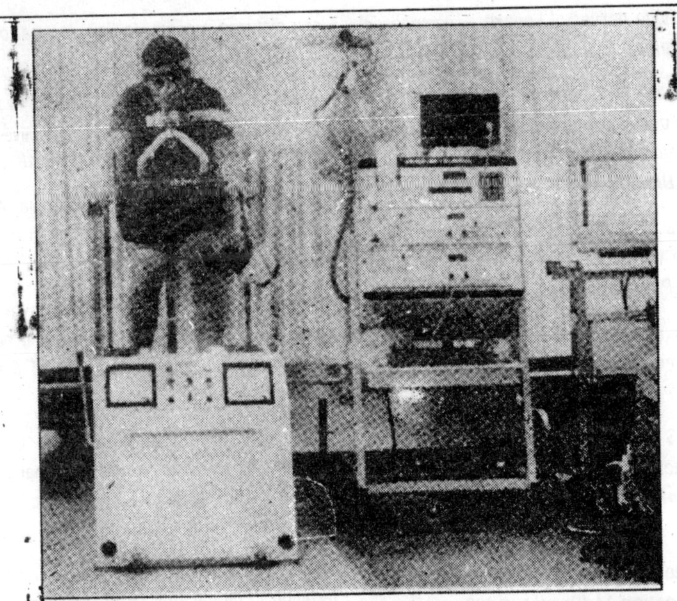

Fig. 1.1 : The equipment used to measure respiratory exchange

spokes. The fan blades displace air as the wheel turns, so the resistance encountered is directly proportional to the pedalling rate. (d) Cycle ergometer that uses hydraulic fluid to vary resistance can produce constant power output independent of pedal rate. As you propel the ergometer, the hydraulic fluid is forced through an opening. Varying the size of the opening allows variation of the resistance against which you propel. The larger the opening, the easier the fluid can flow, thus causing less resistance.

Cycle ergometers are the most appropriate devices for evaluating changes in submaximal physiological function before and after training in people whose weights have changed. Resistance on a cycle ergometer is independent of body weight, but the work performed on a treadmill is directly related to it.

Treadmills generally produce higher peak values for almost all assessed physiological variables such as heart rate ventilation and oxygen uptake. Tethered swimming has provided valuable information about physiological responses, but swimmer's movements are not very natural with this method. The swimming flume, however, allows free swimming and provides results that can be applied to competitive and recreational swimming. When assessing the body's responses to exercise it is essential that the mode of testing be carefully matched to the type of activity a person usually performs. A major area of concern for exercise physiologists is how the body adapts to chronic exposure to exercise or training. These adaptations are highly specific to the type of training you do.

REFERENCES

Banerjee, P. K., Chatterjee, S. P., Chatterjee, P. and Maitra, S. R. (1974) : Aerobic capacity in Bengali young man trained and untrained. ***Indian Journal of Physiology &. Allied Sciençes*** 28 : 91.

Banerjee, S. and Sen R. N. (1955) : Determination of the surface of the body of Indians. ***Journal of Applied Physiology*** 7 : 585-88.

Bhardwaj, K. H., Malhotra, M. S. and Srivastava, K. K. (1973a) : Body composition changes in the plains on descend from high altitude. ***Human Biology*** 46 : 41-56.

Bhardwaj, S., Singh, A. P. and Malhotra, M. S. (1973b) : Body composition of the high altitude natives of Ladakh. A comparison with sea level residents. ***Human Biology*** 45 : 423-434, 1973.

Brahmachari, H. D., Malhotra, M. S. and Joseph, S. (1972a) : Carbohydrate metabolism under environmental stress. Part II : Glucose tolerance under heat, cold and hypoxic stress. ***Indian Journal of Experimental Biology*** 10 : 272-273, 1972.

Brahmachari, H. D., Malhotra, M. S. and Joseph S. (1972b) : Effect of stay at high altitude on the serum proteins of man. ***Indian Journal of Physiology & Pharmacology*** 17 : 365-369.

Banerjee, S. and Sen, R. N. (1958) : Body composition of Indians and its relation to basal metabolic rate. ***Journal of Applied Physiology*** 12 : 29-33.

Banerjee, P. K., Chatterjee, S. and Maitra S. R. 1969; Changes in concentration of serum protein fractions in response to treadmill runners. ***Indian Journal of Physiology & Allied Sciences*** 23 : 26-30.

Bergstrom, J. (1962). Muscle electrolytes in man. Scandinavian, ***Journal of Clinical Investigation*** 14 (Suppl.), 1-100.

Buskirk, E. R. (1992) : from Harvard to Minnesota : Keys to our history, ***Exercise Sports. Science Review*** 20 : 1-26.

Chapman, C. B., and J.H. Mitchell (1965) : The physiology of exercise, ***Scientific American*** 212 : 88-96.

Chatterjee, S., Chatterjee, P. and Maitra S. R. (1978) : Effect of graded workload on the heart of different age groups. ***Digest, ESWBME***, New Delhi, pp 126.

Cooper, K. H. (1968) ***Aerobic***, New York : Evans.

Das, S. K., Chatterjee, S., Chatterjee P. and Maitra, S. R. (1968) : Studies on some aspects of respiration and metabolism in dog under pentothal sodium anaesthesia. ***Indian Journal of Physiology & Allied Sciences*** 22 : 70.

Dey, S. K., Khanna, G. L., Batra, M. (1993) Morphological and physiological studies on Indian National Kabaddi players. ***British Journal of Sports Medicine*** 27(9) 237-41.

Dey, S. K., Khanna, G. L. and Batra, M. (1991) Morphological and physiological study on Indian National Kabaddi player, ***Indian Journal of Physiology & Allied Sciences*** 45 (4), 30-31.

Dill, D. B. (1985) ***The hot life of man and beast***. Springfield. I. L. Charles, C. Thomas.

Dill, D. B. (1938) ***Life, heat and altitude***. Cambridge, MA, Harvard University press.

Fenn, W. O. and H. Rahn eds (1964) ***Handbook of physiology : respiration***, Vol. 1, American Physiology Society, Washington D.C.

Ghosh, A. K., Majumdar, P., Goswami, A. and Khanna, G. L. (1988b) : Aerobic anaerobic transition level of Indian middle and long distance runners. ***Indian Journal of Medical Research*** 88, 10, 371-375.

Ghosh, A. K., Ahuja, A. and Goswami A. Heart rate and blood lactate response in amateur competitive boxing. ***Indian Journal of Medical Research*** 102, 10, 179-183, 1995.

Ghosh, A. K., Goswami, A. and Ahuja, A. (1993) : Evaluation of sports specific training programme in badminton players. ***Indian Journal of Medical Research*** 98 [B], 10, 232-236.

Ghosh, A. K., Majumdar, P., Goswami, A., Ahuja, A. and Puri, T. P. S. (1990b) : Heart rate and blood lactate response in competitive badminton. ***Annals of Sports Medicine*** (USA) 5 85-88.

Ghosh, A. K., Ahuja, A., Khanna, G. L. (19855d), Physical and physiological variables of Indian national soccer players, 3rd ***world congress. of Medical aspects of soccer-USOC Sports Medicine division*** Colorado USA.

Ghosh, A .K., Ahuja, A., Khanna, G. L., Kalley, S. (1985b), Intergroup variation in characteristics of Indian national basketball players. Proc. ***FISU Conference***, Universiade, Kobe pp. 345-346.

Ghosh, A. K., Ahuja, A., Khanna, G. L., (1986a), Physiological status of Indian National Gymnasts., *Congress* ***Scientific de gymnastique Universite de Montreal***, Canada.

Ghosh, A. K., Ahuja, A., Khanna, G. L. (1985c), Pulmonary capacities of some group of sportsmen in India., ***British Journal of Sports Medicine*** 19(4) : 85-88.

Ghosh, A. K., Ahuja, A., Khanna, G. L (1985a), Body composition and maximal aerobic power of Indian national football players. Proc. 3rd. ***International Congress Sports Medicine applied to football***, 2-5 June 1985. Athens, Greece.

Ghosh, A. K., Ahuja, A., Khanna, G. L., (1987a), Distance run as a predictor of aerobic endurance (VO2 max) of sportsmen. ***Indian Journal of Medical Research*** 85 : 680-684.

Ghosh, A. K., Khanna, G. L., Majumdar, P., Mathur, D. N. (1987b), Sex differentiation in the physiological variables of Indian road cyclists at anaerobic threshold level. Pro. ***74th Indian Science Congress***, Bangalore Abstract p. 34.

Ghosh, A. K., Khanna, G. L., Ahuja, A., Mathur, D. N. (1986c) : Comparision of body composition, muscular strength and VO2 max of mute vs. Indian national table tennis players. **XX III *FIMS World Congress on Sports Medicine*.**

Ghosh, A. K., Majumdar, P., Goswami, A., Khanna, G. L. (1988a) Aerobic — Anaerobic transition level of Indian middle and long distance runners, ***Indian Journal of Medical Research*** 1988, pp 371-375.

Ghosh, A. K., Ahuja, A. and Goswami, A. (1991b) : Physical and physiological profile of Indian National Women hockey players. ***NIS Scientific Journal*** 14, 4, 1-9.

Ghosh, A. K., Ahuja, A., Khanna, G. L. (1986b), Intercorrelation of Physical and Physiological parameters of National soccer players. Proc. ***Asian Games Conference***. Seoul, Korea.

Ghosh, A. K., Khanna, G. L., Ahuja, A., Kaul, T. K. (1986d) Cardiorespiratory fitness of Silent Cricketers in India. XX III ***FIMS World Congress on Sports Medicine*** 1986.

Ghosh, A. K., Ahuja, A., Khanna, G. L., (1985e), Physical and physiological determinants of fitness in Indian football players. Paper presented at ***OCA Sports Medicine Symposium***. *Baharaini 10-12 April 1985.*

Ghosh, A. K., Ahuja, A., Khanna, G. L. (1985f) Physiological status of Indian National Gymnasts, Scientific Abstract, Cong. ***Scientifque de Gymnastique***, Montreal, Canada 1985.

Ghosh, A. K., Ahuja, A., Khanna, G. L. (1987c) Physiological variables of Indian national badminton players at anaerobic threshold level — ***World Badminton*** 15(4) : 36.

Ghosh, A. K., Goswami, A., Majumdar, P. and Mathur, D. N. (1991a) : Heart rate and blood lactate response in field hockey. ***Indian Journal of Medical Research*** 94[B], 10, 351-356.

Goswami, A., Mathur, D. N. and Ghosh, A. K. (1995) : Blood lactate removal pattern after submaximal and supramaximal exercises. ***NIS Scientific Journal*** 18, 2, 11-1.

Gupta, S., Goswami, A., Sadhukhan, A. K. and Mathur, D. N. (1996) : Comparative study of lactate removal in short term massage of extremities, active recovery and a passive recovery period after supramaximal exercise sessions. ***International Journal of Sports Medicine*** (Germany) 17, 106-110.

Hill, A. V. (1923) : Muscular exercise, lactic acid and the supply and utilization of oxygen, ***Q. J. Med*** 16 : 135-171.

Khanna, G. L., Majumdar, P., Mandal, M. (1995c) : A secular trend in Maximum aerobic and anaerobic capacity in Indian national endurance sportsmen. ***NIS Scientific Journal*** 4 : 5-13.

Khanna, G. L., Majumdar, P., Saha, M. (1994c) A Comparative study of physiological profile of Indian National And Cuban Olympic boxers. ***Journal of Physical Education & Sports Sciences*** Vol 94 pp. 13-21.

Khanna, G. L., Saha, M. (1992c) Physique and physiological characteristics of Indian national Jr & Sr Swimmers with reference to age. ***NIS Scientific Journal*** 15(3) : 87-94.

Khanna, G. L., Bhatnagar, D. P. and Mathur, D. N. (1992b) Prediction of aerobic and anaerobic capacity from maximal, submaximal and recovery cardiopulmonary responses in children. ***Indian Journal of Sports Science & Physical Education*** Ed. 4(1) : 1-7.

Khanna, G. L., Majumdar, P., Ghosh, A. K., Mathur, D. N. (1986a) : Psycho-Physiological responses of Indian school footballers during graded ergometry. ***NIS Scientific Journal*** 11(2), 1988. 8-12.

Khanna, G. L., Saha, M. (1995b) Effect of four week altitude training on cardiorespiratory variables in national Cyclists. ***Indian Journal of Sports Science & Physical Education*** 7(1) : 1-9.

Khanna, G. L., Majumdar, P., Malik, V., Mandal, M. (1994a) : A study of physiological stress on different positional players in a hockey match. ***Proc. 81st Indian Science Congress*** Part-IV, p. 118(Abstract).

Khanna, G. L., Majumdar, P., Malik, V., Vrinda, T., Mandal, M. (1996d) : A study of physiological responses during match on Indian National Kabaddi Players. ***British Journal of Sports Medicine***. vol. 30, 232-235.

Khanna, G. L., Majumdar, P., Saha, M., Mandal, M. (1993). Cardiorespiratory fitness and body composition of Indian children of 10-16 yrs. ***Medicine and Sports Science*** 43, 132-144.

Khanna, G. L., Ghosh, A. K., Ahuja, A., Mathur, D. N. (1987a) : Recovery oxygen debt analysis in graded maximal and supramaximal exercise. ***Sports Sciences*** 1987 151-156.

Khanna, G. L., Ghosh, A. K., Ahuja, A., Mathur, D. N. (1986b), Recovery oxygen debt analysis in graded maximal and supramaximal exercise. ***2nd National Conference on Physical Education and Sports Science*** February 22-24, 1986. P.4.

Khanna, G. L. (1991) Physiological studies on effect of weight loss on Wrestling performance — a review. ***NIS Scientific Journal*** Vol. 14(4) : 10-16.

Khanna, G. L., Majumdar, P., Vrinda, T., Mandal, M. (1996a) : Assessment of playing heart rate and fractional oxygen utilization in hockey as determining factor in game planning. Presented in the 1996***International Scientific Sports Congress and Exhibition*** held at Bangalore P. 67(Abstract).

Khanna, G. L., Majumdar, P., Lal, P. R., Mandal, M. (1996b) : Comparative study of Iron Status and lipid profile in elite endurance and strength trained athletes. Physical activity, Sports and Health, 1996 ***International Pre-Olympic Scinetific Congress*** USA. P. 124(Abstract).

Khanna, G. L., Ghosh, A. K., Majumdar, P. (1987b) : Assessment of aerobic-anaerobic capacity and aerobic to anaerobic transition point of handball players. Proc. ***74th Indian Science Congress, Bangalore*** Abstract P. 35.

Khanna, G. L., Ghosh, A. K., Ahuja, A. (1986a), Body composition, muscular strength and cardiovascular efficiency of 252 sportsmen of various disciplines, ***SNIPES Journal*** 8 : 45-51.

Khanna, G. L., and Saha, M. (1991) Effect of Six Months training on Cardiorespiratory variables in talented children, ***Indian Journal of Sports Science & Physical Education*** Vol. 45(4) : 31-32.

Khanna, G. L., Ghosh, A. K., Sharma, J. G., Malhotra, M. S. (1983), Physiological status of some judoists in India, ***SNIPES Journal*** 6(2) : 21-27.

Khanna, G. L. and Bhatnagar, D. P. (1991) Physiological profile of aerobic and anaerobic capacities and cardiopulmonary responses in 8-18 years children. ***Indian Journal of Sports Science & Physical Education*** 3(2) : 68-76.

Khanna, G. L., Ahuja, A., Ghosh, A. K. (1985) : Morphophysiological characteristics of Indian basketball players. ***Hungarian Review of Sports Medicine*** 26(4) : 243-249.

Khanna, G. L., Ghosh, A. K., Ahuja, A. and Bhatnagar, S. (1992a). A Comparative study of Physiological variables in Senior and Junior National Cyclists. ***Indian Journal of Sports Science & Physical Education*** 4(2) : 57-60.

Khanna, G. L., Majumdar, P., Mandal, M., Saha, M. (1994b) : Effects of six weeks conditioning training programmes on submaximal and maximal cardiorespiratory variables in National badminton players. ***Indian Journal of Sports Science & Physical Education*** 6(2) : 119-126.

Khanna, G. L., Majumdar, P., Malik, V., Mandal, M. (1995a). Physiological demand of different positional players in women hockey. ***NIS Scientific Journal*** Vol. 18(1) : 5-14.

Khanna, G. L., Saha, M., Majumdar, P. (1993a) Physiological effects of three months training on Indian National volleyballers. ***Indian Journal of Sports Science & Physical Education*** 5(2) : 1993.

Khanna, G. L., Bhatnagar, D. P. (1993b) A Cross-sectional analysis of submaximal and maximal oxygen consumption in Indian Boys. ***NIS Scientific Journal*** 16.

Khanna, G. L., Majumdar, P., Mandal, M. (1996c) : Effect of high altitude training on morphophysiological parameters of middle and long-distance runners. Indian ***Journal of Physiology and Allied sciences*** (Acceped).

La Grange, F. (1889). ***Physiology of bodily exercise***, London : Kegan Paul International Ltd.

Lusk, G. (1928) ***The elements of the science of nutrition***, Philadelphia, WB Saunder.

Maitra, S. R., Chatterjee, S. and Das, S. (1968) : A quantitative information on normal values for respiratory functions in cat. ***Indian Journal of Physiology & Allied Sciences*** 22, 28-33.

Maitra, S. R., Chatterjee, S. and Das, S. K. (1966) : Study on protein concentration in plasma and corpuscular changes of blood in man with minimal, submaximal and maximal work load. ***Proc. Symposium on Human Adaptability to Environments and Physical Fitness***. Ed. Malhotra, M.S. : Defence Institute of Physiology and Allied Sciences, Chennai, India pp 130-140.

Maitra, S. R., Chatterjee, S., Chatter, P., Koyal, S. N., and Das Gupta, S. (1967) : Effect of heavy muscular work of five athletes on exchange of blood lactate, O_2 consumption, hemoglobin, RBC concentration and electrocardiogram. ***Indian Journal of Physiology & Allied Sciences*** 21 : 20.

Majumdar, P., Khanna, G. L., Mandal, M. (1998) : Anthropometric characteristics and Motor function of 8-12 years children in relation to auxological changes. ***Journal of Physical Education & Sports Sciences*** 3, 32-39.

Majumdar, P., Khanna G. L., Malik, V., Sachdeva, S., Arif Md., Mandal, M. (1997) : Physiological analysis to quantify training load in Badminton., ***British Journal of Sports Medicine***, 31 : 342-345.

Majumdar, P., Khanna, G. L., Mandal, M., Ghosh, A. K. analysis of training segment of National badminton players. (1994). ***Proc. 81st Indian Science Congress***. Part-IV p. 120.

Malhotra, M. S. (1971) : Physiological evaluation of Indian elite athletes. ***NIS Scientific Journal***, 5, 2 : 91-96.

Malhotra, M. S., Joseph, N. T., and Sen Gupta, J. (1973) : Physiological assessment of Indian Olympic hockey players. ***Indian Journal of Sports Medicine***. 2 : 5-10.

Malhotra, M. S., Ramaswamy, S. S., Dua, G. L., and Sen Gupta (1966) : Physical work capacity as influenced by age. ***Ergonomics***. 9, 4 : 305-317.

Mathur, D. N. (1970a). Influence of interval training on blood sugar level. ***Track Technique***. 35 : 72-75.

Mathur, D. N. (1970b). The physiological responses and requirements of participation in triple jump. In ***Encyclopaedia of Sports Sciences and Medicine***. Macmillan Press, New York., pp. 312-313.

Mathur, D. N. (1970c). The physiological responses and requirements of participation in Hurdles. In ***Encyclopaedia of Sports Sciences and Medicine***. Macmillan Press, New York., pp. 410-411.

Nair, C. S., Tiwari, O. P., and Malhotra, M. S. (1971a) : Effect of altitude acclimatization and cold on cold pressor response in man. ***Journal of Aerospace Medicine***. 42, 9 : 991-994.

Nair, C. S., Malhotra, M. S. and Gopinathan, P. M. (1971b) : Effect of altitude and cold acclimatization on the basal metabolism in man. ***Journal of Aerospace Medicine***., 42, 10 : 1056-1059.

Mathur, D. N. (1969) : Influence of Interval training on blood sugar level. ***Track Technique***, 35, 72-75.

Railly, T. and Brooks, G. A. (1990). Selective persistence of circadian rhythm in physiological responses to exercise. ***Chronobiology Internal***. 7, 59-67.

Sen, R. N. (1954) : Studies on energy metabolism. ***Masters' Thesis***, Calcutta University, pp. 101.

Sen, R. N. and Banerjee, S. (1958) : Determination of basal metabolic rate and blood concentration of protein bound iodine, cholesterol, and glucose in Indians. ***Indian Journal of Medical Research***, 46, 759-765.

Sen, R. N., Chatterjee, S. K., Saha, P. N., and Subramanian, A. (1964) : Assessment of work load and thermal stress in relation to physiological responses of workers in a cotton textile mill in Bombay. ***Report no. 3, Industrial Physiology Division***, *CLI, Bombay pp.* 27.

Sen Gupta, J., Malhotra, M. S., and Ramaswamy, S.S. (1972) : Exercise dyspnoea and work performance at sea level and at altitude. ***Indian Journal of Physiology and Pharmacology*** 16, 1 : 47-53.

Sen, R. N. (1955) : Fatigue and how to avoid it. Presidency College, ***Physiology Institute Journal*** 5 : 28-32.

Sen, R. N., Chatterjee, S. K., Saha, P. N. (1965) : Physiological stress and physiological strains on workers in a steel rolling mill in Bombay. Paper presented in the international seminar on ***'health productivity'***, Bombay.

Sodhi, H. S. (1980a) Cardiorespiratory fitness and performance on cycle ergometer, ***Journal of Sports Medicine and Physical Fitness*** 20 : 100.

Sodhi, H. S. (1980) A study of morphology and body composition of Indian Basketball players; ***Journal of Sports Medicine and Physical Fitness*** 21 : 50.

2

GENERALIZED CELL AND THE PRINCIPAL ORGANELLES

GENERALIZED CELL AND THE PRINCIPAL ORGANELLES

COMPONENT	STRUCTURE	FUNCTION
Cell membrane	Membrane composed of Phospholipid and protein molecule	Gives form to cell, control passage of materials in and out of cell
Cytoplasm	Fluid, jelly-like substance in which organelles are suspended	Serves as matrix in which chemical reactions occur
Endoplasmic Reticulum	System of interconnected membrane-forming canals and tubules	Smooth endoplasmic reticulum metabolizes nonpolar compounds and stores Ca^{++} in muscles. Rough endoplasmic reticulum assists in protein synthesis
Ribosomes	Granular, particles	Synthesize protein composed of protein and RNA
Golgi apparatus	Cluster of flattened membranous sacs	Synthesizes carbohydrates and packages molecules for secretion : secretes lipid and Glycoprotein
Mitochondria	Membranous sacs with folded inner portions	Release energy from food molecules and transform energy into usable ATP

COMPONENT	STRUCTURE	FUNCTION
Lysosome	Membranous Sacs	Digest foreign molecules
Peroxisome	Spherical Membranous vesicles	Contain certain enzymes form hydrogen peroxide
Centrosome	Nonmembranous mess of two rod like centriole	Helps to organize spindles and distribute chromosomes during mitosis
Vacuoles	Membranous Sacs	Store and excrete various substances within the cytoplasm
Fibrils and Microtubule	Thin hollow tubes	Support cytoplasm and transport materials within the cytoplasm
Cilia and Flagella	Minute cytoplasmic extension from cell	Move particles along surface of cell or move cell
Nuclear membrane	Membrane surrounding nucleus, composed of protein and lipid molecules	Support nucleus and controls passage of materials between nucleus and cytoplasm
Nucleus	Dense membranous mass composed of protein and RNA molecules	Forms ribosomes
Chromatin	Fibrous strands composed of protein and DNA molecules	Controls cellular activity for carrying on life processes

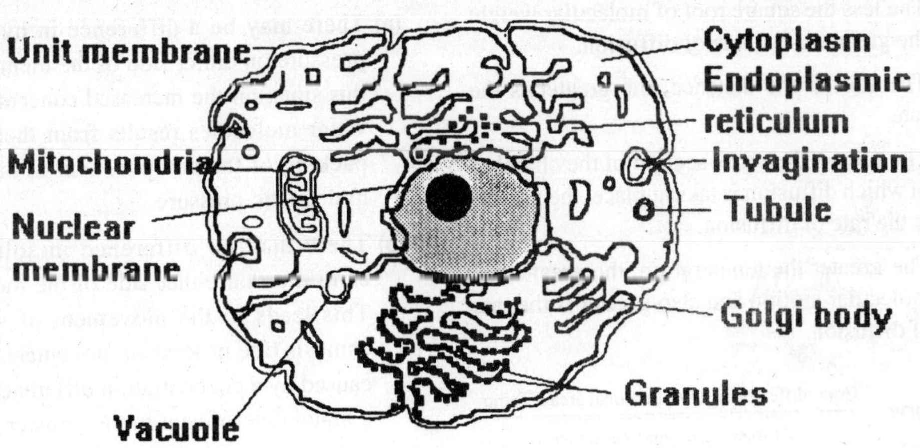

Fig. 2.1 : Schematic diagram of cell structure

FUNCTIONAL SYSTEM OF THE CELL

Ingestion by the cell

Substances can pass through a cell membrane in three separate ways (1) by diffusion through the pores in the membrane or through membrane matrix itself; (2) by active transport through the membrane, a mechanism in which enzyme systems and special carrier substances carry the substances through the membrane and (3) endocytosis, a mechanism by which the membrane engulfs particulate matter or extracellular fluid and its contents.

The fluid inside the cell of the body called intracellular fluid is very different from that outside the cells, called extracellular fluid. Extreacellular fluid, however, contains large quantities of sodium but small quantities of potassium. Exactly the opposite is true of the intracellular fluid. The extracellular fluid contains large quantities of chloride, which intracellular fluid contains very little. The concentrations of phosphates — essentially all of which are organic metabolite intermediates — and proteins in the intracellular fluids are greater than in the extracellular fluid. The difference between the component ECF and ICF are extremely important to the life of the cells.

Diffusion : In a solution the molecules of both solute and solvent are in constant rapid random thermal movement and frequent collisions occur between molecules. This results in the process of diffusion — the movement of solute which occurs when a membrane or boundary separates two fluid at the same hydrostatic pressure but differing in their concentration of solute, i.e., when there is a concentration gradient across the membrane (or within the single solution). If the hydrostatic pressure on the two sides of the membrane are unequal a flow of water and dissolved solutes will occur by filtration.

The following factors affect the rate of diffusion of a substance from one area to another :

(a) The greater the concentration difference, the greater is the rate of diffusion.

(b) The less the square root of molecular weight the greater is the rate of diffusion.

(c) The shorter the distance, the greater is the rate.

(d) The greater the cross-section of the chamber in which diffusion is taking place, the greater is the rate of diffusion.

(e) The greater the temperature, the greater the molecular motion and also greater is the rate of diffusion.

$$\text{Diffusionrate} = \frac{\text{Conc. difference} \times \text{cross sectional area} \times \text{Temp}}{\sqrt{\text{Molecular weight} \times \text{distance}}}$$

The different methods by which substance can diffuse through the membrane are —

1. by becoming dissolved in lipid matrix.
2. by diffusing through minute pores that pass directly through the membrane at wide intervals over its surface.

Bulk flow of water through pores in response to hydrostatic or osmotic pressure gradient. If there exists a difference in the concentrations of water molecules on either side of a membrane there will be a net movement of water through the membrane at a rate determined by the water concentration gradient (Osmotic pressure) and the permeability coefficient of the membrane for water.

Difference in water concentration may arise for two reasons :

(a) There may be a difference in hydrostatic pressure on either side of the membrane. In this situation the increased concentration of water molecules results from their tighter packing of the compartment at the higher hydrostatic pressure.

(b) There may be difference in solute concentration on either side of the membrane. This leads to the movement of water by osmosis (the process of movement of water caused by a concentration difference) and is a major determinant in the transfer of water across the membrane of a living cell.

Active Transport

The cell membrane moves molecule either against a concentration gradient or against an electrical pressure gradient at the cost of energy — the process is called active transport. The energy is delivered to the inside surface of the membrane from high energy substances, principally, ATP inside the cytoplasm of the cell. The transport is carrier mediated, a specific carrier-molecule (or combination of molecules) is required to transport each type of substance or each class of similar substances. A specific enzyme (or enzymes) is required to promote active transport.

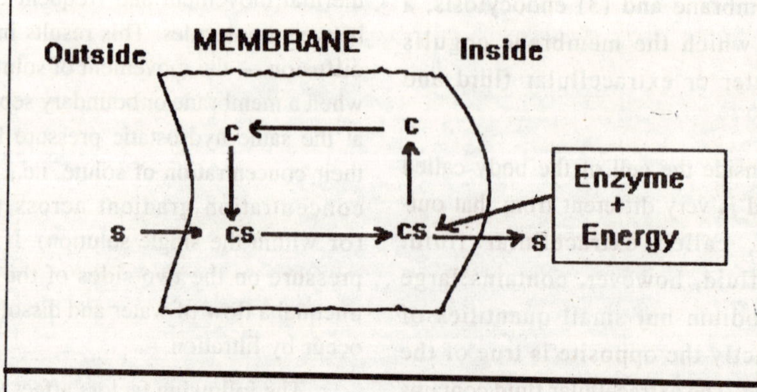

Fig. 2.2 : Basic mechanism of active transport

Fig. 2. 2 shows that the carrier has a natural affinity for the substance and hence combine together. The combination of the two diffuses through the membrane to the inner surface. Here the enzyme catalyzed reaction occurs, utilizing energy from ATP to split the substance away from the carrier. But the released substance, being insoluble in the membrane, cannot diffuse backward through the lipid matrix of the membrane. Therefore it is released to the inside of the membrane while the carrier diffuses back to the outside surface for transport of another molecule of substances in the inward direction.

Transport through intracellular membrane : The permeabilities and specificities for transport are often different but the cellular organelles (mitochondria and endoplasmic reticulum) obey the same law of both diffusion and active transport. Mitochondria has a double membrane. The outer membrane is much more permeable than the inner one. Transport through these membrane plays important role in function of intracellular organelles.

Active transport through cellular sheets : In many places of the body substances must be transported through an entire cellular layer, instead of simply through the cell membrane itself. Transport of this type occurs through the intestinal epithelium, the epithelium of the renal tubules, the epithelium of all exocrine glands, the membrane of the choroid plexus of the brain, and many other membranes. In Fig. 2. 3 shows two adjacent cells in a typical epithelial membrane as found in the intestine, gall bladder etc. on the luminal surface of the cells is a brush border that is highly permeable to water and some solutes, allowing both of these to diffuse from the lumen of the intestine to the interior of the cell. Once inside, some of solutes are actively transported into the lateral space between the cell.

This place is closed at the brush border of the epithelium but is wide open at the base of the cells where they rest on the basement membrane. Furthermore, basement membrane is extremely permeable, therefore, substances transported into this channel between the cells flow toward the connective tissue.

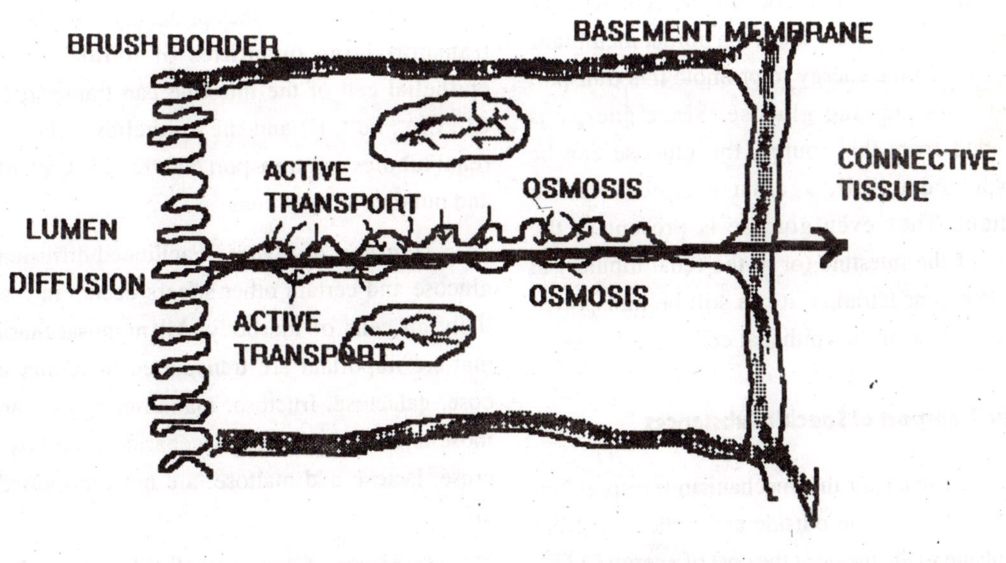

Fig. 2.3 : Basic mechanism of active transport through a layer of cell

One of the most important substances actively transported in this manner is sodium ions (Na^+), when Na^+ are transported into the space between the cells, their positive electrostatic charges pull negatively charged chloride ions (Cl^-) through the membrane as well (principle of electron neutrality). This, in turn, causes osmosis of the water out of the cell and into the intracellular space. In consequence, the Na^+ and Cl^- ions flow along with water into the connective tissue behind the basement membrane, where the water and ion diffuse into the blood capillaries. The same principle of transport apply generally in the intestinal epithelium, the gall bladder epithelium, the renal epithelium and others.

Secondary active transport : Sodium 'Co-transport' of glucose and amino acids

Brush border (luminal lining) is reasonably impermeable to sodium except when sodium combines with a carrier molecules one type of which is called sodium-glucose carrier. When bound with both sodium and glucose the carrier will only then transport both to the interior of the cell. It is the sodium gradient across the brush border membrane that provides the energy to promote this transport of both sodium and glucose. Since energy is provided from this source, the glucose can be transported uphill, against a concentration gradient. Thus even glucose is present in the lumen of the intestine (or in the renal tubules) in very low concentration, it can still be transported to the interior of the epithelial cell.

Active Transport of Specific Substances

The carrier for this mechanism transport Na^+ inside the cell to the outside and potassium from the outside to the inside at the cost of energy (ATP). The carrier is called sodium-potassium ATP ase. The ATP ase is composed of two protein molecules, one is globulin (larger molecule) and the other is glycoprotein. The larger molecule actually binds with both Na^+ and K^+ and also with ATP and smaller molecule (glycoprotein) is necessary to provide some facilitating function. Magnesium ATP binds with $Na^+ - K^+$ – ATP ase at the inside surface of the membrane. The energy released from the ATP causes K^+ to split away from the $Na^+ - K^+$ – ATP ase carrier molecule and, simultaneously, causes Na^+ to bind. At the outside surface of membrane, the Na^+ ion is split away from the carrier while K^+ bind without the need for additional energy. The transport system carries 3 Na^+ ion to the inside of the membrane for each 2 K^+ ion transported to the outside. This gives a net transfer of 50% more positive charges outward through the membrane than inward. $Na^+ - K^+$ pump is called electrogenic pump as it creates negativity inside and positivity outside. $Na^+ - K^+$ pump is important in nerve and muscle fiber for transmission of impulses, various glands for secretion of different substances and prevent cellular swelling.

Active transport of other ion : Ca^{++} and Mg^{++} are transported by all cell membranes, the glandular cell membranes of the thyroid gland can transport large quantities of iodide ion, the epithelial cell of the intestine can transport Na^+, Cl^-, Ca^{++}, Fe^{++}, H^+ and the epithelial cells of the renal tubules can transport Na^+, K^+, Cl^-, Ca^{++}, Mg^{++} and number of other ions.

Transport of sugars : Facilitated diffusion of glucose and certain other sugars occurs in essentially all cells of the body. All monosaccharides that are important are transported including glucose, galactose, fructose, mannose, xylose, arabinose and sorbose, the disaccharides, such as sucrose, lactose and maltose, are not transported at all.

Transport of amino acids : Amino acids are transported inside by facilitated diffusion mechanism, insulin and growth hormone enhances

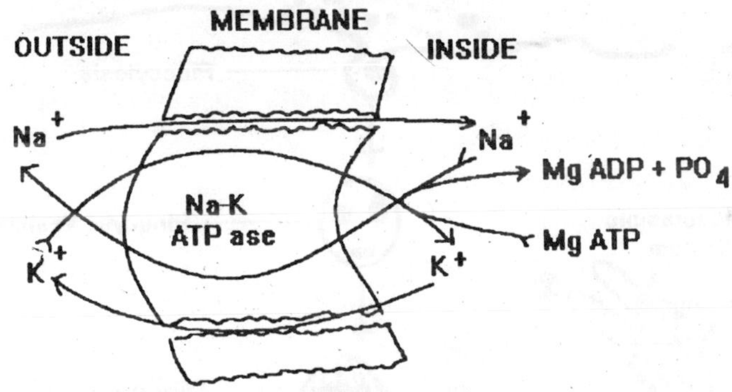

Fig. 2.4 : Postulated mechanism for active transport of sodium and potassium through the cell membrane

this transport of amino acids, similarly glucocorticoid (liver cell) and estradiol (musculature of uterus) help in transporting amino acid.

Endocytosis — phagocytosis and pinocytosis

Phagocytosis means ingestion of large particulate matter, such as bacterium, some other cells or particles of degenerating tissue. Pinocytosis on, the other hand, means ingestion of minute quantities of extracellular fluid and dissolved substance in the form of minute vescicles. Pinocytosis is the only known means by which large molecules, such as proteins, can be transported to the interior of cells.

Digestion of foreign substances in the cell function of lysosome

After formation of pinocytic or phagocytic vesicles inside a cell, lysosomes become attached to the vesicle and empty their hydrolases into the vesicle, which hydrolyzes the proteins, glycogen, lipids, nucleic acid, mucopolysaccharide and other substances in the vesicle. The products of digestion are small molecules of amino acids, glucose, fatty acids, phosphates, that can diffuse through the membrane to the cytoplasm. What is left in the digestive vesicles called the residual body excreted through the cell membrane by a process called exocytosis.

Extraction of energy from nutrients — function of Mitochondria

In the foodstuffs, carbohydrate, protein and fat are converted to its simpler form glucose, amino acids and fatty acids and enter into the cell. The energy released from the nutrients is used to form ATP (adenosine triphosphate). On entry into the cells glucose is subjected to enzymes in the cytoplasm that convert it into pyruvic acid (a process called glycolysis) which is rated as 5% of the total energy, by fat, the major portion of cellular ATP is formed in the mitochondria. The pyruvic acid, fatty acid and amino acid are all converted into the compound acetyl CoA in the matrix of mitochondria.

The substance, in turn, enters into the cyclical chain reaction called Kreb's Cycle or Tricarboxylic acid cycle (TCA cycle). In TCA cycle, acetyl CoA split into its component parts — hydrogen atoms and carbon dioxide (CO_2), CO_2 diffuses out of the mitochondria and eventually out of the cell.

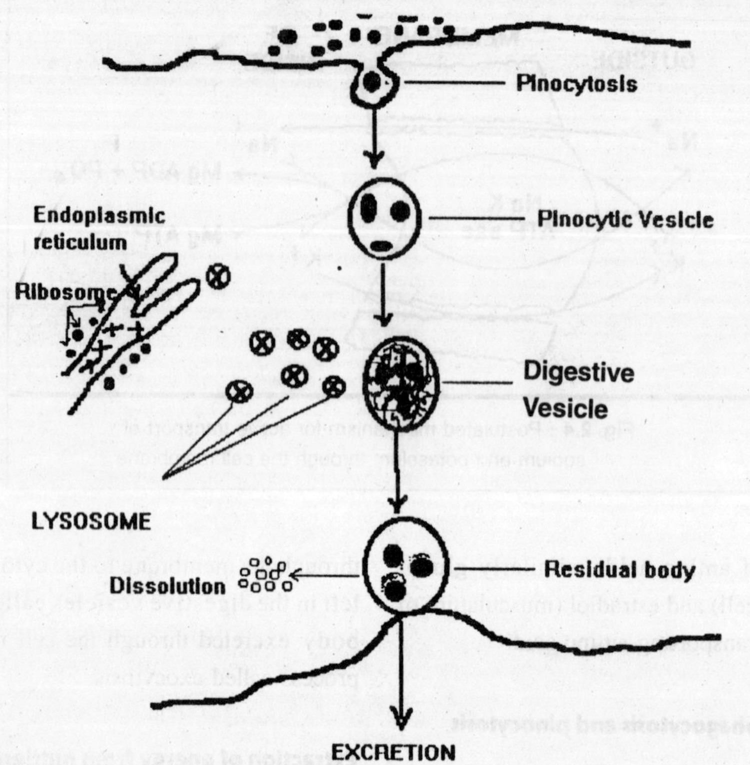

Fig. 2.5 : Digestion of substances in pinocytic vesicles by enzymes derived from lysosome

The hydrogen atoms combine with carrier substances and are carried to the surfaces of the protruding shelves where oxidative enzymes are protruding globules of ATP are attached which catalyzes the conversation of ADP to ATP. The oxidative enzymes, by a series of sequential reactions, cause the hydrogen atoms to combine with oxygen. The enzymes are arranged in such a way that the products of one chemical reaction are immediately relayed to the next enzyme until the complete sequence of reactions has taken place.

During the course of these reactions, the energy released from the combination of hydrogen with oxygen is used to activate the ATP ase and drive the reaction to manufacture ATP. ATP is used to promote three major categories of cellular functions : (a) membrane transport (Na^+ transport). (b) Synthesis of chemical compound throughout the cell by synthesizing protein synthesis by the ribosome. (c) Mechanical work, to supply the energy needed during muscle contraction.

Synthesis and formation of cellular structures by the endoplasmic reticulum and the Golgi complex

These two structures are made of lipid bilayer membranes and their walls are literally loaded with protein enzymes that catalyze the synthesis of most of the substances required by the cell. Most of the synthesis begins in the endoplasmic reticulum and the products formed are then passed on to Golgi complex for further processing prior to release into the cell. The specific products are synthesized in the specific portions of the endoplasmic reticulum and the Golgi complex.

Formation of protein by granular (rough) Endoplasmic Reticulum (ER)

The function of the granular endoplasmic reticulum is to form protein in association with the ribosomes and are secreted by the endoplasmic reticulum and Golgi complex. Some ribosomes are not attached to the endoplasmic reticulum and extrude their protein molecule directly into the cytoplasm.

Synthesis of lipids and other functions of the smooth Endoplasmic Reticulum (ER)

The phospholipid and cholesterol are rapidly incorporated into the lipid bilayer of the endoplasmic reticulum, thus causing the smooth portion of the endoplasmic reticulum to grow continually. Smooth endoplasmic reticulum contains the enzymes that control glycogen when glycogen is to be used for energy. ER contains large number of enzymes which are capable of detoxifying substances that are damaging to the cell, such as drugs. It achieves this by coagulation, oxidation, hydrolysis, conjugation with glucuronic acid and other ways. ER synthesize few carbohydrate molecules that are usually conjugated with protein molecules to form glycoproteins.

Synthetic functions of the Golgi complex

The major function of Golgi complex is the processing of product formeds by ER. It can also synthesize CHO that cannot be formed by ER, viz., sialic acid, fructose and galactose. It can cause the formation saccharide polymers namely hyaluronic acid and chondroitin sulfate. These two substances are the major components of proteoglycans secreted in mucus and other glandular secretions. Chondroitin sulfate and hyaluronic acid are the major components of the ground substance in the interstitial spaces, acting as a filter between collagen fibers and cells — the principal components of the organic matrix in both cartilage and bone.

Processing of endoplasmic secretion by the Golgi complex — formation of intracellular vesicles

As substances are formed in the rough ER, specially protein, they are transported through the tubules towards the portion of smooth endoplasmic reticulum that lie nearest to Golgi complex. At this point small "transport" vesicles of smooth ER continually breakaway and diffuse to the proximal layers of the Golgi complex, carrying inside the vesicles the synthesized proteins and other products. These vesicles instantly fuse with the Golgi complex, and their contained substances enter the vesicular space of the Golgi complex. Here a few additional CHO moieties are usually added to the secretion which may enable to give a compact reticular secretion into highly concentrated packet. As the secretion pass towards the distal layers of the golgi complex the compaction and processing proceed, and, finally, at the distal layer, both small and large vesicles continually breakaway from the golgi complex, carrying with them the compacted secretory substances, and they then diffuse throughout the cell.

Type of vesicles formed by the Golgi complex-secretory vesicles, lysosome — peroxisomes. In a highly secretory cell, the vescicles that are formed by the golgi complex are mainly secretory vesicles, containing specially the protein substances that are to be secreted throughout the surface of the cell. These vescicles diffuse to the surface, fuse with the cell membrane, and empty their substances to the exterior by a mechanism called exocytosis which is, in many cases, stimulated by entry of calcium ion (Ca^{++}).

Specialised portion of Golgi complex form the lysosomes and peroxisomes which form hydrogen peroxide (H_2O_2) by the action of large quantities of the enzyme catalase. Destruction of H_2O_2 is essential to the life of the cell as it is highly toxic for some of the enzyme system use of intracellular vescicles to replenish cellular membrane. Many of the vescicles finally fuse with the cell membrane or membrane of intracellular structure (mitochondria, ER), cell membrane loses much of its substance everytime it forms a phagocytic or pinocytic vescicle and it is vescicles from Golgi complex that continually replenish the cell membrane.

Cell movement

Ameboid motion : Typically, ameboid motion begins with protursion of a pseudopodium from one end of the cell. The outer portion of the cytoplasm is in a gel state called ectoplasm and the central portion of the cytoplasm is in a gel state called endoplasm. In the gel there are numerous contractile microfilaments composed of actomyosin. These filaments contract in the presence of ATP and Ca^{++} ion and there is a continual tendency for the ectoplasm to contract. However, in response to physical or chemical stimulus, the ectoplasm at one end of the cell becomes thin, causing a pseudopodium to bulge outward in the direction of the chemotoxic source. Thus the pseudopodium move progressively forward. The most common cells to exhibit ameboid movement are the WBC moving out of the blood into the tissues in the form of tissue macrophages or microphages. Fibroblast also move into damaged area to help repair the damage, and even some of the germinal cells of the skin will move by ameboid motion towards a cut area to repair the rent, otherwise these are completely senile cells. Finally, ameboid motion is especially important in the development of the fetus, for embryonic cells often migrate long distances from primordial sites of origin to new areas during development of special structures.

Control of ameboid motion (chemotaxis) : The most important factors that usually initiate ameboid motion act presumably by causing potential changes in the cell membrane or by the entry of Ca^{++} ions into the cell which causes the release of chemical substances in the tissues. This phenomenon is called chemotaxis and the substance is known as chemotaxes substances. Most ameboid cells move towards the sources of chemotaxing substance from an area of slower concentration to higher concentration and is called positive chemotaxis. However, some cells move away from the sources called negative chemotaxis.

Movement of cilia : A second type of cellular motion is the movement of cilia on the surface of the cells in the respiratory tract and in the fallopian tubes of the reproductive tract. The cilium is a sharp pointed hair that projects from the surface of the cell. The cilium moves forward with a sudden rapid stroke.

Genetic control of cell function — protein synthesis and cell reproduction

Protein is the most important fabric of the cell. Therefore the synthesis of protein is the most essential function of cell. Deoxyribonucleic acid (DNA) present in the chromosome acts as template or cast. The available raw materials attach in specific sequence of this cast and, with the help of an enzyme ribonucleic acid (RNA) polymerase, they are linked into a polynucleotide chain. This results into the formation of a particular type of RNA, called messenger RNA, which carries the information from DNA. Messenger RNA separates from DNA and passes into the cytoplasm. Within the cytoplasm at the sites of the ribosomes a second kind of RNA (ribosomal RNA) holds the messenger RNA in extended condition from the cytoplasm, a third kind of RNA (transfer RNA) collects amino acids and delivers them to the proper position on the messenger RNA. One kind of transfer RNA can collect only one type of amino acid. Therefore the number of transfer RNA corresponds to the number of available amino acids. Thus different transfer RNAs deliver their amino acids on the specific sites along the entire length of the messenger RNA which remain stretched on the ribosomes. These amino acids unite in a sequence to form a particular protein.

Cell Reproduction

The cell carries the function by a process called cell division. There are three types of cell division (1) Mitosis (2) Meiosis (3) Amitosis. Mitosis involves one nuclear division. It is the chief process of reproduction of body cell, each division ensures duplication of chromosome. As a consequence of mitosis daughter nuclei maintain same number of chromosome. Each human cell contains 46 chromosome arranged in 23 pairs. The general purpose of mitotic division is the material increase of cell number. Synthesis of DNA occurs strictly in the interphase.

Mitosis

Prophase : The first stage of mitosis. It is the largest phase, chromosomes become visible and in due time each appears as paired threads of chromatids. Nuclear membrane disappears and the spindle appears.

Prometaphase : During this stage the nuclear membrane dissolves and microtubules from the forming mitotic apparatus become attached to the chromosomes. This attachment always occurs at the same point on each chromosome at a small condensed portion called kinetochore, located near the centromere where the two chromosomes of each pair are attached to each other.

Metaphase : During metaphase, the centriole pairs are pushed far apart by the growing spindle and the chromosomes are thereby pushed tightly by the attached microtubules to the very center of the cell, lining up in the equatorial plane of the mitotic spindle.

Anaphase : Centromere divides, chromosomes are pulled lengthwise to the opposite poles and since each chromosome material consists of two chromatids — one chromatid of each chromosome moves towards one pole of the spindle.

Telophase : Chromosomes start reassuming the threadlike state by the gradual process of uncoiling, spindles disintegrated daughter nuclei result. Cell pass through the interphase state until further division occurs in the same manner.

Meiosis : Nuclear division occurs thrice in close succession but the chromosomes are duplicated only once. Meiotic division results into four daughter cells. The number of chromosomes in each of these cells is reduced to half (haploid chromosome set) meiosis occurs in the specialized tissues like testis and ovary resulting into sperms ova (reproductive cells), respectively, in sexually reproducing organisms. The resultant cells may be dissimilar (as in the case of Oogenesis). Meiosis is a significant condition for sexual reproduction. The haploid set of chromosomes in gametes fuse to form the diploid zygote and thus the usual chromosome number of the species is maintained. Synthesis of DNA may extend even up to early prophase (1) Transient interphase after the first meiotic division is devoid of synthetic phase.

A. Prophase (1st)

This is also the longest phase as in mitosis but is much more complicated. The entire phase has been subdivided into following (1) leptotene (2) zygotene (3) pachytene (4) diplotene (5) diakinesis.

The characteristics events are — chromosomes become discrete, visible and oriented in a polarized way. The homologous chromosomes become entwined. These paired chromosomes are now termed bivalent. Now each chromosome in the bivalent splits into two chromatids. This is followed by breaking and rejoining of chromatid segments resulting into exchange of genetic material between the homologous chromosomes (crossing over). This is accompanied by chiasma formation.

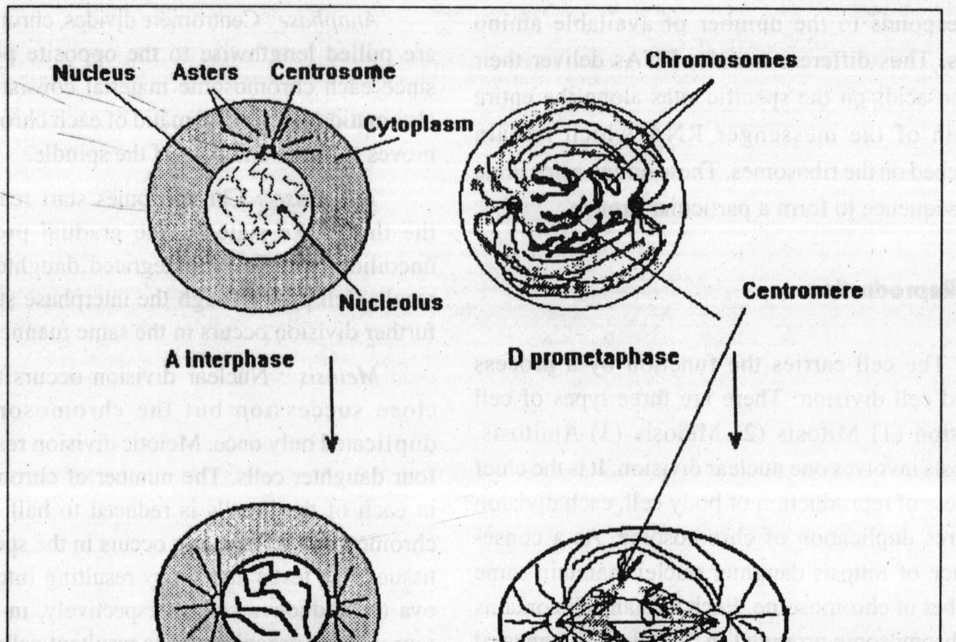

Fig. 2.6 : Process of Mitosis — (A-F) Stages of mitosis — A. Interphase. B. Early prophase, C. Late Prophase, D. Prometaphase, E. Metaphase, F. Early anaphase. The circle drawn in Fig. E to indicate equatorial plane is imaginary. It never appears during cell division

Chiasma is the cytological equivalent of the crossing over. The bivalent now begin to orient themselves on the spindle. Each has two centromeres. Interchange of chromosomal material involving genetic exchange renders evolution its dynamicity.

B. Metaphase 1

Centromeres get attached with spindle fibers. Bivalent orient themselves at the equator in such a way that each of the homologous chromosomes can move to the reserve pole.

C. Anaphase (1st)

Characteristic feature of meiotic anaphase (1) is that it results in the segregation of homologous chromosomes to the opposite poles. Each of these parting members of the homologous set (with its new genetic make-up resulting from crossing over) may eventually participate in the genetic constitution of two individuals of the next generation through fertilization of the resultant sex cells. The phenomenon has definite importance from the point of view of evolution.

D. Telophase (1st)

Two daughter nuclei (and eventually cells) are formed in the same way or the two sets of chromosomes may enter directly into the second meiotic divisions.

Duration of the entire meiotic division is usually much longer in comparison to that of mitosis. The second meiotic division involves two daughter nuclei or cells. The characteristics are (i) centromere splits so that at anaphase (II) the chromatids can move to the two poles (ii) At telophase (II) nuclear membrane forms around each mass

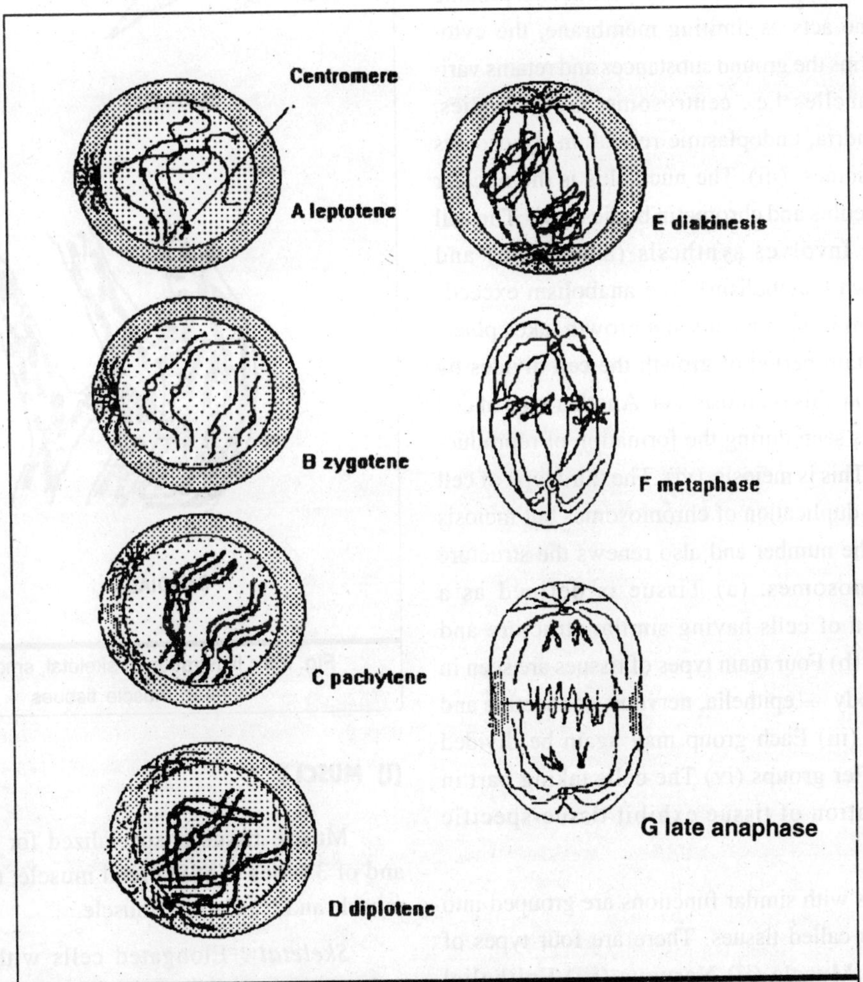

Fig. 2.7 : Stages of first meiotic division

of chromosomal materials. Four nuclei (and cells after cytokinesis) result, each containing only one set of homologous chromosomes.

Amitosis : Several instanc·· the nucleus divides without the disappearance of nuclear membrane and formation of spindle apparatus. Such direct division of nucleus is known as amitosis. Some intranuclear mechanism help for equal distribution of chromosome.

Summary

(i) The cell is the unit of living body. It contains (a) cell membrane (b) cytoplasm and (c) nucleus. (ii) The cell membrane/plasma membrane acts as limiting membrane, the cytoplasm forms the ground substances and retains various organelles i.e., centrosome, Golgi bodies, mitochondria, endoplasmic reticulum, lysosomes and ribosomes. (iii) The nucleolus is the nuclear sap, nucleolus and chromatin bodies. (iv) The cell function involves synthesis (anabolism) and breakdown (catabolism). The anabolism exceeds catabolism in young cells and growth takes place. After certain period of growth the cell divides by duplication, this is mitosis. (v) Another type of cell division is seen during the formation of reproductive cell. This is meiosis. (vi) The third type of cell results in duplication of chromosomes but meiosis reduces the number and also renews the structure of chromosomes. (a) Tissue is defined as a collection of cells having similar structure and function. (b) Four main types of tissues are seen in human body — epithelia, nervous, connective and muscular (iii) Each group may again be divided into smaller groups (iv) The cells taking part in the formation of tissue exhibit tissue-specific affinity.

Cells with similar functions are grouped into categories called tissues. There are four types of tissue (i) Muscle (ii) Nervous (iii) Epithelial (iv) Connective.

TISSUE

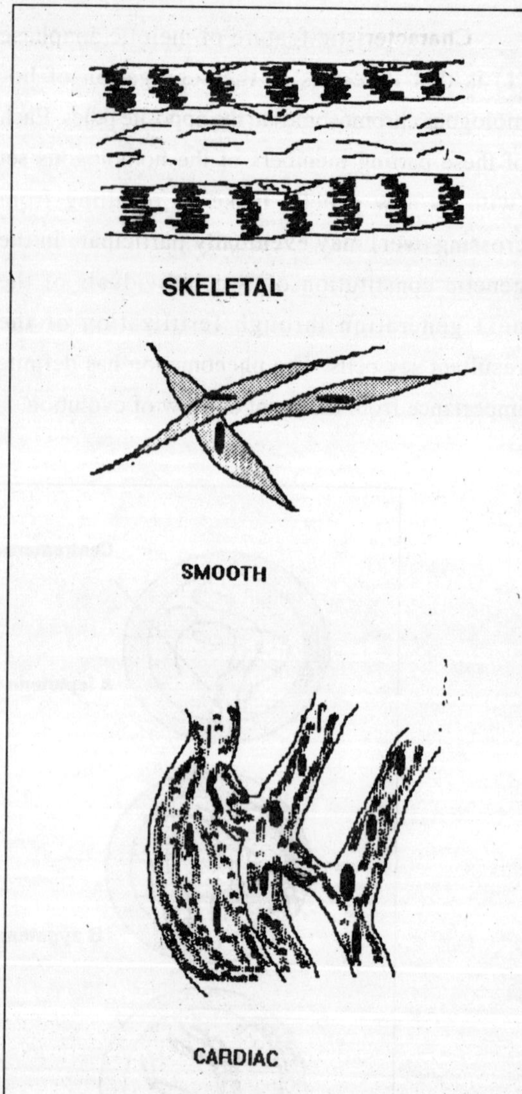

Fig. 2.8 : Illustration of skeletal, smooth & cardiac muscle tissues

(i) MUSCLE

Muscle tissue is specialized for contraction and of 3 types : (a) Skeletal muscle, (b) Smooth muscle and (c) Cardiac muscle.

Skeletal : Elongated cells with striation, voluntary in nature, contain alternate dark and light bands and form striation. Muscle fibers are parallely arranged and to be controlled individually vary the strength of the whole muscle's contraction.

Smooth : Non-striated, absence of light and dark band, involuntary, spindle-shaped, contain one nucleus, absence of sarcolemma. Found in alimentary canal, urinary bladder, blood vessels. Rhythmic contractions of circular and longitudinal layers of muscle produce peristalsis — a process that pushes food from one end of digestive tract to the other.

Cardiac : Modified striated, involuntary, absence of sarcolemma, contain number of nucleus, muscle fibers are interconnected by strand — syncytium.

(ii) NERVOUS TISSUE

Nervous tissue consists of 3 parts (a) Cell body, which contains the nucleus and serve as metabolic center. (b) Dendrites : highly branched cytoplasmic extensions — Receive input from other neurons or from receptor cells. (c) Axon : single cytoplasmic extension specialized for conducting nerve impulses from cell body to another neuron. Neuroglial cells bind neurons together and influence the nourishment and electrical activity of neurons. Neuroglial cells are about 5 times more abundant than neurons and maintain a limited ability to divide by mitosis.

TYPE	STRUCTURE & FUNCTION	LOCATION
SIMPLE EPITHELIA	Single layer of cells; diffusion and filtration	Covering visceral organ linings of lumina and body cavities
A. Simple squamous epithelium	Single layer of flattened tightly-bound cells; diffusion and filtration	Capillary walls; air sacs of lung, covering visceral organs; Lining of organs; Lining of body cavities.

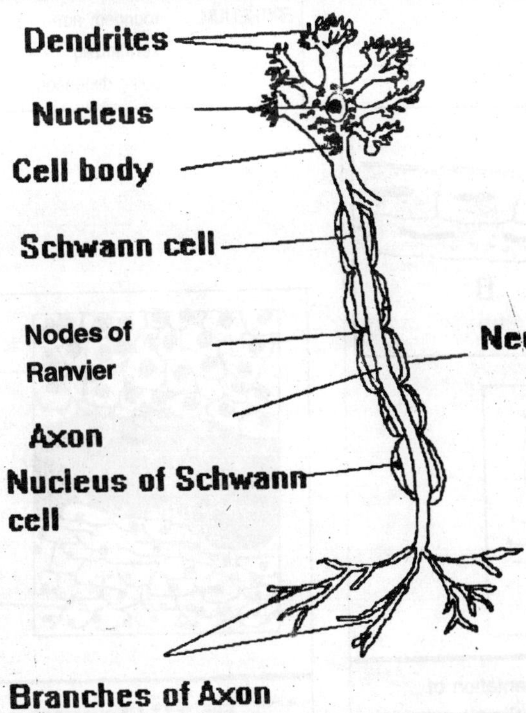

Fig. 2.9 : Schematic representation of nervous tissue

TYPE	STRUCTURE & FUNCTION	LOCATION
B. Simple cuboidal epithelium	Single layer of cube-shaped cell; excretion, secretion or absorption	Surface of ovaries, Lining of kidney tubules; salivary ducts and pancreatic duct.
C. Simple columnar epithelium	Single nonciliated	Lining of digestive tract layer of fall columnar shaped
D. Simple ciliated columnar epithlium	Single ciliated layer of columnar shaped cell. Trans; portive role trhough ciliary motion	Lining of the uterine tube lumen.
E. Pseudo-stratified ciliated columnar epithelium	Single layer of ciliated irregularly shaped cells	Lining of respiratory passage ways, and ciliary movement of many goblet cell.

TYPE	STRUCTURE & FUNCTION	LOCATION
STRATIFIED EPITHELIUM	Two or more layers of cells; protection, strengthening or distention	Epidermal layer of skin lining of body openings layer of skin; ducts, urinary bladders.
Stratified squamous epithelium (Keratinized)	Numerous layers contain keratin outer layers flattened and dead; Protection	Epidermis of skin
Stratified squamous epithelium (Non keratinized)	Numerous layers, lack keratin, outer layer moistened and alive; protection and pliability	Linings of oral and nasal cavities
Stratified cuboidal Epithelium	Usually two layers of cube-shaped cells. Strengthen luminal walls	Larger duct of sweat glands, salivary glands, and pancreas
TRANSITIONAL EPITHELIUM	Numerous layers of rounded, non-keratinized cells; distention	Luminal walls of ureters & urinary bladder

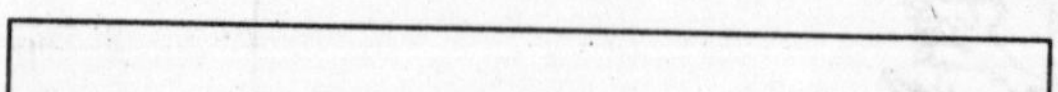

Fig. 2.10 : Schematic representation of A. Simple squamous epithelium, B. Simple cuboidal epithelium, C. Simple columnar epithelium.

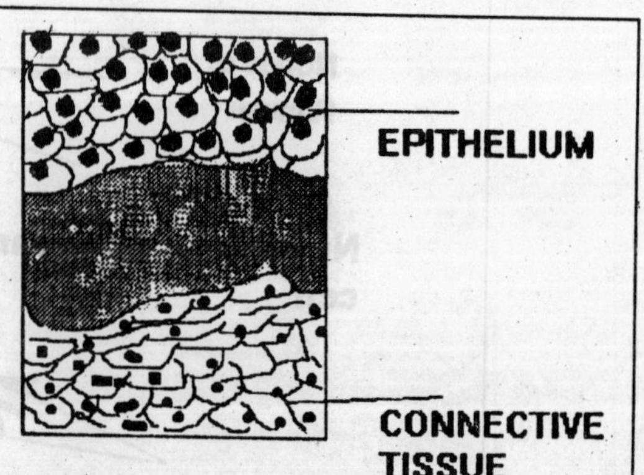

Fig. 2.11 : Schematic representation of non-keratinized squamous tissue

1. CONNECTIVE TISSUE PROPER

TYPE	STRUCTURE & FUNCTION	LOCATION
Loose connective tissue (Areolar)	Predominantly fibroblast cells with lesser amounts of collagen and elastin cells, binds organs; hold tissue fluids; diffusion	Surrounding nerves and vessels, between muscles, beneath the skin
Dense fibrous connective tissue	Densely packed collagen fibers; provides strong flexible support	Tendons, ligaments
Elastic connective tissues	Predominantly irregularly arranged elastic fibers; supports, provide framework	Large arteries, lower respiratory tract
Reticular connective tissues	Reticular fibers, forming supportive network, stores phagocytic vescicles	Lymph nodes, liver, spleen, thymus, bone marrow
Adipose connective	Adipose cells, Protects, stores fat, insulates	Hypodermis of skin surface of heart, kidney, surrounding joints

CARTILAGE

Cartilage consist of group of cells in a matrix (condrocytes) tough and elastic covered by a membrane — perichondrium.

TYPE	STRUCTURE & FUNCTION	LOCATION
Hyaline cartilage	Chondrocyte surrounded by a semi-solid ground substance supportive action: Gives thick coating	It forms end of ribs, nose, larynx, trachea and bronchial tubes
Fibrous cartilage	Chondrocytes surrounded by fibrous tissues. Tolerate greater strength, serves as a strong flexible connective material between bones	Bone joints
Elastic cartilage	Chondrocytes surrounded by elastic tissue fibers strengthen and maintain shape of these organs	Epiglottis, cartilages of the larynx, auditory tube and external ear

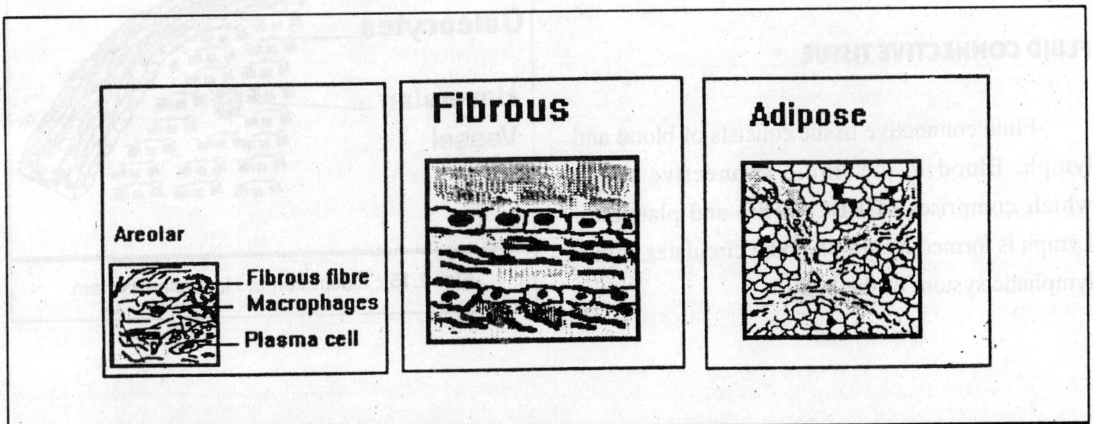

Fig. 2.12 : Schematic representation of connective tissue proper — Areolar, Fibrous, Adipose tissues

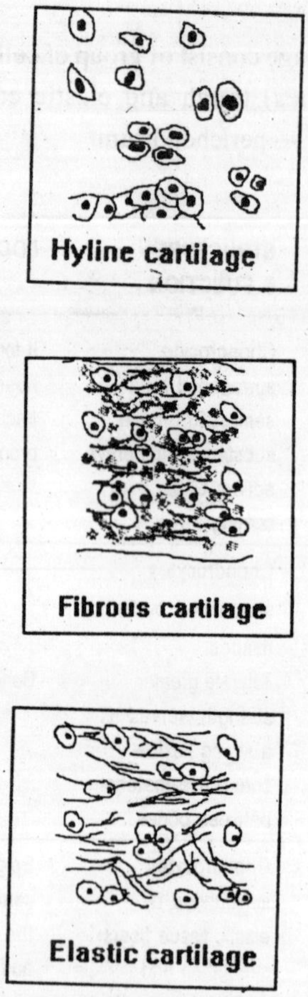

Fig. 2.13 : Schematic representation of cartilage tissues

SKELETAL TISSUE (BONE)

Layer of calcified material laid around blood vessels. Bone forming cells or osteoblast surrounded by their calcified products, become trapped within cavities called lacunae. The trapped cell (osteocyte) is nourished by the cytoplasm extended from the cell to the blood vessels in canaliculi. Blood vessels lie within central canals surrounded by concentric rings of bone lamellae with their trapped osteocyte called Haversian systems.

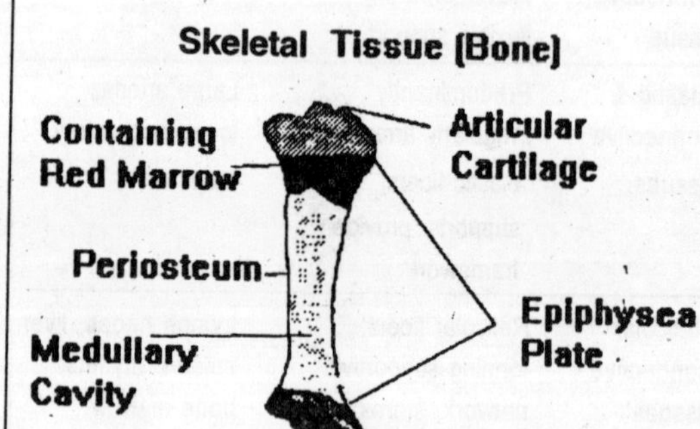

Fig. 2.14 : Illustration of Skeletal tissue

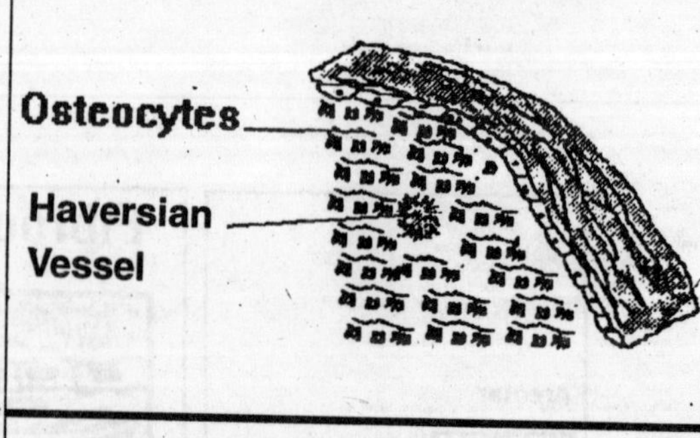

Fig. 2.15 : Illustration of Haversian system

FLUID CONNECTIVE TISSUE

Fluid connective tissue consists of blood and lymph. Blood is the liquid connective tissue which comprises of RBC, WBC and plateletes. Lymph is formed by lymph node; circulates within lymphatic system of the body.

3

CONTROL OF THE INTERNAL ENVIRONMENT

Homeostasis is defined as maintenance of a constant or unchanging normal internal environment. The term steady state is also defined as a constant internal environment but this does not necessarily mean that the internal environment is completely normal. When the body is in a steady state, a balance has been achieved between the demand placed on the body and the body's response to those demands.

A biological control is a series of interconnected components that serve to maintain a physical and chemical parameter of the body at a near constant value. The system is composed of a receptor, an integrating center and an effector. Most control systems act by way of negative feedback (**Asterita, 1985; Gareia & Sainz, 1991**). An example of negative feedback can be seen in the respiratory system's regulation of the CO_2

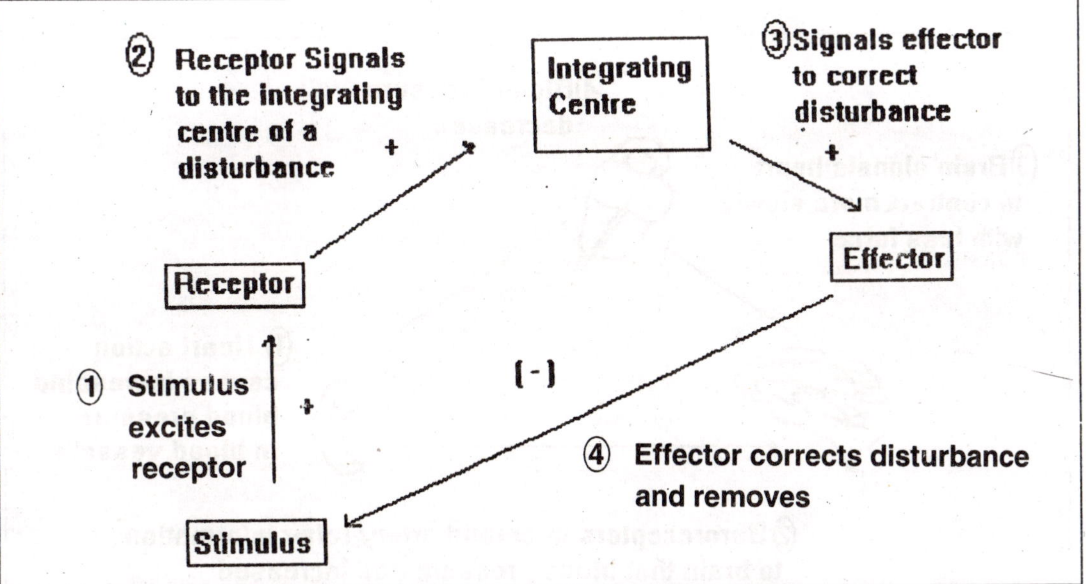

Fig. 3.1 : Schematic diagram of the components that compose a biological control system

concentration in extracellular fluid. In this case an increase in extracellular CO_2 above normal levels triggers a receptor which sends information to the respiratory control center (integrating center) to increase breathing. The effectors in this example are the respiratory muscles. The increase in breathing will lower extracellular CO_2 concentration back to normal, thus reestablishing homeostasis. The reason that this type of feedback is termed negative is that the response of the control system is negative (opposite) to the stimulus.

The precision with which a control system maintains homeostasis is termed the gain of the system :

$$\text{Gain} = \frac{\text{Amount of correction needed}}{\text{Amount of abnormality that exists after correction}}$$

$$\text{Feedback gain} = \frac{22° - 0°C}{37° - 36°} = \frac{22}{1} = 22$$

A control system with a large gain is more capable of maintaining homeostasis than a system with a low gain.

Example of homeostatic control

Regulation of arterial blood pressure : An excellent illustration of homeostatic control that uses negative feedback is the "baroreceptor system" which is responsible for the regulation of blood pressure. The baroreceptors are pressure sensitive receptors located in the carotid arteries and the arch of the aorta. When arterial blood pressure increases above the normal levels, these baroreceptors are stimulated and nerve impulses are transmitted to the cardio-vascular control center in the medulla of the brain. In turn, the cardio-vascular control center decreases the number of impulses transmitted to the heart, which lowers the amount of blood pumped by the heart, and causes arterial pressure to return to normal.

In contrast, a reduction in arterial pressure reduces the number of impulses transmitted from the baroreceptor to the brain, which causes the cardiovascular control center to increase the number of impulses transmitted to the heart to produce an increase in blood pressure (Fox, S 1996).

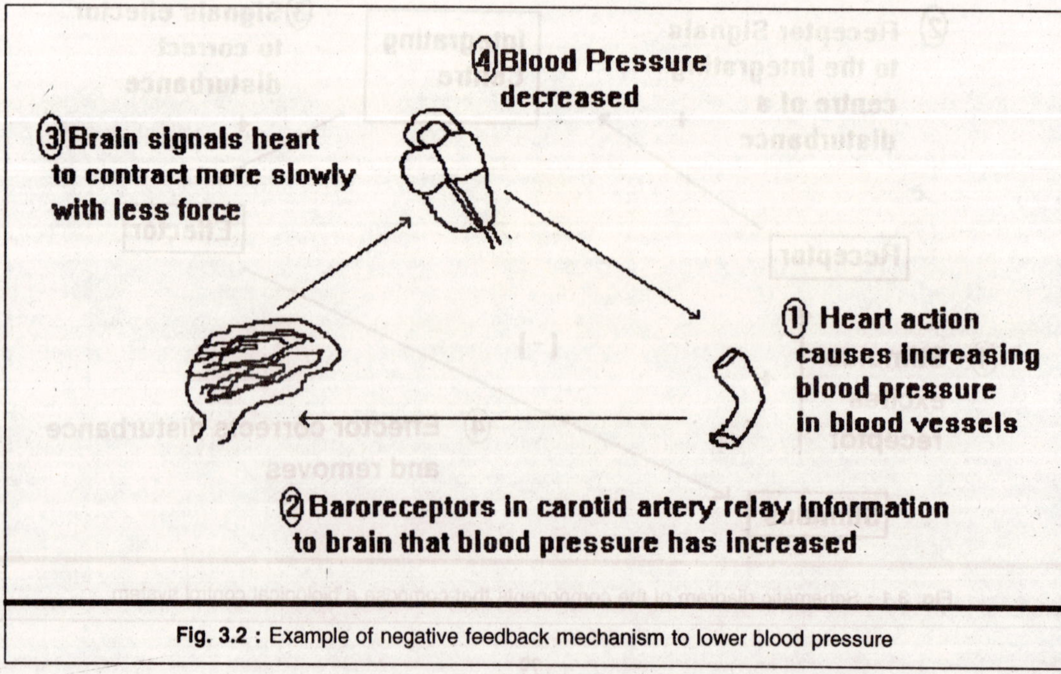

Fig. 3.2 : Example of negative feedback mechanism to lower blood pressure

Regulation of blood glucose

Homeostasis is also a function of the endocrine system. The body contains eight major endocrine glands, which synthesize and secrete bloodborne chemical substances called hormones. Hormones are transported via the circulatory system through out the body as an aid to regulate circulatory and metabolic functions (**Asterita M. 1985, Hill & Wyse 1989**). The hormone insulin regulate cellular uptake and the metabolism of glucose and is, therefore, important in the regulation of blood glucose concentration. After a large carbohydrate meal, the blood glucose level increases above normal. The rise in blood glucose signals the pancreas to release insulin, which then acts to lower blood glucose by increasing cellular uptake. Failure of the blood glucose control system results in the disease called diabetes.

Exercise : A test of Homeostatic control

Heavy muscular exercise produces large of amount lactic acid which causes an increase in intracellular and extracellular activity (**Edwards 1983, McCully K et al 1991, Vollestad & O Sejersted 1988**). The increase in acidity represents a serious challenge to the body's acid base control system (**Brooks and Fahey 1984, Fox S 1996**). Additionally, heavy exercise results in large increases in muscle oxygen requirement and large amount of CO_2 is produced. These changes must be countered by increase in breathing and blood flow to increase oxygen delivery to the exercising muscle and remove metabolically produced CO_2. However, intense exercise or prolonged work in a hostile environment (i.e., high temperature/humidity) may exceed the ability of a control system to maintain a steady state and severe disturbances in homeostasis may occur.

REFERENCE

Asterita, M. (1985) : ***Physiology of Stress***, New York, Human Sciences Press.

Brooks, G. and Fahey, T. (1984) : ***Exercise Physiology*** : Human Bioenergetics and its application. New York, John Willey and Sons.

Edwards, R. H. T. (1983) : Biochemical basis of fatigue in exercise performance : catastrophe theory of muscular fatigue. ***In biochemistry of exercise*** eds. H. Kunttagen, J. Vogal and J. Poortmans. Champaign IL Human Kinetics.

Fox, S. (1996) : ***Human Physiology***, Dubugue IA WMC Brown.

Gracia Sainz J. (1991) : Cell responsiveness and protein kinase C — receptor G proteins and membrane effectors, ***News in physiological sciences*** 6 : 196-73.

Hill, R. and G. Wyse (1989) : ***Animal Physiology***, New York, Harper and Row.

Iyengar, S. (1984) : ***Computer modelling of complex biological system*** Boca Raton Fl. CRC Press.

McCully, K. et al. (1991) : Biochemical adaptation to training. Implications for resisting muscle fatigue, ***Canadian Journal of Physiology and Pharmacology*** 69 : 274-278.

Toates, F. (1975) : ***Control theory in biological and experimental Physiology***, London, Hutchinson Education.

Vollestad, N. and O. Sejersted (1988) : biochemical correlates of fatigue, ***European Journal of Applied Physiology*** 57 : 336-37.

4

CARDIOVASCULAR SYSTEM

STRUCTURE OF HUMAN HEART

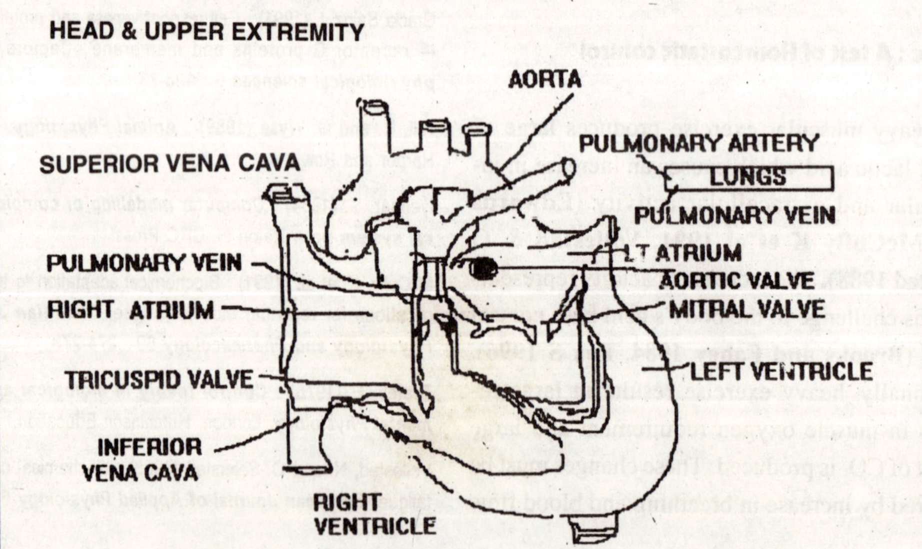

Fig. 4.1 : Structure of human heart

Heart is situated in the thoracic cavity between the lungs towards left side. Heart has four chambers — right auricle, right ventricle and left auricle, left ventricle. The upper chambers (auricles) are separated by a partition known as intraauricular septum, similarly the lower chambers (ventricles) are separated by the intraventricular septum. It is an hollow organ formed by cardiac muscles (myocardium) which are striated and involuntary. It is covered by a thin layer, namely pericardium. The inner layer of the heart is known as endocardium. The heart is composed of three major types of cardiac muscle — atrial muscle, ventricular and a specialized excitatory and conductive muscle fibers. Both atrial and ventricular muscles contract in the same way as the skeletal muscle fiber. On the other hand, specialized excitatory muscle fibers contract feebly because they contain few contractile fibrils; instead, because of their rhythmical properties and their rapidity of conduction, they provide an excitatory system for the heart and a transmission system for rapid conduction of impulses throughout the heart. Myocardium differs from skeletal muscle in one important way — the cardiac muscle fibers are anatomically interconnected end to end by interconnected disks. These disks have desmosome, which are structures that anchor the individual cell together, so they do not pull apart during contraction, and gap junctions which allow rapid transmission of the impulse signalling contraction. These features allow the myocardium in all four chambers to act as one large muscle fiber. All fibers contract together. Because of the syncytial nature of cardiac muscle, stimulation of any single atrial or ventricular muscle fiber causes the action potential to travel over the entire atrial and ventricular muscle mass, respectively, if the AV bundle is intact, the action potential passes also from the atria to the ventricle. This is called the 'all or none' principle.

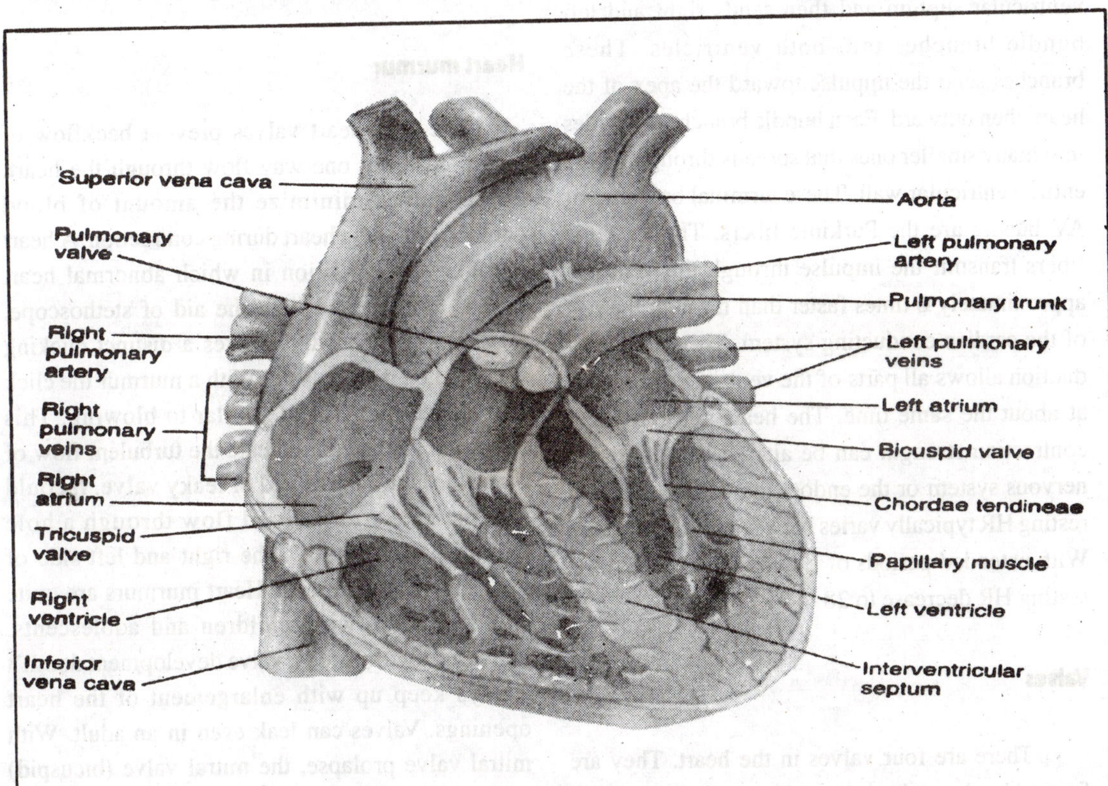

Fig. 4.2 : Anatomy of human heart

Cardiac tissue is capable of auto-conduction and has its own conductivity system. It imitates its own pulse with neural control. The impulse for heart conduction is initiated in the SA node, a group of specialized cardiac muscle fibers located in the posterior wall of the right atrium. This tissue generate the impulse, typically at a frequency of about 60-80 bpm (sinus rhythm). The electrical impulse generated by the SA node spreads through both atria and reaches AV node located in the right atrial wall, near the center of the heart. As the impulse spreads through the atria, the atria contract.

The AV node conducts the impulse from the atria into the ventricle. The impulse is delayed by about 0.13s as it passes through AV node, then it enters AV bundles. This delay allows the atria to fully contract before the ventricles do, maximizing ventricular filling. The AV bundles travels along ventricular septum and then sends right and left bundle branches into both ventricles. These branches send the impulse toward the apex of the heart, then outward. Each bundle branch subdivides into many smaller ones that spreads throughout the entire ventricular wall. These terminal branches of AV bundle are the Purkinje fibers. The Purkinje fibers transmit the impulse through the ventricle approximately 6 times faster than through the rest of the cardiac conducting system. This rapid conduction allows all parts of the ventricle to contract at about the same time. The heart rate (HR) and contraction strength can be altered by autonomic nervous system or the endocrine system. Normal resting HR typically varies between 60 and 85 bpm. With extended periods of Endurance Training, the resting HR decrease to 28 to 35 bpm.

Valves

There are four valves in the heart. They are formed by the endocardium. They allow the blood to pass only in one direction.

(i) Right atrioventricular valve (Tricuspid valve) is situated between the right auricle and right ventricle. It has three flaps or cusps which allow the blood flow from the right auricle to the right ventricle only.

(ii) Left atrioventricular valve (Bicuspid valve or Mitral valve) is situated between the left auricle and left ventricle. It has two strong cusps or flaps which allow blood to pass from the left auricle to the left ventricle only.

(iii) Pulmonary semilunar valve is situated between the right ventricle and pulmonary artery. It allows the blood to pass from the right ventricle to the lungs through the pulmonary artery.

(iv) Aortic semilunar valve is situated between the left ventricle and the aorta which allows blood to pass from the left ventricle to all parts of the body through aorta.

Heart murmur

The four heart valves prevent backflow of blood, ensuring one-way flow through the heart. These valves minimize the amount of blood pumped out of the heart during contraction. A heart murmur is a condition in which abnormal heart sounds are detected with the aid of stethoscope. Normally a heart valve makes a distinct clicking sound when it snaps shut. With a murmur the click is replaced by a sound similar to blowing. This abnormal sound can indicate the turbulent flow of blood through a narrowed or leaky valve. It could also indicate errant blood flow through a hole in the wall separating the right and left side of the heart (septal defect). Heart murmurs are quite common in growing children and adolescents. During growth periods, valve development doesn't always keep up with enlargement of the heart openings. Valves can leak even in an adult. With mitral valve prolapse, the mitral valve (bicuspid) regurgitate some blood to flow back into the left atrium during ventricular contraction. This disorder, common to adults (6% to 17% of the population) including athletes, usually has little clinical significance unless there is significant back flow. Most murmurs in athlete are benign affecting neither the heart's pumping nor the athletes performance. But heart murmurs can indicate diseased valves, such as those with stenosis, in which the valve is narrowed and often thickened and rigid. This condition can require surgical replacement of the valve.

During contraction, when blood is forced our of the left ventricle under high pressure, the aortic semilunar valve is forced open. When this valve opens, its flaps block the entrance of blood into coronary arteries. As the pressure in the aorta decreases, the semilunar valve closes and these entrances are exposed, so blood can then enter the coronary arteries. This design ensures that the coronary arteries are spared the very high blood pressure created by contraction of the left ventricle, thus protecting these vessels from damage.

BLOOD CIRCULATION

In human body, blood is circulated either by systemic or pulmonary circulation.

Systemic circulation

In this circulation oxygenated blood is supplied to the various parts of the body and deoxygenated blood returns to the heart. Left ventricle receives the oxygenated blood from the left auricle through the mitral valve and from there the blood passes through aorta and its branches to all parts of the body. Deoxygenated blood from all parts of the body reaches through superior and inferior vena cava to the right auricle.

Pulmonary circulation

The right ventricle receives deoxygenated blood from the right auricle through the tricuspid valve and from there the blood passes to the lungs through the pulmonary arteries for oxygenation. This oxygenated blood returns to the left auricle through the pulmonary veins.

Return of blood to the heart

Cardiovascular system requires assistance to overcome the force of gravity when returning blood from the lowest part of the body back to the heart. 3 mechanisms assist the process : (a) breathing, (b) the muscle pump, and (c) valves. Each time when we inhale and exhale, pressure changes in the abdominal and thoracic cavities assist blood return to the heart. As they contract, the skeletal muscles in the legs or abdomen share this function. During breathing and skeletal muscle contraction, the veins in the immediate vicinity are compressed and blood is pushed upward toward the heart. These actions are aided by a series of valves in the veins that allow blood to flow in only one direction, thus preventing backflow and pulling down of the blood in the lower body.

Distribution of blood

At rest under normal condition, the most metabolically active tissues receive the greatest blood supply. The liver and kidney receive almost half the blood being circulated (27% and 22%, respectively) whereas resting skeletal muscles receive only 15%. During exercise (heavy endurance) muscles receive up to 80% or more of the available blood. Similarly, after a heavy meal, digestive system receives more blood than at rest. Distribution of blood to various areas is controlled primarily by the arterioles. These vessels have a strong muscular wall that can significantly alter vessel diameters. They also respond to the mechanisms that control blood flow through autoregulation and extrinsic neural control.

As exercise begins, the active skeletal muscles rapidly experience an increased need for blood supply. This need is met through a generalized sympathetic stimulation of vessels in those areas in which blood flow is to be reduced (viz. digestive system, kidney). This causes contraction of vessels in those areas and thus diverts blood flow to the skeletal muscles where it is needed. In contrast, the skeletal muscles' sympathetic stimulation to the constrictor fibers in the vessel's wall is reduced and sympathetic stimulation to the vasodilator fiber is increased. Thus these vessels dilate and additional blood flow to the active muscles. The metabolic rate of the muscle tissue rises during exercise, as a result metabolic waste products begin to accumulate. Increased metabolism causes an increase in acidity, CO_2 and temperature in muscle tissue. These local changes trigger vasodilatation through autoregulation, increasing blood flow through the local capillaries. Auto-regulation is also triggered by the low partial pressure of O_2 (PO_2) in the tissue (increased O_2 demand), the act of muscle contraction and, possibly, other vasoactive substances released as a result of contraction.

Competition for blood supply

Mikirman et al (1991) studied the effects of feeding versus fasting on the distribution of blood flow during exercise on pigs. The pigs were divided into 2 groups. One group fasted for 14-17 hours. The other group ate their morning ration distributed in 2 feedings — half feed 90-120 mins before exercise and half feed 30 to 45 mins before exercise. Both groups of pigs were run at 65% of their VO_2 max. Blood flow to the hinder limb muscles during exercise was 18% lower in the feeding group than in the fasting group. Gastro Intestinal (GI) blood flow was increased 23% in the fed group. **Waaler et al (1990)** reported similar results in humans, concluding that the redistribution of GI blood flow to the working muscles is less marked after a meal than before a meal. This suggests that athletes should be very careful in timing their meals before competition, because they want as much blood flow as possible available to the active muscles during exercise.

Cardiovascular drift

Exercise in hot-humid condition results a reduction of blood volume by a loss of water through sweating and generalized shifting of fluid out of the blood into the tissues (edema). The total blood volume gradually decreases as the duration of exercise increases and with a redistribution of more blood to the periphery for cooling, comes a reduction in pressure for cardiac filling. This causes decreased venous return which, in turn, reduces SV (EDV is decreased). The HR compensates for the decreased SV by increasing, in an effort to maintain cardiac output (Q) these alterations are referred to as cardio-vascular drift. This response enables one to continue exercise at low to moderate intensity. However, human body is unable to fully compensate for decreased SV at high intensities because the heart rate attains its maximal value at a much lower exercise intensity, thus limiting the maximal performance capacity.

Redistribution of venous blood

The majority of blood is located in the venous return channels — about 64% (vein, venules, venous sinuses). Thus the venous system provides a large reservoir of blood readily available to meet an increased need. When this need arises sympathetic stimulation of the venules and veins constricts these vessels. This causes rapid distribution of blood from peripheral venous circulation back to the heart, and then out of those areas that have greater needs. Not only is blood diverted away from other tissues but more blood is sent into arterial circulation from the venous system — thereby ensuring a substantial increase of blood flow to a needy area.

Heart (7%) → Arteries (13%) → Arterioles & capillaries (7%) → Veins (64%) → Pulmonary (9%)

CARDIOVASCULAR REGULATION

Regulation of Heart Rate

During exercise the quantity of blood pumped by the heart must change in accordance with the elevated skeletal muscle oxygen demand. Since SA node controls heart rate, changes in heart rate often involves factors that influence the SA node. The two most prominent factors that influence heart rate are the parasympathetic and sympathetic nervous systems. The parasympathetic fibers that supply the heart arise from neurons in the cardiovascular control center in the medulla oblongata and make up a portion of the vagus nerve. Upon reaching the heart, these fibers make contact with both SA node and the AV node. There they cause a decrease in the activity of both the SA and AV node due to hyperpolarization. The end result is the reduction of heart rate. Even at rest the vagus nerve carry impulses to the SA and AV node **(Fox, 1987, Gurton, 1986)**. This is referred to as 'Parasympathetic tone'. As a consequence a decrease in parasympathetic tone to the heart activity causes a slowing of heart rate.

Studies revealed that the initial increase of HR up to approximately 100 beats/minute is due to a withdrawal of parasympathetic tone **(Rowell, 1986)**. At a higher work rates, stimulation of the SA and AU nodes by the sympathetic nervous system is responsible for increases in heart rate **(Rowell, 1986)**. Sympathetic fibers reach the heart by means of the cardiac accelerator nerves, which innervate both the SA node and the ventricle. Ending of these fibers release norepinephrine upon stimulation which causes an increase in both heart rate and the force of myocardial contraction.

At rest, a normal balance between parasympathetic tone and sympathetic activity to the heart is maintained by the cardiovascular control center in the medulla oblongata. An increase in resting blood pressure above normal stimulates pressure receptors in the common carotid artery and the arch of aorta, which, in turn, send impulses to the cardiovascular control center. In response the cardiovascular control centre increases parasympathetic activity to the heart to slow the heart rate and reduce cardiac output. This reduction in cardiac output causes blood pressure to decline back towards normal.

Another regulatory reflex involves pressure receptors located in the right atrium. An increase in right atrial pressure signals the cardio-vascular control center that an increase in venous return has occurred, hence in order to prevent a back up of blood in the systemic venous system, an increase in cardiac output must result. The cardiovascular control center responds by sending sympathetic accelerator nerve impulse to the heart, which increases heart rate and cardiac output. The end result is that the increase in cardiac output lowers right atrial pressure back to the normal and venous blood pressure is reduced. A change in body temperature can influence heart rate. An increase in body temperature above normal results in an increase in heart rate, while a lowering of body temperature below normal causes a reduction in heart rate **(Brengelmann, 1983, Kenny, 1988, Rowell, 1974, Rowell et al, 1976, Rubin, 1987)**.

Regulation of blood flow (Auto-regulation)

Auto regulation refers to the vessels' ability to self-regulate their own blood flow depending on the immediate needs of the tissues they supply. The arterioles undergo vasodilatation, opening up to allow more blood to enter an area in need. Oxygen demand appears to be the strongest stimulus. As the tissue's oxygen need increases, available oxygen is diminished in local arterioles and it dilates to allow more blood, and then more oxygen, to perfuse that area. Other chemical changes that can provide stimuli are decrease in

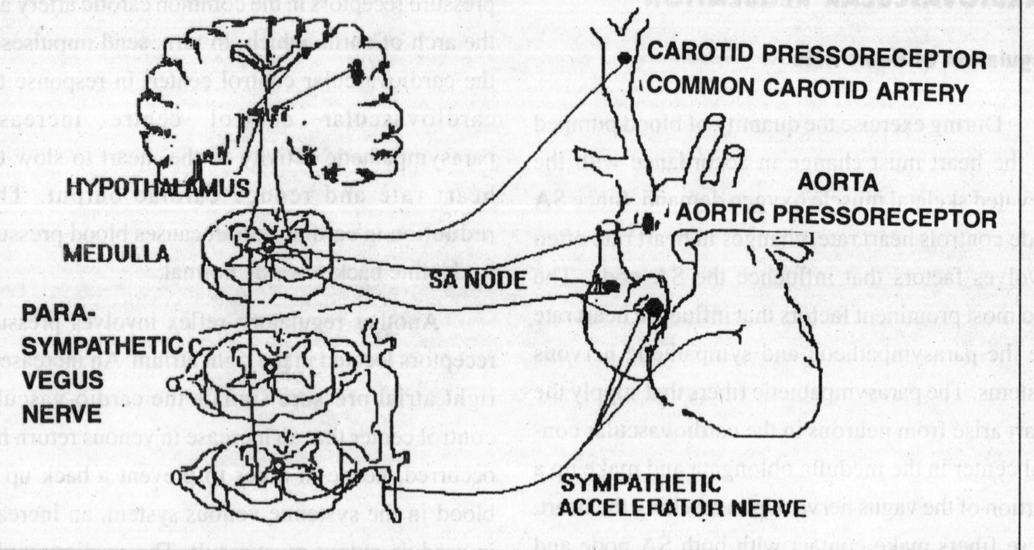

Fig. 4.3 : Neural pathway controlling cardiovascular function

other nutrients and increases in byproducts (CO_2, K^+, H^+ and lactic acid) or inflammatory chemicals. Increased blood supply can either bring in needed substances or clear out harmful ones.

Extrinsic Neural Control

Under normal conditions, the sympathetic nerves transmit impulses continuously to the blood vessels, keeping the vessels in a state of moderate constriction to maintain adequate blood pressure. This state of partial constriction is referred to as vasomotor tone. When sympathetic stimulation increases, further constriction of the blood vessels in a specific area decreases blood flow into that area and allows more blood to shift elsewhere. But if sympathetic stimulation decreases below that needed to maintain tone, contraction of vessels in that area is lessened, so the vessels dilate, increasing blood flow in that area. Therefore, sympathetic stimulation will cause vasoconstriction in most vessels, but blood flow is altered by either increasing or decreasing the amount of vasoconstriction relative to the normal vasomotor tone. The sympathetic system can also directly cause vasodilatation through some of its fibers. A different type of sympathetic fiber supplies some blood vessels in skeletal muscle and in the heart. This system functions during the classic flight or fight response and increase blood flow into skeletal muscles and the heart. This response is also active during exercise, when skeletal muscles and the heart are working harder, requiring much more blood than when at rest.

CARDIAC CYCLE

Cardiac cycle includes all events occurring between two consecutive heart beats. In mechanical terms it consists of all heart chambers undergoing relaxation phase (diastole) and a contraction phase (systole). During diastole, the chambers fill with blood. During systole the chambers contract and expel their contents. The diastolic phase is longer than the systolic phase. For a normal individual with a heart rate at 74 bpm the entire cardiac cycle takes 0.815 to complete (60/74 beats). Of the total cardiac cycle at this rate, diastole accounts for 0.5s or 62% of the cycle and systole accounts for 0.31s or 38%. As the heart rate increases, these absolute time intervals shorten proportionately.

Events of cardiac cycle

Venous blood from superior and inferior vena cava → Rt. Atrium

Oxygenated blood through pulmonary vein → Lt. Atrium

Atrio-Ventricular valve open < Rt. Atrium — Tricuspid Valve Lt. Atrium — Mitral Valve

Blood flows freely to the ventricle., Both semi-lunar valve close

Atrial systole : Filling is more complete (0.2 Sec) (0.3 Sec)

Ventricular systole : Rising pressure exceeds the atrial pressure

Atrio ventricular valve close (1st Heart sound)

Closure of all the valves, no blood pumped; ventricle is in isometric contractile state

Pressure increased and exceeding the pressure of pulmonary artery & aorta

Both semilunar valve open and ejection starts

Ventricle contract (Isotonic contraction)

Ventricle relax (0.5 Sec)

Intraventricular pressure below the pressure of pulmonary artery and aorta

Both semilunar valve close (2nd heart sound)

Complete relaxation of ventricle and pressure drops below the atrial pressure

Atrial diastole (0.7 Sec); AV valve open

Refilling of blood in diastasis (3rd heart sound)

BLOOD

Composition of Blood

BLOOD

- **Plasma (55%)**
  - Solid (8-9%)
    - Inorganic Constituent (0.9%)
      - Na^{+}, K^{+}, Ca^{++}, Mg^{++}, P_4, Fe^{++}, Cu^{++}
    - Organic Constituent (7.5%)
      - Proteins
        - Prothrombin
        - Albumin
        - Globulin
        - Fibrinogen
      - Non protein Nitrogenous substance
        - Urea, Uric acid, Xanthine, Creatine, Creatinine, Ammonia, Amino acid
      - FAT
        - Natural Fat (Phospholipid, Cholesterol)
      - Glucose, Fructose etc.
      - Antibodies and various enzymes viz. : Amylases, Protease, Lipase, Phosphatase
  - Water (91-92%)
- **Blood Corpuscles (45%)**
  - RBC
  - WBC
  - Platelet

White blood cell (WBC)

WBC

- GRANULOCYTE
  - Neutrophil (60-70%)
  - Eosinophil (1-4%)
  - Basophil (0-1%)
- AGRANULOCYTE
  - Lymphocytes (25-30%)
  - Monocytes (5-10%)

Blood and lymph are the substances that transport materials to and fro from body tissues. Fluid from the plasma enters the tissues, becoming interstitial fluid. Most interstitial fluid returns to the capillaries, but some enters the lymphatic system as lymph, eventually returning to the blood. Blood is about 55% to 60% plasma and 40-45% formed elements. RBC constitute 99% of the formed elements volume, WBC and platelet together account for less than 1%. The percentage of the total blood volume composed of RBC is referred to as hematocrit. It typically varies between 40% and 45%. Oxygen is primarily transported bound to the haemoglobin (Hb) in RBC. Each RBC contain approximately 250 million Hb molecules, each able to bind 4 O_2 molecules. So each RBC can bind up to a billion molecules of oxygen. There are an average of 15 gm of Hb per 100 ml of whole blood. Each gram of Hb can combine with 1.33 ml of oxygen. So as much as 20 ml of O_2 can be bound for each 100 ml of blood.

Exercise and blood response

The changes that occur in the blood during exercise demonstrate that the blood is carrying out its necessary tasks. Here the major changes are seen. This happens because the venous oxygen concentration decreases during exercise, reflecting increased extraction of oxygen from the blood for use by the active tissues. The oxygen content drops, approaching zero in the active muscles, but the mixed venous blood in the right atrium of the heart rarely drops below 2-4 ml of oxygen per 100 ml of blood.

Plasma volume decreases during exercise. The fluid is pushed out of the capillaries by increases in hydrostatic pressure as blood pressure increases and is drawn into the muscles by the increased osmotic pressure that result from waste accumulation. However, with prolonged exercise or exercise in hot environments, increasingly more plasma fluid is lost through sweating, in an attempt to maintain body temperature and placing the person at risk of dehydration — a 10% to 20% or greater reduction in plasma volume can occur in prolong workout. Similar 15% to 20% decreases in plasma volume have been observed in one minute bout of exhaustive exercise (**Sejersted et al, 1986**). With resistance training the plasma volume loss is proportional to the intensity of effort, which loses off 7.7% when exercising at 40% of one repetition maximum, up to 13.9% when training at 70% (**Carlsten & Grimby, 1966**). A reduced plasma volume will likely impair performance.

For long duration activities in which heat loss is a problem, the total flow of blood to active tissue, must be reduced to allow increasingly more blood to be diverted to the skin in an attempt to lose body heat.

Reduced plasma volume also results in increased blood viscosity, which can impede blood flow and thus limit O_2 transport, especially if the hematocrit exceeds 60%. Hemoconcentration occurs as plasma fluid (water) is lost. Although the actual number of RBC might not increase, the net effect of this process is to increase number of RBC per unit of blood, which increase oxygen-carrying capacity. The hemoconcentration increases RBC concentration substantially by up to 20% to 25%. Hematocrit increases from 40% to 50%. This substantially increases oxygen-carrying capacity, which is advantageous during exercise.

Blood pH can change significantly during exercise, becoming more acidic as it moves from slight alkaline resting value of 7.4 down to 7.0 or lower. The muscle pH decreases even further. The decrease in pH primarily results from increased blood lactate accumulation during increased exercise intensity. As exercise intensity increases above 50%, pH start to decrease and blood become more acidic. Blood pH value of 7.0 or lower have been reported following maximal sprint training. The pH in active muscle drops more — to 6.5 or lower.

Functions of blood

1. Transport of respiratory gases : CO_2 & O_2.
2. Transport of nutrients : Carbohydrate, protein and fat, minerals and vitamins.
3. It acts as a vehicle : Through which hormones and vitamins are brought to their place of activity.
4. Drainage for waste products : Waste products of cellular activity are being carried out through the organ of excretion.
5. Maintenance of water balance :

   Factors involved —

   (i) endocrine (a) From Posterior pituitary vasopressin and oxytocin are secreted which reabsorb water from distal convoluted tubules and fluid loss maintained. (b) Adrenal cortex secretes aldosterone which stimulates ADH and causes retention of urine. (c) Adrenal medulla releases adrenaline which increases renal circulation and retains volume of urine.

   (ii) autonomic nervous system controlling ADH through hypothalamus.

   (iii) vasomotor system — circulation is regulated through vasoconstrictor and vasodilator nerves.

   (iv) lung and skin.
6. Maintenance of acid-base equilibrium — buffering power helps to maintain a constant reaction of the body.
7. Regulation of body temperature — high specific heat absorbs large amount of heat which prevents sudden change in body temperature. High conductivity results in quick distribution of heat, high latent heat of evaporation causes heat loss through skin and lungs.
8. Maintenance of ion balance Na^+, K^+, Cl^-, Ca^{++} between cell and its surrounding.
9. Defensive action — WBC's phagocytic properties engulf bacteria from foreign body, lymphocyte's T cell and B cell provide cell-mediated immunity.
10. Property of coagulation guards against hemorrhage.
11. Plasma protein. Albumin — Maintains colloidal osmotic pressure — transport fatty acid.

    Alfa 1 Globulin — Transportation of lipid, thyroxine, adrenal, cortical hormone

    Alfa 2 globulin — lipids, copar

    Beta Globulin — lipids iron (hemes : antibody activity)

    Gama Globulin — most of the circulating antibodies.

    Fibrinogen — Blood-clotting
12. Regulation of blood pressure by changing volume and viscosity.

CARDIAC FUNCTION

Stroke volume

During systole, a certain volume of blood is ejected from the left ventricle. This amount is the stroke volume (SV) of the heart. To understand stroke volume, consider the amount of blood in the ventricle before and after contraction. At the end of diastole, just before contraction, the ventricle has completed filling. The volume of blood it now contains causes the end diastolic volume, or the EDV. At the end of systole, just after contraction, the ventricle has completed its ejection phase. The volume of blood remaining in the ventricle is called the end systolic volume of ESV. Stroke volume is the volume of blood that was ejected, and is merely the difference between EDV and ESV.

In the figure (Fig. 4.4) stroke volume increases to maximal value during submaximal exercise (40-50% of VO_2 max at a heart rate range of

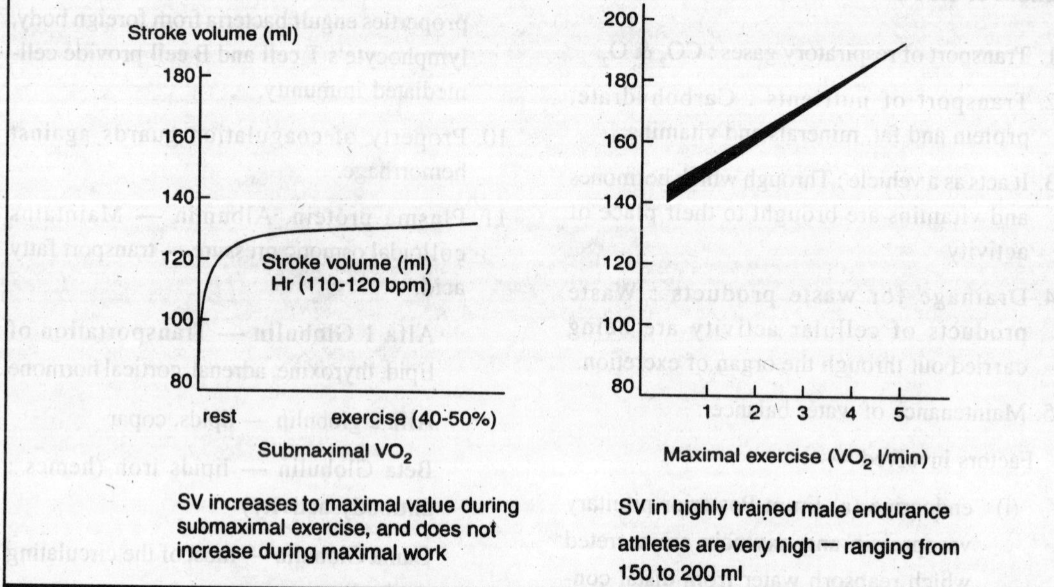

Fig. 4.4 : Exercise response on Stroke Volume

110-120 beats per minute) and does not increase during maximal work. Stroke volume in highly trained male endurance athletes are very high ranging (150-200 ml). Increase of SV is due to increase in venous return during diastole. According to Starling's law, greater the initial length of cardiac muscle fiber, the stronger is the myocardial contraction resulting in increment of stroke volume. Muscle pumping action results in increased filling of atria which, in turn increase the length of myocardial fiber. The filling of ventricles is increased, as a result ventricular contraction is increased, and stroke volume increase.

Ejection fraction

The proportion of blood pumped out of the left ventricle in each beat is the ejection fraction (EF). It is determined by dividing the stroke volume by the end diastolic volume.

$$EF = SV/EDV = 60/100 = 60\%.$$

Thus 60% of the blood in the ventricle at the end of diastole is ejected with the next contraction and 40% remains.

Cardiac output (Q°)

Cardiac output is defined as the amount of blood pumped by the left ventricle in one minute. It is the product of stroke volume and heart rate. SV at rest averages between 60 to 80 ml of blood.

$$Q° = SV \times HR;\ 75\ ml \times 70\ beats/min = 5{,}250\ ml/min.$$

Cardiacoutput' Fick's Principle'

$$= \frac{\text{Oxygen consumption/min (ml/min)}}{\text{Arterial } O_2 \text{ content} - \text{venous } O_2 \text{ content} (mlO_2\, 100\ ml\ blood)} \times 100$$

$$Q° = 200/20 - 16 \times 100 = 5{,}000\ ml$$

Cardiac output (Q°) Untrained :

Resting : 5,000 ml = 70 bpm × 71.4 ml

Maximal exercise :

22,000 ml = 195 bpm × 113 ml

Trained :

Resting : 5,000 ml = 50 bpm × 100 ml

Maximal exercise :

35,000 ml = 195 bpm × 179 ml

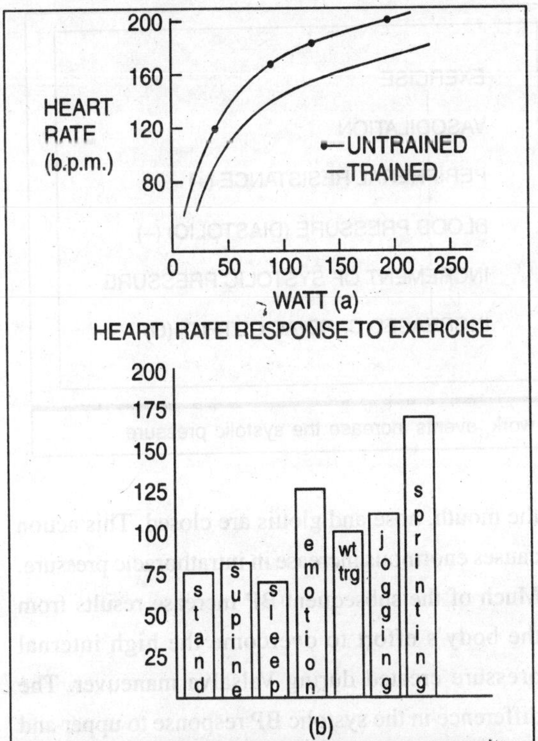

Fig. 4.5 : (a) Heart rate response during exercise in trained and untrained subject. (b) Maximum heart rate in various sports and events

Heart rate

Fig. 4.5 indicates some selected factors affecting heart rate :

(i) *Posture* — from recumbent to standing — variation of heart rate is evident from 10-12 beats per minute.

(ii) *Sex* — females have higher resting heart rate than males. Adult female 84 beats per minute, adult male 78 beats per minute.

(iv) *Emotion* — rise of heart rate (anticipatory rise) due to psychological reason.

(iii) *Age* — maximum heart rate decrease with age.

(v) *Environmental factors* — temperature, humidity etc. affect the heart rate. Fig. 4.5 also denotes that trained individuals can perform similar task at lower heart rate (economy of effort). Heart rate is influenced by either increase in body temperature, or fall in blood oxygen content.

Control of heart rate

Pressure afferent sources causing the elevation of heart rate :

(i) Proprioceptive reflexes originating in the working muscle and joints.

(ii) Impulses arising in the chemoreceptor of the carotid body and the aortic body as a result of decreased pH or increased CO_2.

(iii) Impulses arising from cerebral cortex prior to athletic event cause anticipatory increase in heart rate.

(iv) Impulses arising in the adrenal medulla & discharge epinephrine& norepinephrine through sympathetic stimulation.

Depressure afferent sources decrease the heart rate :

(i) Stimulation of parasympathetic nerve (vagus) causes the release of acetylcholine (Ach.) which slows down the rate of impulse formation in SA node.

(ii) Stretch receptors in the carotid sinus & aortic arch decrease the HR.

BLOOD PRESSURE

Blood pressure is the lateral pressure exerted on the wall of the blood vessels. When the pressure is measured during ejection phase of the heart, it is known as systolic blood pressure; the pressure being gauged during relaxation phase is known as diastolic blood pressure. Systolic blood pressure is the highest pressure within the vascular system. Diastolic BP is the lowest pressure on the vessel wall.

An approximation of mean arterial pressure is :

Mean arterial pressure = Diastolic pressure + [0.333 (Systolic BP — Diastolic BP)].

To illustrate, with a systolic pressure of 120 mm Hg and diastolic pressure 80 mm Hg. The mean arterial pressure = 80 + [0.333 × (120 — 80)] = 93 mm Hg. Note that this relationship is not a simple average of systolic average of systolic and diastolic values. Heart is in diastole longer than in systole, so arteries experience diastolic pressure longer than systolic — that is factored into the equation.

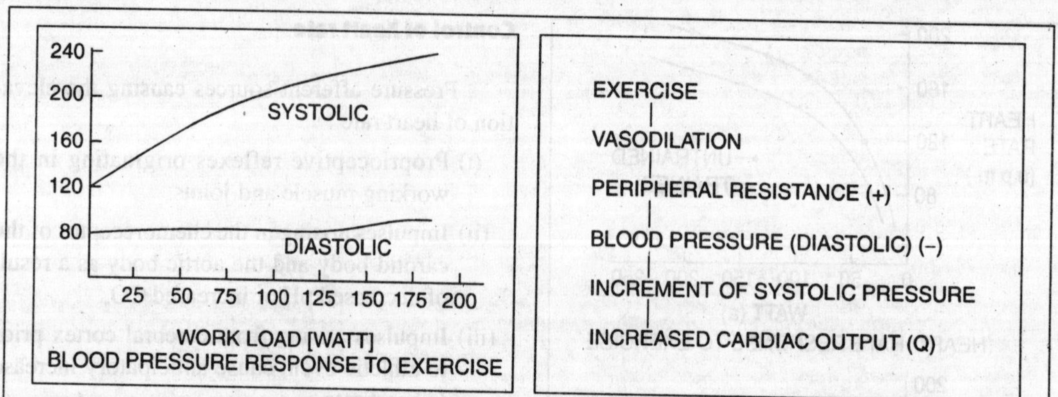

Fig. 4.6 : Blood pressure response in dynamic work, events increase the systolic pressure

With endurance type whole body activity, systolic BP increases in direct proportion to increased exercise intensity. Systolic pressure of 120 mm Hg at rest can exceed 200 mm Hg at exhaustion. Systolic pressure 240-250 mm Hg have been reported in normal, healthy, highly trained athletes at maximum levels of exercise. Increased systolic pressure results from the increased Q that accompanies increasing rate of work. Diastolic BP changes little during endurance exercise, regardless of the intensity. Increases in diastolic pressure of 15 mm Hg or more are considered abnormal response to exercise and should stop the workout. Blood pressure reaches a steady state during submaximal steady state endurance exercise. As work intensity increases so does systolic BP. If steady state exercise is prolonged, the systolic pressure might start to decrease gradually due to increased arteriole dilatation in the active muscle which decreases the total peripheral resistance, but diastolic pressure remains constant.

Blood pressure responses to resistant exercise viz., weight lifting — BP can exceed 480/350 mm Hg (**Mac Dougall et al, 1985**). In such exercise, use of the Valsalva maneuver is quite common. The maneuver occurs when a person tries to exhale while the mouth, nose and glottis are closed. This action causes enormous increase in intrathoracic pressure. Much of the subsequent BP increase results from the body's effort to overcome the high internal pressure created during Valsalva maneuver. The difference in the systolic BP response to upper and lower body exercise has important implications for the heart. Myocardial O_2 uptake or myocardial blood flow are directly related to the product of HR and systolic BP. This value is referred to as double product (DD = HR × Systolic BP). With static or dynamic resistances exercise or upper body work, the DP is elevated indicating a much higher cost of the heart.

CARDIOVASCULAR RESPONSE TO EXERCISE

As exercise intensity increases, heart rate increases. The heart pumps blood more often, thus speeding up circulation. Stroke volume also increased with exercise, so the amount of blood ejected with each contraction increases. SV is determined by 4 factors : (i) the volume of venous blood return to the heart (ii) ventricular distensibility, or the capacity to enlarge the ventricle (iii) ventricular contractility (iv) aortic and pulmonary artery pressure.

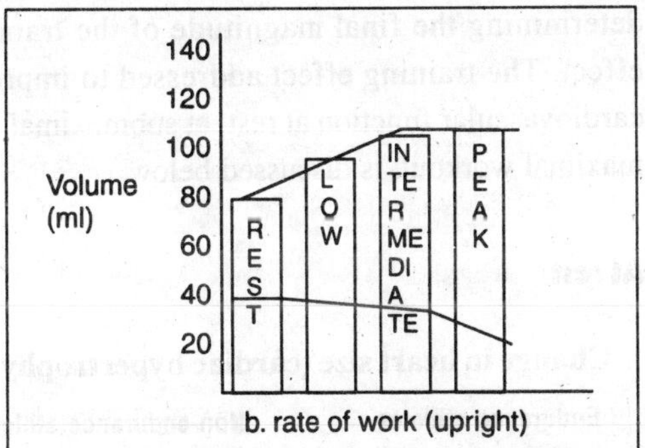

Fig. 4.7 : Stroke volume changes with exercise

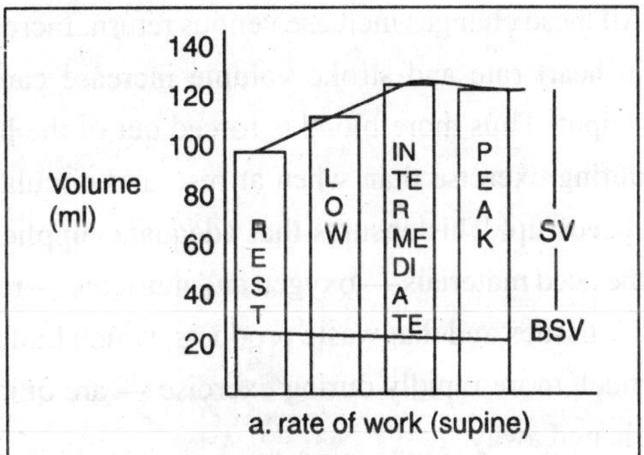

Fig. 4.8 : Stroke volume and end diastolic volume at rest

Most researchers agree that stroke volume increases with increasing rate of work, but only up to exercise intensity between 40% and 60% of maximal capacity. Several studies have found a plateau in SV at approximately 50% of VO_2 max with little or no change occurring with further increases (**Crawford et al, 1985, Higginbotham et al, 1986**). However, several other studies have shown that SV continues to increase beyond this rate (**Ekblom & Hermansen, 1968, Harmensen et al, 1970; Scruggs et al, 1991**).

When the body is in upright position, SV almost doubles from resting to maximal values. For example, in active untrained person it increases from 50-60 ml at rest to 100 to 120 ml at maximal exercise. In highly endurance trained athlete volume can increase from 80-110 ml at rest to 160-200 ml at maximal exercise. During supine exercise such as swimming, SV increase by only about 20% to 40% because in supine position blood does not pool in the lower extremities and blood returns more easily to the heart, which means that resting SV values are much higher in the supine position than in upright position. Thus the increase in SV with maximal exercise is not as great in supine position as in the upright position.

In one study participants were tested during both supine and upright cycle ergometry under 4 conditions : 1. Rest 2. A low work rate 3. An intermediate work rate 4. A peak work rate. An increase in left ventricular EDV (greater filling) would indicate that the Frank-Starling mechanism is operating, and a decrease in the left ventricular ESV (greater emptying) would indicate an increased degree of contractility. The results indicate that both the Frank-Starling mechanism and increased contractility are important in increasing SV. The Frank-Starling mechanism appears to have greatest influence at the lower rates of work, and contractility has its greatest effects at the higher rates of work. Several other studies supported this interpretation. The plateau or small decrease in left ventricular EDV could be caused by reduced ventricular filling time which was reduced from about 500-700 ms at rest to about 150 at higher heart rates (about 150 to 200 bpm) (**Turkevich et al, 1922**). So with increasing work rate, approaching maximum HR, the diastolic filling time could be shortened enough to limit filling. As a result, EDV might plateau or start decreasing.

For Frank-Starling mechanism to work, the amount of blood entering the ventricle must increase. For this to occur, venous blood return to the heart must increase. This can happen rapidly with redistribution of blood by sympathetic activation of arteries and arterioles in inactive areas of the body and general sympathetic activation of the venous system. The muscles are more active during exercise. So their pumping action increases. In addition, respiration increases. So intrathoracic and intrabdominal pressure changes are increased.

All these changes increase venous return. Increases in heart rate and stroke volume increase cardiac output. Thus more blood is forced out of the heart during exercise than when at rest, and circulation speeds up. This ensures that adequate supplies of the need materials — oxygen and nutrients — reach the tissues and that waste products, which build up much more rapidly during exercise — are quickly cleared away.

During the initial stages of exercises, increased Q is due to an increase in both HR and SV. When level of exercise exceeds 40% to 60%, the SV has either plateaued or begun to increase at a much slower rate. Thus further increases in Q are largely the result of increase in HR. It is important to realize that there are very specific responses to each of these modes.

Table 1 : Changes in heart rate, stroke volume and cardiac output in 3 activities.

Activity	Condition	Heart Rate (bpm)	Stroke Vol ml. beat^{-1}	Cardiac Output L min^{-1}
Running	Resting	60	70	4.2
	Max. Exercise	190	130	24.7
Cycling	Resting	60	70	4.2
	Max. Exercise	185	120	22.2
Swimming	Resting*	55	95	5.2
	Max. Exercise	170	135	22.9

*Measurement taken in supine position. It is important to realize that there are very specific responses to each of these modes.

CARDIOVASCULAR ADAPTATION TO METHODICAL TRAINING

The effect of training are influenced by many factors. Generally, the optimum intensity, frequency and duration of the training program leads to a greater improvement in most functions. The training effects are specific to the type of training program. Genetic limitations are also influential in determining the final magnitude of the training effect. The training effect addressed to improve cardiovascular function at rest, at submaximal and maximal workout, is discussed below.

At rest

Change in heart size (cardiac hypertrophy)

Endurance athletes	Non-endurance athletes
1. A large ventricular cavity.	1. A normal sized ventricular cavity.
2. Normal thickness of ventricular wall.	2. A thicker ventricular wall.
3. Filling of blood in the ventricle during diastole is more and greater than non-endurance athletes.	3. Ventricular force of contraction is more compared to their endurance counterpart.
Events : Long distance runners, Swimmers, Marathon runners	Events : Power events, Wrestling, Throwing

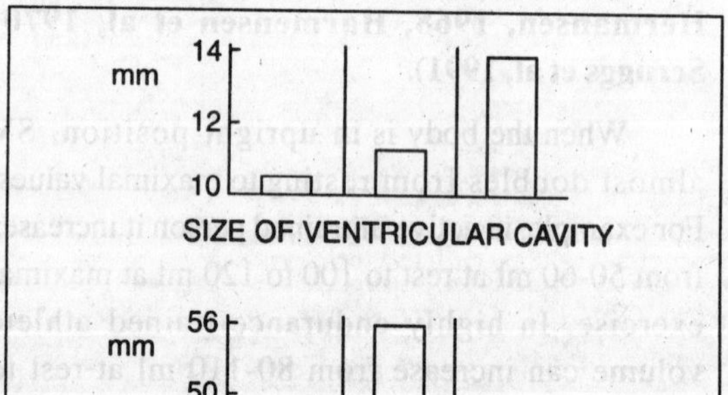

Fig. 4.9 : Diagrammatic representation of ventricular wall thickness, size of ventricular cavity, size of left ventricle of endurance athletes, power athletes and normal population (Morganroth et al, 1975, Nutter et al, 1975)

Heart volume is not genetically dependent (**Klissouras et al, 1973**). An intensive training can improve the heart volume (**Frick et al, 1963**). In endurance activity due to prolong effort, cardiac output sustained at high level (**Fox and Costill, 1972**) causes volume stress resulting in cardiac hypertrophy through an increase in the size of ventricular cavity. In power activity, intermittent elevation of arterial pressure causes pressure stimulus which, in turn, results in hypertrophy through thickening of ventricular wall.

Decreased heart rate

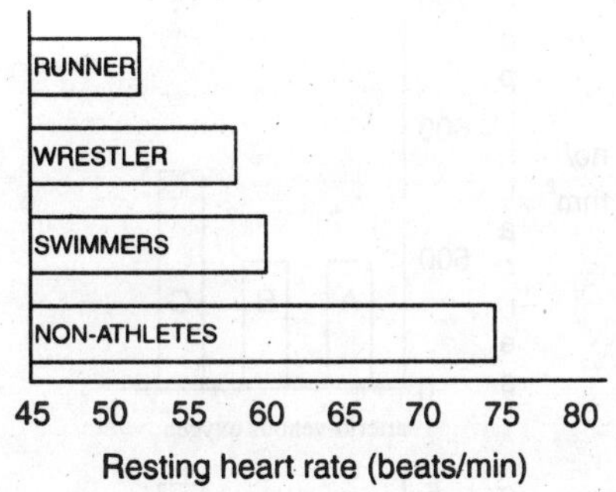

Fig. 4.10 : Diagrammatic representation of resting bradycardia in various sports and events

Resting bradycardia resulting from training it is evident when athletes and non-athletes are compared and less evident but still clear when sedentary subject undergo training program; less evident when athletes are studied in the untrained versus trained state (**Frick et al, 1967**). Resting bradycardia is dependent upon (a) long time period of intensive training, and (b) inversely proportional to the level of fitness. What causes the training bradycardia? It may be due to parasympathetic inhibition (increased vagal tone), decreased sympathetic influence or combination of both. The evidence indicates that resting bradycardia due to physical training is a result of a parasympathetic inhibition (**Bolter et al, 1973 & Scheuer et al, 1974**).

Increased stroke volume

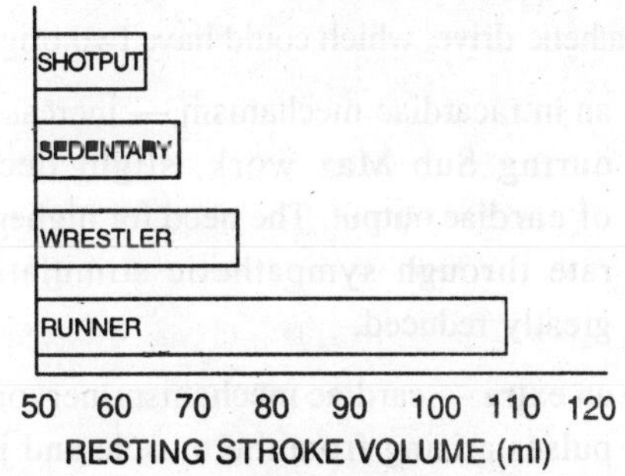

Fig. 4.11 : Diagrammatic representation of resting stroke volume in various sports and events

Increased stroke volume (SV) is more pronounced in endurance athletes due to increased ventricular cavity. More blood refilling during diastole increases SV. Long term intensive training program increases myocardial contractility. Pronounced increment of SV is observed when athletes are compared with non-athletes (**Penparg Kul & Scheuer, 1970**).

Changes in blood volume and hemoglobin

The total blood volume and haemoglobin increase with training (**Kjellberg et al, 1949; Oscai et al, 1968**). The increased haemoglobin and blood volume improve the oxidative capacity and is thus correlated with VO_2 max. Decreased heart rate during submaximal exercise following training (**Ekblom et al, 1968, Fox et al, 1973; Fox et al, 1975; Frick et al, 1967; Frick et al, 1963; Saltin et al, 1969**).

At submaximal exercises

No change or slight decrease in cardiac output.

Increased stroke volume.

Increased ventricular cavity.

Greater amount of blood filling.

Decreased heart rate or bradycardia during submaximal exercise caused by a decreased sympathetic drive, which could have two origins —

(a) an intracardiac mechanism — increased SV during Sub Max work, slight decrease of cardiac output. The need for higher heart rate through sympathetic stimulation is greatly reduced.

(b) an extra — cardiac mechanism-nervous impulses arising from the muscle and joints, descending impulses from the motor cortex, both can modify sympathetic stimulation to the heart. A reduced heart rate from this kind of modification means — primary change is in the muscle, secondary training effect is on the heart.

Changes in muscle blood flow

Blood flow/kg of working muscles is lower in trained than in untrained individuals at submaximal exercise, this is compensated by a greater a-VO_2 differences (**Saltin, 1969**). It may be related to the increased enzymatic activity for production of energy in the muscle. All the changes induced by training tend to reduce the relative stress imposed on oxygen transport and related systems.

At maximal exercise

1. Increased stroke volume through cardiac hypertrophy & myocardial contractility.
2. Increased cardiac output.
3. No changes or slight decrease in maximum heart rate :

   (a) An increased heart volume.

   (b) A decreased sympathetic drive.

   (c) No change in muscle blood flow.
4. Blood flow to the total working musculature is greater during maximal work following training. Increased blood flow is distributed over a larger muscle mass — thus making blood flow/kg of muscle mass constant.
5. Improvement of peripheral hemodynamics by endurance training improve capillarization, i.e., increase in capillary area due to endurance training (**Brodal, 1976**). Improved capillarization is by enlargement of existing capillaries and opening up of reserve capillaries (**Saltin et al, 1977**). Muscle biopsy studies have shown a mean increase in the capillary area of 36% due to endurance training (**Schon et al, 1978**).

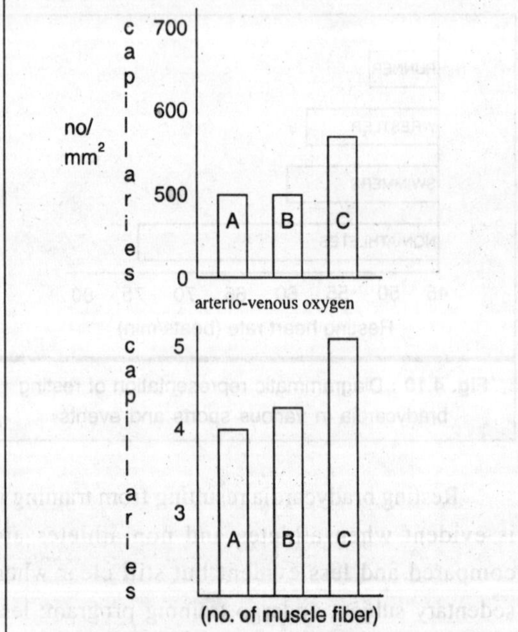

Fig. 4.12 : Diagrammatic representation of capillarization in Physically Inactive, Active and Endurance athletes

Collateral improvement : A more efficient intramuscular blood distribution. Blood flow characteristics are improved by endurance training with an improvement in the elasticity of the erythrocyte membrane which results in an increase the ability of the erythrocytes to change their shape in the capillaries (**Hollmann et al, 1988**).

IMPORTANCE OF HEART RATE MONITORING

Heart rate monitoring of actual game condition and training work out supply an objective picture of the exercise. For this reason alone it makes sense to register heart rate regularly. By analyzing heart rate records it appears that many mistakes are made during workout. It is often difficult to estimate the right intensity of the exercise in specific training addressed to develop endurance. Heart rate records provide an excellent means to teach the athlete the correct subjective feeling for a given intensity which enables him to have optimal benefits of his training by which performance level may rise.

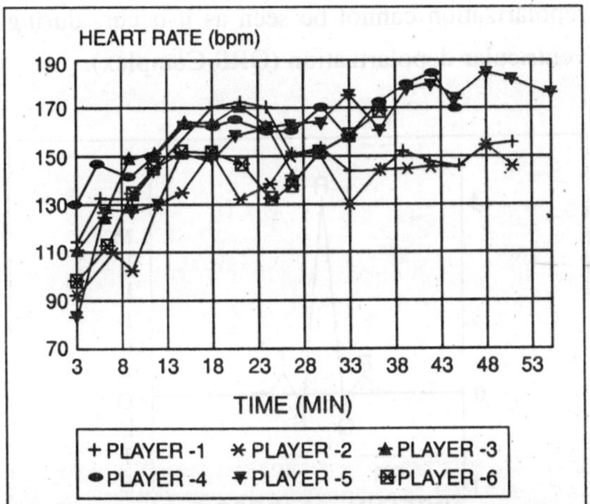

Fig. 4.13 : Heart rate response of Badminton game situation

Speed-Heart Rate relationship

Conconi's Principle

Conconi found that with very intense exercise heart rate/intensity relationship is no longer linear. The straight line deflects at high intensities. In other words, the intensity may be increased but the increase of heart rate lags at a certain point depicted in the figure. This point is the heart rate deflection point. The exercise intensity corresponding to this point is the maximum activity that can be done with aerobic energy supply.

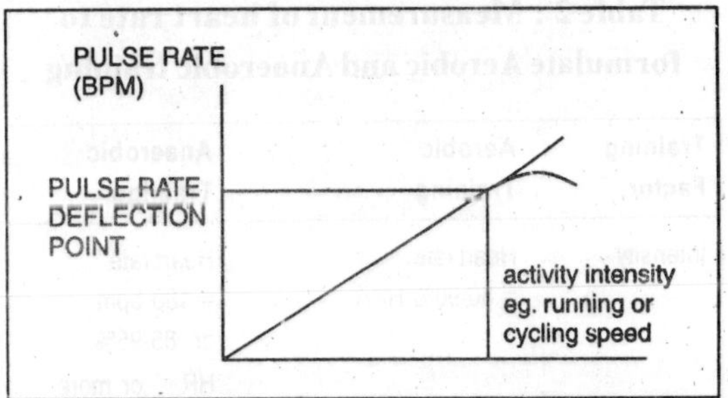

Fig. 4.14 : Graphical display of heart rate deflection point by Conconi's principle

The deflection in the curve marks the exercise intensity beyond which the athlete obtains a large amount of energy via anerobic pathway. The deflection point marks the maximum speed that can be maintained for a long period of time. It is the highest speed or heart rate that can be supported aerobically.

Interpretation : Five repetition of running workout with graded intensity to be given to athlete. In each repetition athlete is supposed to maintain a steady pace and the heart rate to be recorded. The recorded heart rate of each intensity effort is plotted against the performance score. The deflection point is termed critical heart rate or threshold heart rate. The same heart rate can act as a training tool for developing endurance.

For endurance training programs, training intensity can be judged from the heart rate response to exercise. The target heart rate (THR) should be between 80 and 90 percent of the maximal heart rate reserve (HRR) plus the resting heart rate (HR rest) or between 85 and 95 percent of the maximal heart rate (HR max).

The HRR is defined as the difference between the HR max and the HR rest. The HR max may be estimated from the equation. HR max = 220 – age. The HR rest may be determined by palpation of an artery, such as the carotid, in the neck.

Table 2 : Measurement of heart rate to formulate Aerobic and Anaerobic training

Training Factor	Aerobic Training	Anaerobic Training
Intensity	Heart rate = 80-90% HRR	Heart rate = 180 bpm or, 85-95% HR_{max} or more
Frequency	4-5 days per week	3 days per week
Session/day	one	one
Duration	12-16 weeks or longer	8-10 weeks
Distance /Workout	3-5 miles (km.)	1.5-2 miles (km.)

Method of assessment of heart rate

During ventricular contraction blood is ejected into the arteries with a pressure and this pressure wave is transmitted throughout the arterial system which can be felt easily in superficial artery. The number of pressure waves per minute felt at the arteries is called pulse rate. Normally it is about 70 to 80 per minute. In trained person it is found to be as low as 40 to 50 beats per minute. Measurement of heart rate can be done by the following way : (a) Stethoscope, (b) by pulse, (c) through electrocardiogram and (d) by radio-telemetric devise.

Stethoscope

It is a simple instrument which can magnify the sound generated by the heart. By counting the number of heart sounds per min heart rate can be found out. Pulse — Radial artery is commonly used to measure the pulse since it is easily accessible and lies against bone. The other arteries used to measure pulse are common carotid, brachial, femoral and dorsalis pedis. Method of measurement of radial pulse — Keep tips of the first three fingers over the wrist (Thumb side, lateral side). Number of pulsation, per minute are counted.

Electrocardiogram (ECG)

The ECG is a recording of the heart's electrical functioning. An exercise ECG may reveal underlying cardiac disorders. Three components of the ECG represent aspect of cardiac function. The P wave, the QRS complex and the T wave. The P wave represents atrial depolarization and occurs when an electrical impulse travels from SA node through the atria to the AV node. The QRS represents ventricular depolarization and occur as the impulse spreads from the AV bundle to the Purkinje fibers and through the ventricle. The T wave represents ventricular repolarization. Atrial repolarization cannot be seen as it occurs during ventricular depolarization (QRS Complex).

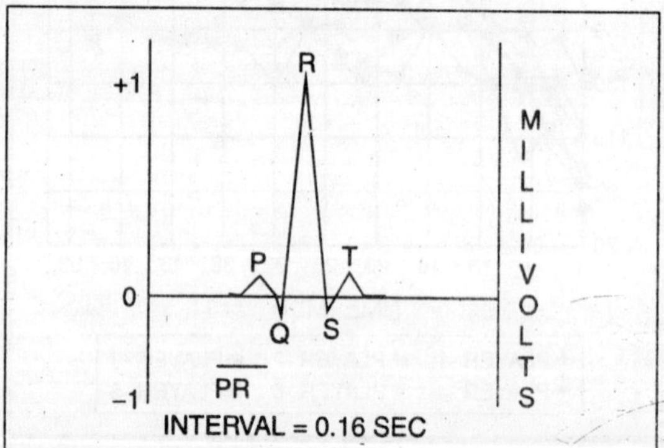

Fig. 4.15 : Electrical components of the ECG represent aspects of cardiac function

Radiotelemetry

Nowadays this method is commonly used for recording the heart rate in the field. In this method electrodes are attached along with a transmitter and are received by a receiver. The receiver is connected to a recorder or a heart rate monitor. The heart rate can also be stored in the memory of a microcomputer which can be carried on the wrist as a watch (Sports tester-PE3000).

Table 3 : Example of training programs adopted for speed endurance

Training Recovery HR (beats.min^{-1})	Duration of Intensity activity (sec)	No. of HR repetition (beats.min^{-1}) in set	Duration of rest in between repetitions (sec)	Recovery HR in between rest (bpm)	Rest between sets (min)
Shadow 105-130	40-50 153-190	6-8	40-50	150-165	2
Multishuttle 104-170	40-50 165-185	3-4	60-120	130-173	5

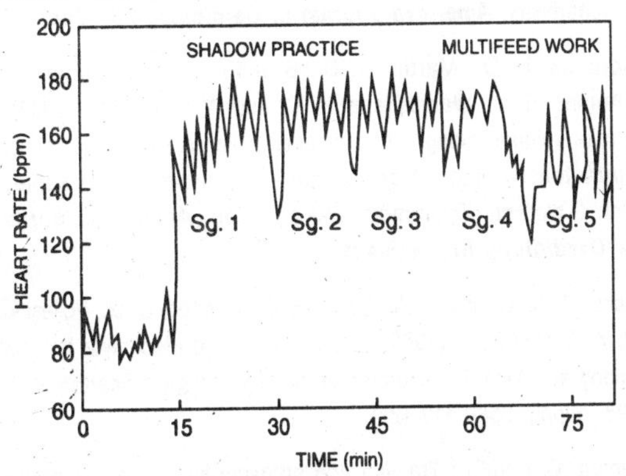

Fig. 4.16 : Monitoring of training in Badminton

REFERENCE

Bevegard, S., Holmgren, A. and Jonsson, B. (1963) : Circulatory studies in well trained athletes at rest and during heavy exercise with special reference to stroke volume and the influence of body postion, ***Acta Physiological Scandenavia*** 57 : 26-50.

Bolter, C. et al, (1973) : Intrinsic rate and cholinergic sensitivity of isolated atria from trained and sedentary rates, ***Proc. Society Experimental, Biology Medicine*** 144 : 364.

Brengelmann, G. (1983) : Circulatory adjustments to exercise and heart stress, ***Annual Review of Physiology*** 45 : 191-212.

Brodal, P. et al, (1976) : Capillary supply of skeletal muscle fibers in untrained and endurance trained men. ***Acta Physiologica Scandinavica*** (Suppl.) 440.

Carlsten, A. & Grimby, G. (1966) ***: The Circulatory Response to Muscular Exercise in Man***, Springfield I L, Charles C Thomas.

Crawford, M. H., Petru, M. A. and Rabinowitz, C. (1985) : Effect of isotonic exercise training on left ventricular volume during upright exercise, ***Circulation*** 72 : 1237-1243.

Ekblom, B., Astrand, P., Saltin, B., Stenberg, J. and Walstrom B. (1968) : Effect of training on circulatory response to exercise, ***Journal of Applied Physiology*** 24 (4) : 518-528.

Ekblom, B. and Hermansen, L. (1968) : Cardiac output in athletes, ***Journal of Applied Physiology*** 25 : 619-625.

Fox E., and Costill D. (1972) : Estimated cardiorespiratory responses during marathon running, ***Arch. Environment and Health*** 24 : 315-324.

Fox, S. (1987) Human Physiology, Dubuque, Ia : Wm, C. Brown Guyton, a (1986) ***Text Book of Medical physiology***, Philadelphia WB Saunder Company.

Fox, E., Bartels, R., Billings, C., O'Brien, R., Bason, R. and Mathews, D. (1975) : Frequency and duration of interval training programs and changes in aerobic power ***Journal of Applied Physiology*** 38(3) 481-484.

Fox, E., Barteis, R., Billings, C., Mathews, D., Bason, R. and Webb, W. (1973) Intensity and distance of interval training programs and changes in aerobic power, ***Medicine and Science in Sports*** 5(1) 18-22.

Frick, M., Kowttiner, A. and Sarayas, S. (1963) : Effects of physical training on circulation at rest and during exercise, ***American Journal of Cardiology*** 12 : 142-147.

Hermansen L., Ekblom B., and Saltin B. (1970) Cardiac output during submaximal and maximal treadmill and bicycle exercise, ***Journal of Applied Physiology*** 29 : 82-86.

Higginbotham, M. B., Marris, K. G., Willioms, R. S., McHale, P. A., Coleman, R. E. and Cobb, F. R. (1986) Regulation of stroke volume during submaximal and maximal upright exercise in normal man, ***Circulation Research*** 58 : 281-291.

Hollmann, W., Frenkl, R., Bertean, P. & Rost, R. (1988). The cardiovascular systems, ***The Olympic Book of Sports Medicine,*** (ed) Dirix A., Knuttgen, H. G. and Tittes, K., Blackwell Scientific Publications pp 40-48.

Kenny, W. L., (1988) Control of heat induced cutaneous vasodilatation in relation to age, ***European Journal of Applied Physiology*** 57 : 120-25.

Kjellberg, S., Rudhe, U. and Sjostrand, T. (1949) : Increase of the amount of haemoglobin and blood volume in connection with physical training, ***Acta Physiologica Scandinavia*** 19 : 146-151.

Klissoweas, V., Piray, F. and Petit, J. (1973) : Adaptation to maximal effort, genetics and age, ***Journal of Applied Physiology*** 35 (2) : 288-293.

Mac Dougall, J. D., Tuxen, D., Sale, D. B., Morz, J. R. and Sutton, J. R. (1985) Arterial BP response to heavy resistance exercise, ***Journal of Applied Physiology*** 58 : 785-790.

Mckirnan, M. D., Gray, C. G. and White, F. C. (1991) : Effects of feeding on muscle blood flow during prolonged exercise in miniature swine, ***Journal of Applied Physiology*** 70 : 1097-1104.

Morganroth, J., Maron, B., Henry, W. and Epstein, S. (1975) : Comparative left ventricular dimensions in trained athletes, ***Annals International Medicine*** 82 : 521-524.

Nutter, D., Gilbert, C., Heymsfield, S., Perkins, J. and Schlant, R. (1975) : Cardiac hypertrophy in the endurance athletes, ***Physiologist*** 18(3) : 336.

Oscai, L., Williams, B and Hertis, B. (1968) : Effect of exercise on blood volume, ***Journal of Applied Physiology*** 24(5) : 622-624.

Rowell, L. (1974) ***: Human Circulation Regulation During Physical Stress*** New York : Oxford press.

Rubin, S. (1987) : Core temperature regulation of heart rate during exercise in humans, ***Journal of Applied Physiology*** 62 : 1997-2002.

Saltin, B., Blomqvist, G., Mitchell, J., Johnson, R. (1968), Wildenthal, K. and Chapman, C : Response to exercise after bed-rest and after training, ***Circulation*** Supply 7.

Saltin, B., Hartley, L., Kilbom, Å and Åstrand, I. (1969) : Physical training — sedentary middle aged and older men II, Oxygen uptake, heart rate and blood lactate concentrations at submaximal and maximal exercise, ***Scandinavian Journal of Clinical Lab Investigation*** 24 : 323-334.

Saltin, B., and Karlsson, J. (1971) : Muscle glycogen utilization during work of different intensities. In Pernow B. and Saltin B. (eds), ***Muscle Metabolism During Exercise*** New York, Plenum Press pp 289-299.

Saltin, B. et al, (1977) : Fiber types and metabolic potentials of skeletal muscles in sedentary man and endurance runners, ***Annal New York Academy of Science*** 301 : 3.

Saltin B (1969) : Physiological effects of physical conditioning, ***Medicine Science Sports***. 1 : 50.

Schan, F. A., Hollmann, W., Liesen, H. and Waterloh, E. (1980) : Elektronen-mikroskopische Befunde am M. Vastur lat von Untrainlerten und Marathon Laufern Sowice iwea Beziehug zur relativen maximalen Sarerstoffanfnahme und laktatproduktion, ***Dtsch Z., Sportmed*** 31 (12) 343.

Scheuer J. et al, (1974) : Experimental observations on the effects of physical training upon intrinsic cardiac physiology and biochemistry, ***American Journal of Cardiology*** 33 : 744.

Scruggs, K. D., Martin, N. B., Broader, C. E., Hofman, Z., Thomas, E. L., Wambsgans, K. C. and Wilmore, J.H. (1991) : Stroke volume during submaximal exercise in endurance trained normotensive subject and in untrained hypertensive subject with ß-blocked (Propranolo and pindolol), ***American Journal of Cardiology*** 67 : 416-421.

Schon, I. A., Hollmann, W., Leser, H. & Sejersted, O. M., Vollestad, N. K. & Medbol, I. (1986) : Muscle fluid and electrolyte balance during and following exercise, ***Acta Physiologica Scandinavica*** 128 (supply. 5560 119-127).

Tipton, C. (1965) : Training and bradycardia in rats, ***American Journal of Physiology*** 209 : 1089-1094.

Tipton, C., Barnard, R. and Tcheng, T. (1969) : Resting heart rate investigations with trained and non-trained hypophysectoismed rats, ***Journal of Applied Physiology*** 26 (5) 585-588.

Turkevich, D., Micco, A. and Reeves, J. T. (1988) : Non-invasive measurement of the decrease in left ventricular filling time during maximal exercise in normal subjects, ***American Journal of Cardiology*** 62 : 650-652.

Wailer, B. A., Eriksen, M. and Jonbu, T. (1990) : The effect of a meal on cardiac output in man at rest and during moderate exercise, ***Acta Physiologica Scandinavica*** 140 : 167-173.

Waterloh, E. (1980) : Elektronen Nickroskopische Befunde asslafern sowie hire Beziehug Zwe relative maximalen Sanerstoffanfanahme and Laktatproduktion, ***Dtsch Z. Sportmed*** 31 (12), 343.

5

RESPIRATION

The word respiration can be divided into two separate but related subdivisions : (a) External respiration and (b) Internal respiration. (a) The sequence of events in the external (pulmonary ventilation) phase includes — air entering the lungs, and O_2 leaving the lungs and entering the pulmonary blood. Blood transporting O_2 to all the cells of the body, O_2 being utilized by the cells while CO_2 is being produced. Blood transporting CO_2 to the lungs. CO_2 leaving the blood and entering the lungs. CO_2 leaving the lungs. (b) Internal (cellular) phase includes — utilization of oxygen by cell, production of CO_2 and other metabolites by the cell.

The external and internal respirations are linked by circulatory system. In this chapter we will discuss the component of respiration.

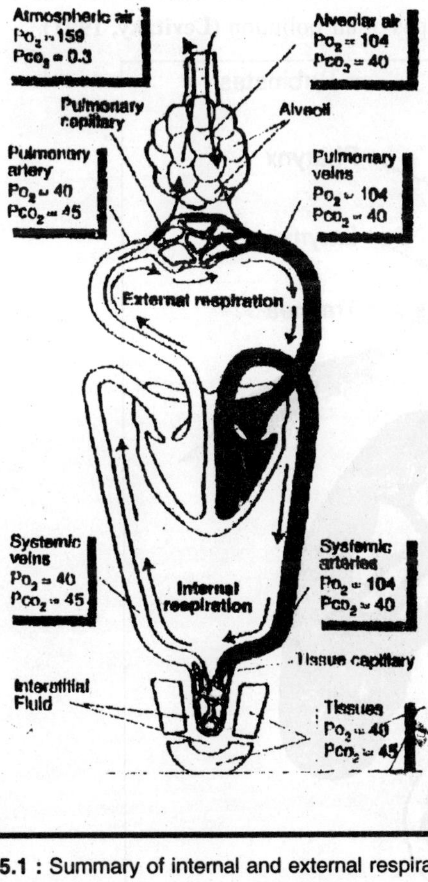

Fig. 5.1 : Summary of internal and external respiration

ANATOMY

The lungs are not directly attached to the ribs. Rather, they are suspended by the pleural sacs. These envelop the lungs and contain a thin layer of pleural fluid that reduces friction during respiratory movements. The visceral pleura adheres to the outer surface of the lung, whereas the parietal pleura lines the thoracic walls and the diaphragm. These sacs are connected to the lungs and the inner surface of the thoracic cage, causing the lungs to take the shape and size of the cage as the chest expands and contract, the pressure in the pleural cavity (intrapleural pressure) is less than the atmospheric and becomes even lower during inspiration, causing air to inflate the lungs. The fact that intrapleural pressure is less than atmospheric pressure is important since it prevents the collapse of the fragile air sacs within the lungs. These relationships between the lungs, the pleural sacs, and the thoracic cage determine air flow in and out of the lungs. Respiratory system consists of a pair of lungs and the passage leading to the lungs.

Respiratory passage includes nasal cavities, pharynx, larynx, trachea and bronchi. Nasal cavities play important role in filtration, warming and moistening of air (**Levitzky, 1991**). This warming and humidification of air serves to protect body temperature and prevents the delicate lung tissue from drying out. Filtration and cleaning process are achieved via two principal means. First, mucus secreted by the cells of the conducting zone serves to trap small inhaled particles. This mucus is moved towards the oral cavity via tiny finger-like projections called cilia. These cilia move in a wavelike fashion, which propels the mucus at a rate of 1-2 centimeters/minute. When a particle becomes trapped in the mucus, it is moved towards pharynx via ciliary action, where it can be either swallowed or expectorated. A second means of protecting the lung from foreign particles is by the action of cells called macrophages that reside primarily in the alveoli (**Reynolds, 1991**). These macrophages literally engulf particles that reach the alveoli. The cleansing action of both cilia and macrophages has been shown to be hindered by cigarette smoke and certain types of air pollution (**Levitzky, 1991**).

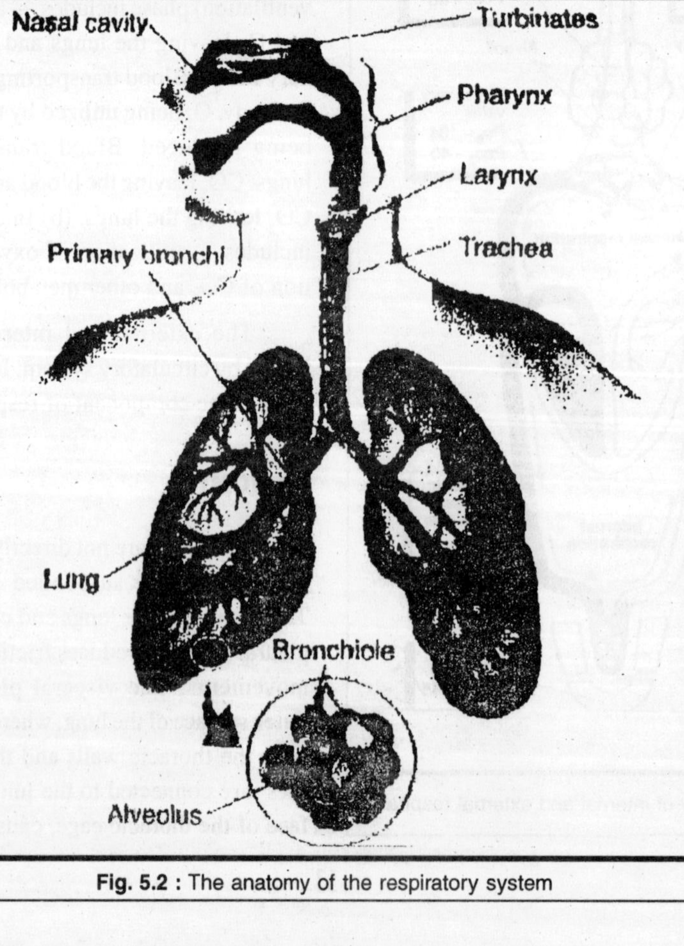

Fig. 5.2 : The anatomy of the respiratory system

Pharynx is divided in two parts; nasopharynx allows air to pass into the larynx and oropharynx which allows food into the oesophagus. Larynx (Voice box) traps dust and other particles and allows air to pass downward by opening epiglottis. In general, humans breathe through the nose until ventilation is increased to approximately 20-30 liters per minute, at which time the mouth becomes the primary passage-way for air (**Dempsey and Fregosi, 1985**). Trachea conduct air between larynx and the lungs. Bronchi is divided into terminal bronchiole and respiratory bronchiole. Terminal bronchiole divides and redivides and leads to alveolar sacs whereas respiratory bronchiole may or may not divide.

The region of the lung where gas exchange occurs is labelled as respiratory zone and includes the respiratory bronchiole and alveolar sacs.

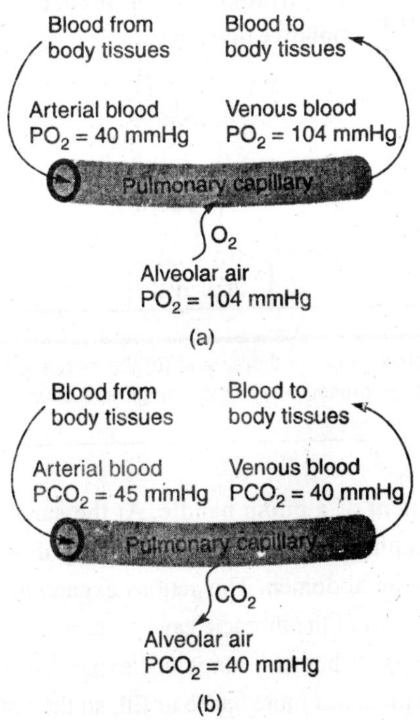

Fig. 5.3 : (a) Partial pressure of oxygen in blood moving through a pulmonary capillary. (b) Partial pressure of carbon dioxide in blood moving through a pulmonary capillary

Inspiration is an active process through which the diaphragm and the external intercostal muscles increase the dimensions — and thus the volume — of the thoracic cage. This decreases the pressure in the lungs and draws air in.

The PO_2 of air at standard atmospheric pressure is 159 mm Hg. But this drops to 100 to 105 mm Hg when air is inhaled and enters the alveoli. The inhaled air mixes with the air in the alveoli and the alveolar air contains a lot of water vapour and carbon dioxide that contribute the total pressure there. The blood — stripped of much of its oxygen by the tissue — typically enters the pulmonary capillaries with a PO_2 of 40 to 45 mm Hg. This is about 55 to 65 mm Hg less than the PO_2 in the alveoli. The pressure gradient for oxygen across the respiratory membrane is typically between 55 to 65 mm Hg that derives the oxygen from the alveoli into the blood to balance the pressure of the oxygen on each side of the membrane. The PO_2 in the alveoli stays relatively steady at about 104 mm Hg at the arteriole end of the capillary, just as exchange begins the PO_2 in the blood is only about 40 mm Hg. But as the blood moves further to the venous end of the capillary the PO_2 across the membrane equilibrate rapidly so that both the alveoli and capillary blood have PO_2 values of 104 mm Hg. Thus blood leaving the lungs through the pulmonary veins to return to the systemic side of the heart has a rich supply of oxygen to deliver to the tissues.

Carbon dioxide exchange moves along the pressure gradient. The blood passing to the alveoli has a PCO_2 of about 40 mm Hg. The pressure gradient of 5 mm Hg is more than adequate as the carbon dioxide's membrane solubility is 20 times greater than oxygen. So carbon dioxide can diffuse across the respiratory membrane much more rapidly.

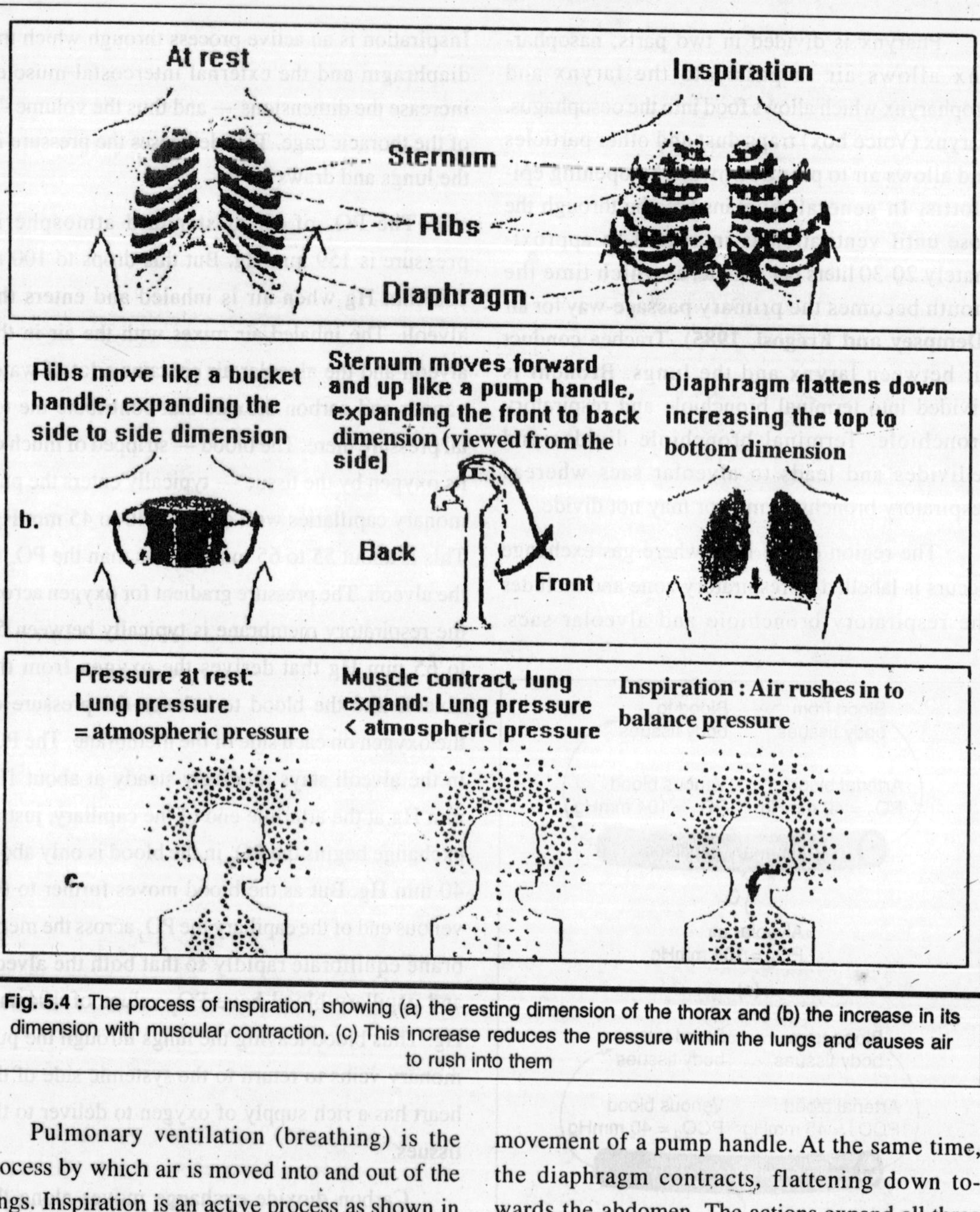

Fig. 5.4 : The process of inspiration, showing (a) the resting dimension of the thorax and (b) the increase in its dimension with muscular contraction. (c) This increase reduces the pressure within the lungs and causes air to rush into them

Pulmonary ventilation (breathing) is the process by which air is moved into and out of the lungs. Inspiration is an active process as shown in Fig. 5.4. Fig. 5.4a shows the resting dimensions of the lungs and the thoracic cage. Fig. 5.4 indicates the movements that occur during inspiration. The ribs and sternum are moved by the external intercostal muscles. The muscles swing up and out, much like the movement of a bucket handle. The sternum swings up and forward, much like the movement of a pump handle. At the same time, the diaphragm contracts, flattening down towards the abdomen. The actions expand all three dimensions of the thoracic cage, in turn expanding the lungs. When the lungs are expanded the air within them has more space to fill, so the pressure within the lungs decreases than the pressure of the air outside the body and air moves into the lungs to reduce the pressure difference. Thus air is brought into the lungs during inspiration.

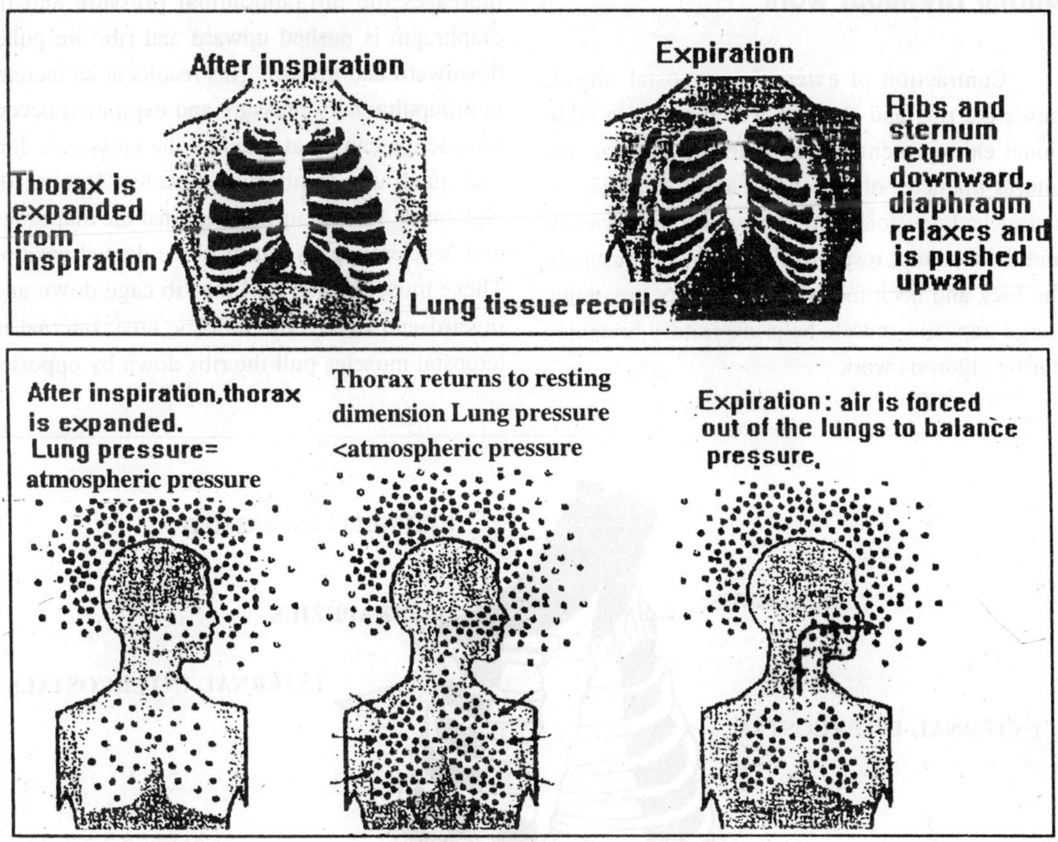

Fig. 5.5 : The process of expiration (a) returning the thorax to its resting dimensions and (b) forcing air out of the lungs

During forced or labored breathing, such as during heavy exercise, inspiration is further assisted by the actions of other muscles, which help to raise the ribs even more than during regular breathing. During inspiration at rest the intrapulmonary pressure decreases by only 3 mm Hg. However, during maximal respiratory effort, such as during exhaustive exercise, the intrapulmonary pressure may decrease by 80 to 100 mm Hg. At rest expiration is usually a passive process involving the relaxation of the respiratory muscles and elastic recoil of the lung tissue. This is depicted in Fig. 5a. As the diaphragm relaxes, it returns to its normal upward arched position. As the external intercostal muscle relaxes, the ribs and sternum lower back into their resting positions. While this happens, the elastic nature of the lung tissue causes it to recoil to its resting size. As shown in Fig. 5b, this increases the pressure to the thorax, so air is forced out of the lungs, thus expiration is accomplished. During forced breathing, expiration becomes a more active process and is assisted by muscles which pull the rib cage down.

RESPIRATORY MUSCLES

Muscles for inspiration

When the Diaphragm contracts the bottom of the thorax flattens. This increases vertical diameter and, as a result, the domed area is lowered.

During strenuous work

Contraction of external intercostal muscle raises the ribs and sternum which result in additional enlargement of the antero-posterior and lateral diameter of the chest cavity. Scalene and sternocleidomastoid help to raise the first two ribs and the sternum, respectively. Extensor muscle of the back and neck facilitate inspiratory breathing. Large trapezius muscle help inspiratory breathing during vigorous work.

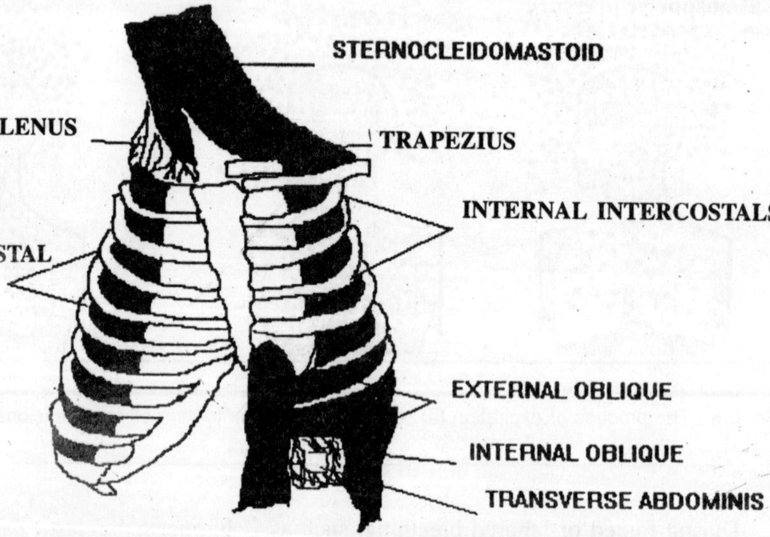

Fig. 5.6 : Various muscles involved in inspiration and expiration

Muscles for expiration

Passive progress : Elastic recoil of the inspiratory muscles (diaphragm and external intercostal).

During exercise

The most important muscles involved in expiration are those found in the abdominal wall which includes the rectus abdominus and the internal oblique. When these muscles contract, it increases the intraabdominal pressure and the diaphragm is pushed upward and ribs are pulled downward and inward. This results in an increase in intrapulmonary pressure and expiration occurs. This action can be assisted by the latissimus dorsi and quadratus lumborum muscles, forcing the abdominal viscera upward against the diaphragm and accelerating its return to the domed position. These muscles also pull the rib cage down and inward and reduce the thoracic area. Internal intercostal muscles pull the ribs down by opposing the external intercostal muscles and bring them closer. This action can be assisted by the latissimus dorsi and quadratus lumborum muscles.

BLOOD FLOW TO THE LUNG

The pulmonary circulation is a low pressure system due to low vascular resistance in the pulmonary circulation. During exercise, pulmonary blood flow increases, the resistance in the pulmonary vascular system falls due to distension of vessels and recruitment of previously unused capillaries. This decrease in pulmonary vascular resistance allows lung blood flow to increase during exercise with relatively small increases in pulmonary arterial pressure. In a standing position, most of the blood flow to the lung is distributed to the base of the lung due to gravitational force. At rest about 23 ml of oxygen diffuse into the pulmonary blood each minute for each 1 mm Hg of pressure difference. During maximal effort, oxygen uptake can increase to 45 ml kg-1 min-1 in untrained people and to as high as 80 ml kg-1 min-1 in elite endurance athletes. The increase in oxygen diffusion capacity from rest to exercise is due to relatively inefficient sluggish circulation through the lungs at rest, which results primarily from limited perfusion of the upper regions of the lung due to gravity. During maximal exercise, however, blood flow through the lungs is greater — primarily due to elevated blood pressure, thereby increasing lung perfusion.

Athletes with large aerobic capacity often also have greater oxygen diffusion capacities. This is likely the combined result of increased cardiac output, increased alveolar surface area, and reduced resistance to diffusion across respiratory membranes. The a-VO_2 difference increases from a resting value of about 4-5 ml to 100 ml of blood during intense exercise. This increase reflects an increased extraction of oxygen from arterial blood by active muscle, thus decreasing the oxygen content of the venous blood.

VENTILATION-PERFUSION RELATIONSHIPS

Efficient gas exchange between the blood and the lung requires proper matching of blood flow to ventilation (called ventilation-perfusion relationships). The ideal ratio of ventilation to perfusion is 1 since this ratio implies a perfect matching of blood flow to ventilation. At rest, the ventilation in the upper region of the lung is estimated to be 0.24 liters/min, while the blood flow is considered to be 0.07 liters/min. Thus the ratio (V/Q) is 3.3. A large V/Q ratio represents a disproportionately high ventilation relative to blood flow, which results in poor gas exchange. Ventilation at the base of the lung is 0.82 liters/min, with a blood flow of 1.29 liters/min (V/Q ratio = 0.82/1.29 = 0.63). A V/Q ratio less than 1 represents a greater blood flow than ventilation to the region. In most cases V/Q ratios greater than 0.50 are adequate to meet the gas exchange demand at rest. In exercise, light exercise may improve V/Q relationship, while heavy exercise results in V/Q inequality, and thus an impairment of gas exchange (**Hammond et al, 1986**). It is still unclear whether the inequality is due to mismatch in ventilation or perfusion.

STATIC LUNG VOLUME

Tidal Volume : The volume of air inspired or expired with each normal breath (500 ml).

Inspiratory Reserve Volume : Extra volume of air that can be inspired over and beyond the normal tidal vol. (3,000 ml).

Expiratory Reserve Volume : The amount of air that can still be expired by forced expiration beyond the normal tidal expiration (1,100 ml).

Residual Volume : Volume of air remaining in the lung after forced expiration (1,200 ml).

Inspiratory Capacity : Amount of air a person can breathe beginning at the normal expiratory level and distending his lungs to the maximum amount (TV + IRV) (3,500 ml).

Functional Residual Capacity : Amount of air remaining in the lung at the end of normal expiration (ERV + RV) (2,300 ml).

Vital Capacity : The amount of air expelled during forced expiration (IRV + IC) (4,600 ml).

Total Lung Capacity : Maximum vol. to which lungs can be expanded with the greatest possible inspiratory effort.

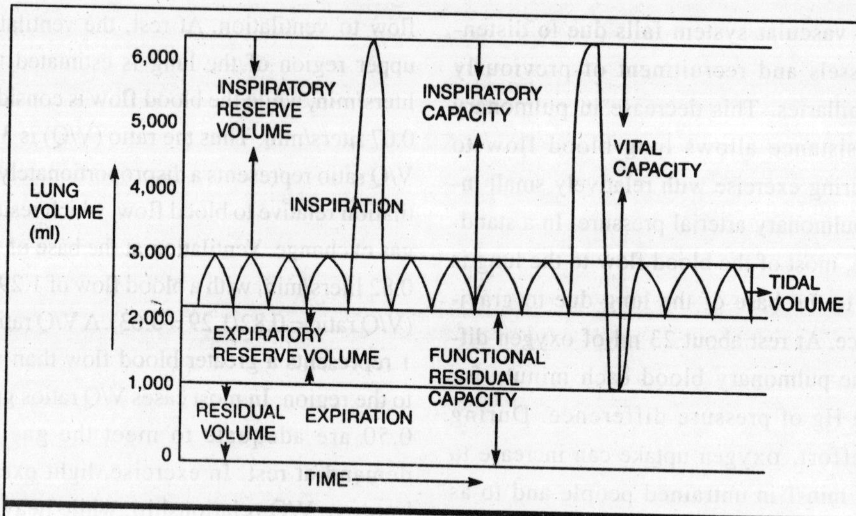

Fig. 5.7 : Graphical expression of various lung volumes and lung capacities

DYNAMIC LUNG VOLUME

Dynamic lung volumes dependent on the maximum stroke volume (VC) of the lung and the speed with which the volume can be moved. The velocity of air flow depends upon the resistance offered by the respiratory passage to the smooth flow of air, and the resistance offered by both the chest and the lung tissue to a change in shape during breathing. To obtain a more dynamic measure percentage (%) of vital capacity (VC) has coined in for lung diagnosis :

Force Expiratory Volume in 1 Second (FEV 1.0) is introduced. (Amount of air expired forcefully in 1 sec.) FEV 1.0 Provides an indication of respiratory power (expiratory) and overall resistance to air movement in the lung (Normal 80% of VC).

Maximum Voluntary Ventilation : Total amount of air inspired on expired with maximum effort in one min (Normal 80-120 liters). MVV is usually about 25% higher than the ventilation volume during max. exercise. It indicates that the ventilatory system is not stressed maximally in exercise.

LUNG FUNCTION AND EXERCISE PERFORMANCE

Little use in predicting fitness on performance if the values fall within the normal range. No difference was noted in the average vital capacity values of Olympic wrestlers and trained middle distance athletes and in those of untrained healthy subject (Newman F. et al, 1961). Players from a professional football team averaged only 94% of their predicted vital capacity, with the defensive backs achieving only 83% of values predicted 'normal' for their body size (Wilmore and Haskell 1972). In swimming and diving, the inspiratory muscles are probably strengthened as the work against additional resistance caused by the weight of water compressing the thoracic cage. Relatively large vital capacities have been reported for skin-divers (Carey et al, 1955) and competitive swimmers (Newman et al, 1961).

Significant improvement in vital capacity following swim training has been reported (Bachman and Harvath 1968). This may be due to an improved inspiratory capacity as well as to a reduced residual lung volume due to more complete exhaustion. The lung volumes of Olympic speed-skaters tended to be larger than those of

untrained healthy individuals. The inability to predict exercise performance through lung function test : When lung volumes and capacities were normalized for body size there was essentially no relationship between lung function and various track performances including marathon run (**Kaufmann et al, 1974**). Larger than normal lung volumes and breathing capacities of some athletes is genetically endowed and may reflect strengthened respiratory muscles as a result of specific exercise training. It is evident that the normal capacity for pulmonary ventilation does not limit exercise performance.

PULMONARY VENTILATION

Pulmonary ventilation refers to the movement of gas into and out of the lungs. The amount of gas ventilated per minute is the product of the frequency of breathing (f) and the amount of gas moved per breath (tidal volume). VE = TV × f. In a 70 kg man VE at rest is generally around 7.5 liters/minute, with a tidal volume of 0.5 liters and a frequency of 15. During maximal exercise ventilation may reach 120-175 liters per minute, with a frequency of 40-50 and a tidal volume of approximately 3-3.5 liters.

Ventilation : Response at rest and during exercise

Adult male

Rest : Normal range of VE = Tidal volume × Respiratory frequency

4 - 15 1/min = 400 - 600 ml * 10 - 23 breaths/min

Exercise : 70 - 135 1/min = 2,000 - 3,000 ml * 35 - 45 breaths/min

Olympic speed-skating (male)

200 1/min = 2.63 1/min * 76 breaths/min

Olympic speed-skating (female)

160 1/min = 2.66 1/min * 60 breaths/min.

Ventilatory responses in submaximal exercise and in maximal exercise :

Changes before exercise

Anticipation of the ensuing exercise bout stimulate cerebral cortex which results in ventilation to be increased before exercise bout.

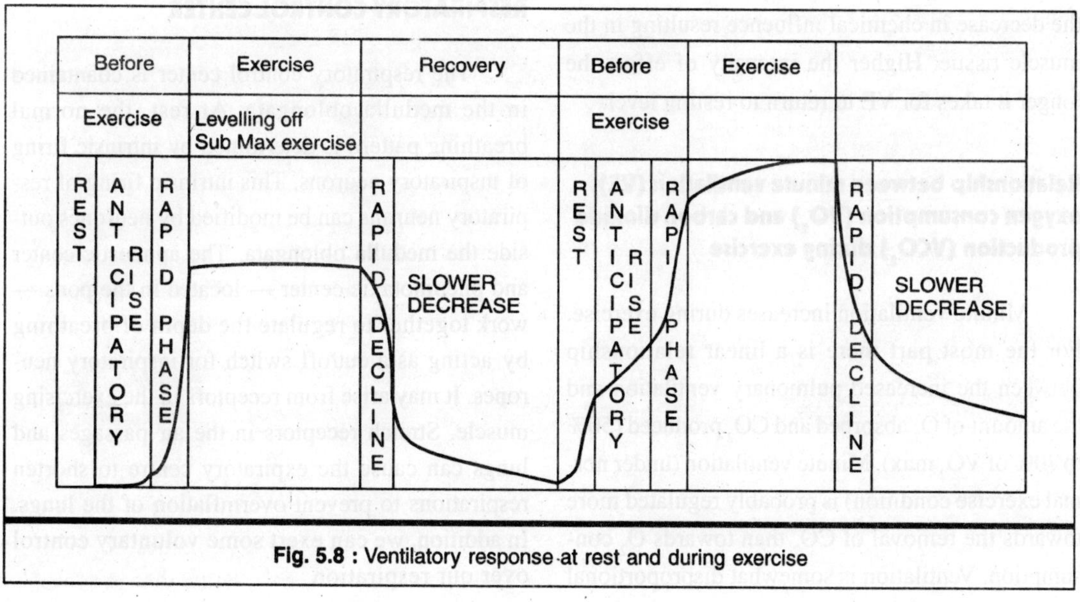

Fig. 5.8 : Ventilatory response at rest and during exercise

Changes during exercise

A very rapid increase within only a few seconds of start of exercise. This is related to stimulation arising from the joints resulting from the movement generated by the working muscles. In submaximal exercise, the rapid rise in ventilation soon ceases and is replaced by a slower rise (level off) tend to reach a steady state value. Arterial PO_2 and PCO_2 are maintained relatively constant during this type of exercise. In maximal exercise ventilation continues to increase until the exercise is terminated. These changes are thought to be stimulated by chemical stimuli mainly from the CO_2 in the blood produced during exercise. During prolonged exercise in a hot/humid environment, ventilation 'drifts' upward due to the influence of rising body temperature on the respiratory control center.

Changes during recovery

Immediately after exercise a sudden decrease in VE is due to the cessation of motor activity from the muscle and joints. The gradual slower decrease in VE toward resting values is probably related to the decrease in chemical influence resulting in the muscle tissue. Higher the intensity of effort the longer it takes for VE to return to resting level.

Relationship between minute ventilation (VE), oxygen consumption (VO_2) and carbon dioxide production (VCO_2) during exercise

Minute ventilation increases during exercise. For the most part there is a linear relationship between the increased pulmonary ventilation and the amount of O_2 absorbed and CO_2 produced (50% to 70% of VO_2 max). Minute ventilation (under normal exercise condition) is probably regulated more towards the removal of CO_2 than towards O_2 consumption. Ventilation is somewhat disproportional to O_2 uptake at or near 80-85% of VO_2 max. value and begins to rise exponentially. This ventilatory inflection point has been called the ventilatory threshold (**Hagberg et al, Power et al, 1983**). Untrained subjects have lower working capacities as well as lower respiratory efficiencies. The trained subjects have a smaller VE at a given VO_2 than do the untrained subjects.

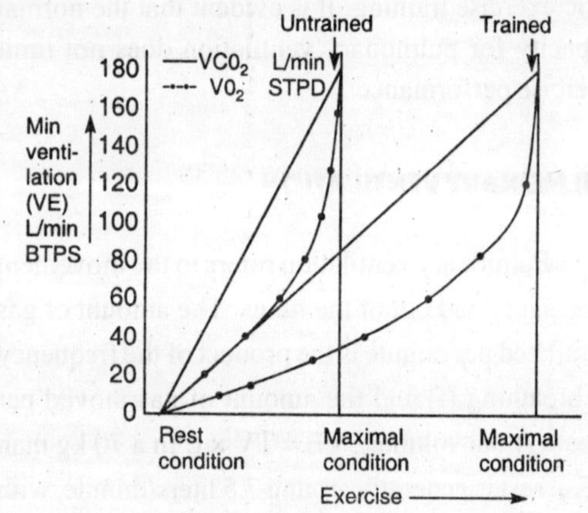

Fig. 5.9 : Relationship between minute ventilation, oxygen consumption and carbon dioxide production during exercise

RESPIRATORY CONTROL CENTER

The respiratory control center is coantained in the medulla oblongata. At rest, the normal breathing pattern is determined by intrinsic firing of inspiratory neurons. This intrinsic firing of respiratory neurons can be modified by neurones outside the medulla oblongata. The apneustic center and pneumotaxic center — located in the pons — work together to regulate the depth of breathing by acting as a cut/off switch for inspiratory neurones. It may arise from receptors in the exercising muscle. Stretch receptors in the air passages and lungs can cause the expiratory centre to shorten respirations to prevent overinflation of the lungs. In addition, we can exert some voluntary control over our respiration.

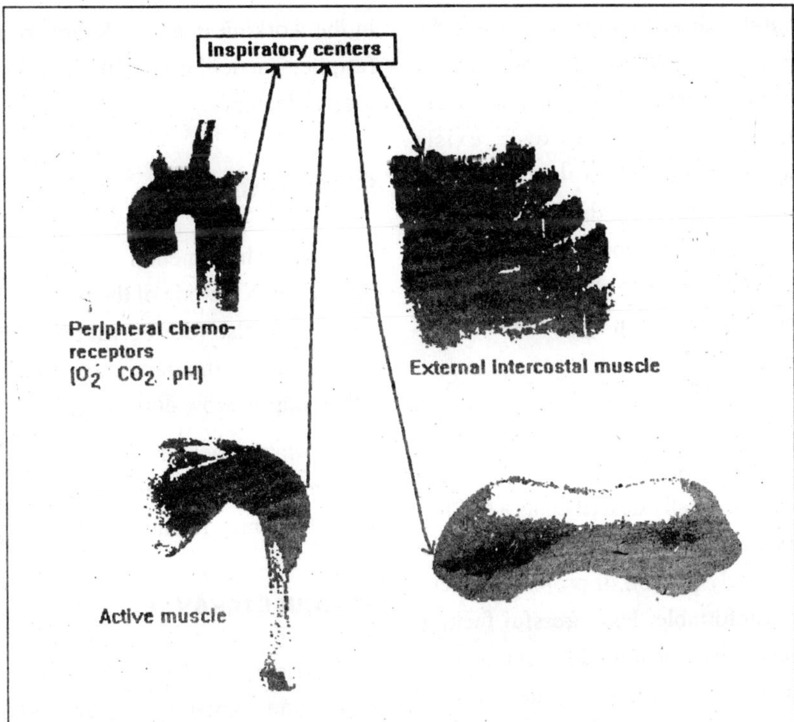

Fig. 5.10a : The process involved in inspiratory regulation

Humoral input may arise from central chemoreceptors in the brain which responds to changes in the concentrations of CO_2 and H^+. When either of these rise, the inspiratory center increases respiration. Peripheral receptors in the arch of aorta and the bifurcation of the common carotid artery respond primarily to changes in blood oxygen levels, but also to changes in CO_2 and H^+ levels. If oxygen levels drop too low, or if the other level rises, these chemoreceptors relay their information to the inspiratory center, which, in turn, increases respiration. There is evidence (**Green and Sheldon, 1983, Green and Schmidt, 1984**) that specialized chemoreceptors sensitive to CO_2 are located in the lungs, which send a message to the respiratory control centre to increase the ventilation. The primary drive to increase ventilation during exercise probably comes from neural afferents and/or efferents.

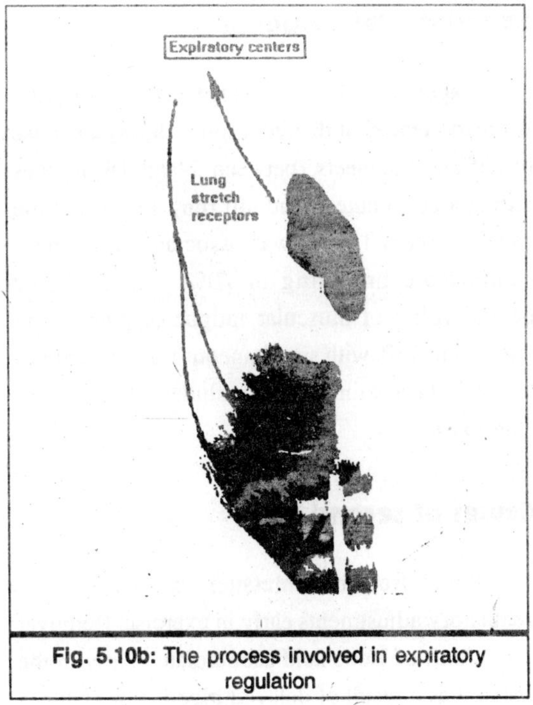

Fig. 5.10b: The process involved in expiratory regulation

The humoral role in this process is for the chemoreceptor to 'fine tune' ventilation to match metabolism, which serves to closely regulate arterial PCO_2. Controversy, however, exists concerning the mechanism to explain the linear rise in ventilation (ventilatory threshold) during incremental exercise test. It appears that the rise in blood H^+ concentration provides the principal stimulus to increase ventilation via stimulation of the carotid bodies.

SECOND WIND

Second wind is usually described as a sudden transition from an ill-defined feeling of distress or fatigue during an early portion of prolonged exercise to a more comfortable, less stressful feeling later in the exercise. This apparent distress is sensed in a variety of ways viz intense breathlessness (dyspnea), rapid shallow breathing, chest pain, throbbing headache or vertigo, pain in various muscles.

Experimental evidence

Experimental finding suggests second wind was experienced at different times during exercise by different subjects (between 2 and 18 minutes during a 20 minutes treadmill run). In 90% of the subjects, second wind was associated with more comfortable breathing in 70% with relief or partial relief of muscular fatigue or pain in the legs and in 35% with simultaneous relief from both leg and chest pain. This concludes second wind does exist.

Causes of second wind

Relief from breathlessness caused by slow ventilatory adjustments early in exercise. Removal (oxidation) of lactic acid accumulated early in the exercise as a result of delayed blood flow changes in the working muscles. Relief from local muscle fatigue, particularly of the diaphragm. Psychological factors.

Stitch in the side

This phenomenon is usually described as a sharp pain in the side of the rib cage. It occurs early during exercise (during running and swimming). In some cases the pain is severe and individuals either stop or slow down exercise altogether.

Cause : Lack of oxygen (hypoxia) in the diaphragm and intercostal muscle due to insufficient blood flow may result in stitch.

GASEOUS EXCHANGE

Gaseous exchange at the alveolar capillary and tissue capillary membranes is primarily dependent on the partial pressure gradients of the gas involved. Partial pressure of a gas depends on both barometric pressure and the tractional concentration of the gas. Consider the air we breathe, it is composed of 79.04% nitrogen (N_2), 20.93% oxygen (O_2), and 0.03% carbon dioxide (CO_2). At sea level, the atmospheric pressure is approximately 760 mm Hg, which is referred to as standard atmospheric pressure. This is considered the total pressure or 100%. We assume atmospheric pressure is 760 mm Hg, then the partial pressure of nitrogen (PN_2) in air is 600.7 mm Hg (79.04% of the total 760 mm Hg pressure). Oxygen's partial pressure (PO_2) is 159.0 mm Hg (20.93% of 760 mm Hg) and carbon dioxide's partial pressure (PCO_2) is 0.3 mm Hg (0.03% of 760 mm Hg).

Gases in our bodies are dissolved in plasma. According to Henry's law, gases dissolve in liquid in proportion to their partial pressures, depending also on their solubilities in the specific fluids and on the temperature. A gas's solubility in blood is constant, and blood temperature also remains relatively constant.

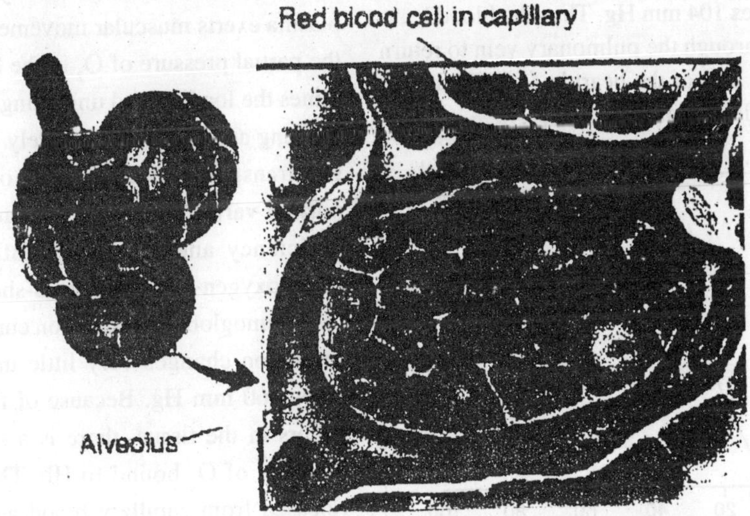

Fig. 5.11 : The Alveolus and the RBC in alveolar capillary

Factors affecting gaseous exchange

1. The length of the diffusion path.
2. The number of Red cells or their Hb concentration.
3. The surface area available for diffusion.

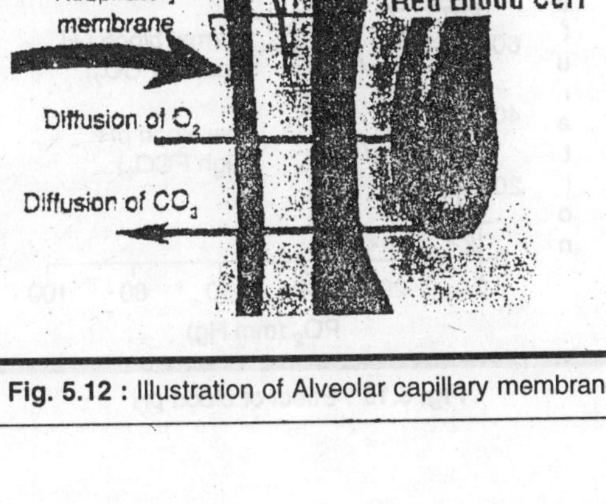

Fig. 5.12 : Illustration of Alveolar capillary membrane

During exercise, opening of more alveoli and capillaries results in surface area to be increased. Diffusion capacity increased. Athletes have large aerobic capacities, often also have greater oxygen diffusion capacities. This is likely the combined result of increased cardiac output, increased alveolar surface area and reduced resistance to diffusion across respiratory membranes.

Transport of oxygen

The PO_2 of air at standard atmospheric pressure is 159 mm Hg. But this drops to 100-105 mm Hg when air is inhaled and enters the alveoli. The blood, stripped of much of its oxygen by the tissues enter pulmonary capillaries with a PO_2 of 40-45 mm Hg. This is about 55-65 mm Hg less than the PO_2 in the alveoli and is the pressure gradient that drives the oxygen from the alveoli into the blood to balance the pressure on each side of the membrane. The PO_2 in the alveoli stays relatively steady at about 104 mm Hg. At the arteriole end of the capillary, the PO_2 of the blood is only about 40 mm Hg. As the blood moves more exchange occurs and at the venous end of the capillary the PO_2 achieves 104 mm Hg. Thus the blood leaving the lungs through the pulmonary vein to return to the systemic side of the heart has a rich supply of oxygen to deliver to the tissues.

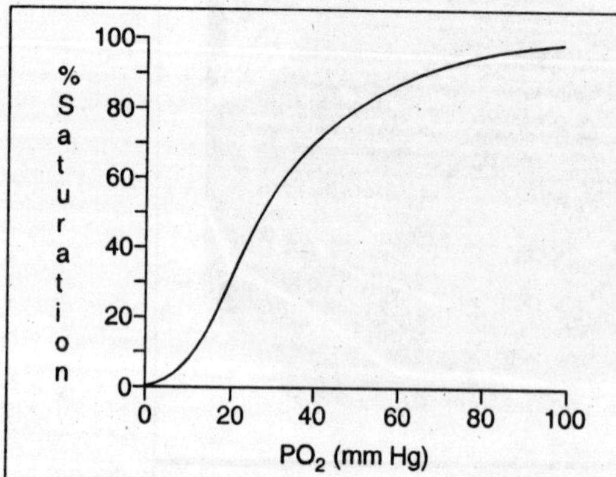

Fig. 5.13 : Normal oxygen dissociation curve

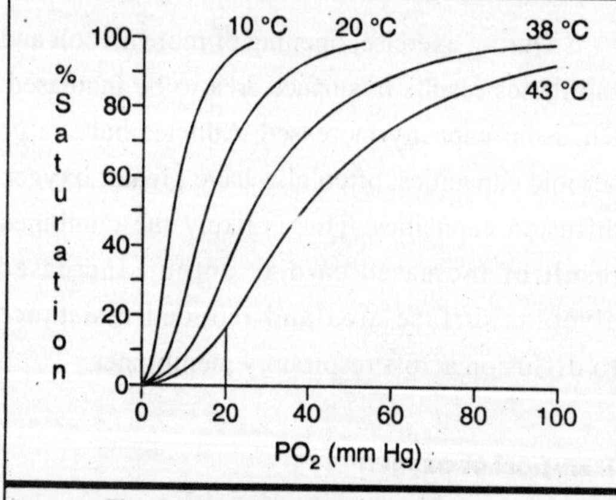

Fig. 5.14 : Effect of blood temperature

Hemoglobin — the iron protein pigment in the RBC — increases the oxygen-carrying capacity of whole blood about 65 times of that carried in physical solution dissolved in the plasma. Oxygen diffusion capacity increases as you move from rest to exercise. At rest, about 23 ml of oxygen diffuse into the pulmonary blood each minute for each 1 mm Hg of pressure difference. During maximal effort, oxygen uptake can increase to 45 ml kg^{-1} min^{-1} in untrained people to as high as 80 ml kg^{-1} min^{-1}.

The small amount of oxygen dissolved in plasma exerts muscular movement and establishes the partial pressure of O_2 in the blood. This determines the loading and unloading of hemoglobin at the lung and tissue, respectively. The blood's oxygen transport capacity varies only slightly with normal variations in Hb content. However, iron deficiency anemia significantly decreases the blood oxygen-carrying. The S-shaped nature of the oxy-Hemoglobin dissociation curve shows that Hb saturation changes very little until the PO_2 falls below, 60 mm Hg. Because of this, low pressure occurs in the tissue, there is a sharp drop in the quantity of O_2 bound to Hb. Thus O_2 is rapidly released from capillary blood and flows into the tissue in response to the cell's metabolic demands. So cell can rapidly obtain O_2 when the metabolic demands increase suddenly. Increase in acidity, temp. and CO_2 concentration and 2, 3 DPG in RBC causes an alteration in the molecular structure of Hb, thereby reducing its effectiveness to hold oxygen. Because these factors are accentuated in exercise, the release of O_2 to the tissue is further facilitated. In skeletal and cardiac muscle, the iron-protein pigment myoglobin releases its oxygen at low O_2 pressure and facilitates O_2 transfer to the mitochondria, especially during strenuous exercise when cellular PO_2 decreases considerably.

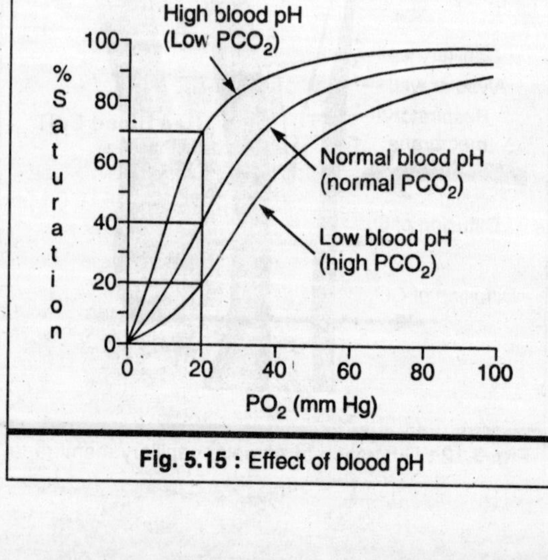

Fig. 5.15 : Effect of blood pH

Table 1 : Difference in myoglobin content in athletes and sedentary group

Myoglobin content (mg g^{-1} wet muscle)			
Exercise	1.90	2.17	0.73
Sedentary	1.05**	1.20**	0.70

Transport of carbon dioxide

Carbon dioxide is transported by the blood and moves along a pressure gradient. The blood passing through the alveoli has a PCO_2 of about 45 mm Hg. In the alveoli, air has a PCO_2 of about 40 mm Hg, so the pressure gradient is only 5 mm Hg. The pressure gradient for carbon dioxide exchange is less than for oxygen exchange, but carbon dioxide's membrane solubility is 20 times greater than that of oxygen. So carbon dioxide crosses the membrane easily, even without a large pressure gradient.

As bicarbonate

CO_2 diffuses into tissue capillary blood and reacts with water in plasma and RBC to form carbonic acid $CO_2 + H_2O = H_2CO_3$. In plasma, carbonic anhydrase is absent, but in RBC it is highly concentrated. Therefore, the formation of carbonic acid takes place principally within the RBC. Once carbonic acid is formed most of it ionizes to hydrogen (H^+) ion and bicarbonate ions (HCO_3).

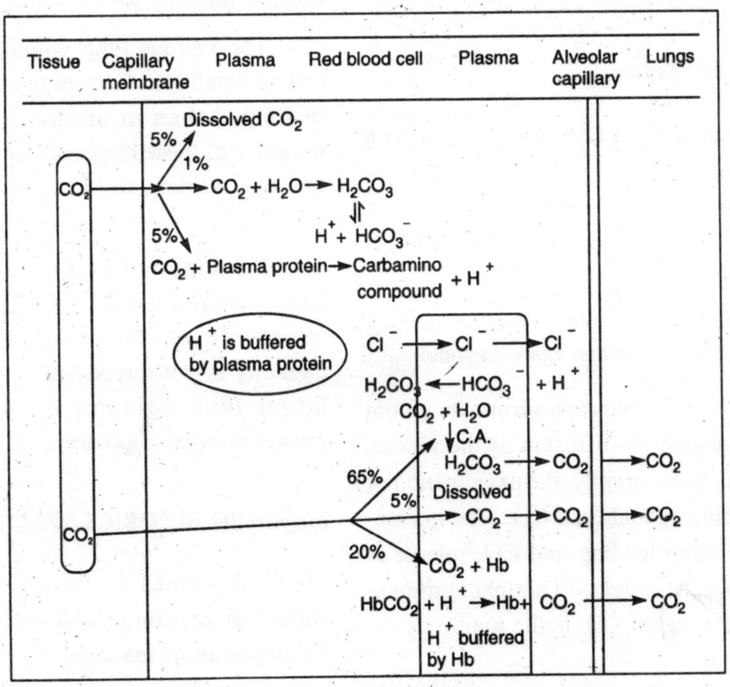

Fig. 5.16 : Schematic representation of CO_2 transport

$$CO_2 + H_2O = H_2CO_3 \xrightarrow{\text{Carbonic Anhydrase}} H^+ + HCO_3$$

The H^+ is then buffered by the protein portion of Hb to maintain the pH of blood within relatively narrow limit. Due to higher solubility, HCO_3^- diffuses from the RBC into the plasma in exchange for the chloride ion (Cl^-) that moves into the RBC to maintain ionic equilibrium (chloride shift). 80% of the total CO_2 is carried as plasma bicarbonate. As PCO_2 increases in the tissue carbonic acid is rapidly formed. In the lung CO_2 leaves the blood and plasma PO_2 is lowered. This disturbs the equilibrium between carbonic acid and the formation of bicarbonate ion. As a result, H^+ recombine to form carbonic acid. In turn, CO_2 and water re-form and CO_2 exits through the lung.

$$H^+ + HCO_3 \xrightarrow{\text{Carbonic Anhydrase}} H_2CO_3 \longrightarrow CO_2 + H_2O$$

As carbaminohemoglobin

At the tissue level, CO_2 reacts directly with the amino molecules of blood proteins to form carbamino-compounds. This is specially true for the globin portion of Hb that carries about 20% of the body's carbon dioxide as follows

$$\underset{\text{(Hemoglobin)}}{CO_2 + NBNH} \longrightarrow \underset{\text{(Carbaminohemoglobin)}}{NBNHCOOH}$$

In the lungs, CO_2 splits apart from the globin and enters the alveoli by diffusion as the plasma PCO_2 is lowered. Concurrently, the oxygenation of Hb reduces its binding ability of CO_2. The interaction between oxygen loading and CO_2 release is termed the 'Haldane Effect'. This phenomenon facilitates the removal of CO_2 in the lung.

Transport in solution

About 5% of CO_2 produced during energy metabolism is carried as free CO_2 in solution in the plasma. Although this quantity is relatively small, it is the random movement of dissolved CO_2 molecule that establishes the PCO_2 of the blood.

ADAPTATIONAL CHANGES IN THE RESPIRATORY SYSTEM TO PHYSICAL TRAINING

Maximum minute ventilation is increased following training. The increase in ventilation should be considered secondary to the increase in maximum VO_2. Increment is brought about by increase in both tidal volume and breathing frequency.

Training causes an increased ventilatory efficiency. The amount of air ventilated at the same O_2 consumption level is lower in trained athletes as compared to their untrained counterparts. Since the O_2 cost of ventilation increases greatly with increasing ventilation causing a greater ventilatory efficiency, particularly over a prolonged effort (e.g., the marathon), it would result in less oxygen to the respiratory muscles and more to the working skeletal muscles.

The various lung volumes measured under resting conditions (except tidal volume) are larger in trained than in untrained individuals. The majority of these changes can be attributed to the fact that training results in improved pulmonary function and, therefore, in larger lung volumes.

Athletes tend to have larger diffusion capacities at rest and during exercise than do non-athletes (e.g., endurance runners). Diffusion capacity is not directly affected by training, but larger lung volumes of athletes provide a greater alveolar-capillary surface area.

MAXIMUM AEROBIC CAPACITY (VO_2 max)

It is defined as the volume of oxygen consumed at maximum effort in the last 30 sec breathing air of sea-level.

Table 2 : Comparison of VO_2 max in trained and untrained persons

Untrained		Trained	
Male	Female	Male	Female
2-3.5 1/min	1.72-2.5 1/min	3.0-5.0 1/min	2-3.5 1/min
36-50 ml /kg/min	30-45 ml /kg/min	45-75 ml /kg/min	45-65 ml /kg/min

Aerobic capacity or VO_2 max is related to body size, lean body mass, diffusion capacity, the functional capacity of cardiovascular system, the cellular metabolic process and cardiac output.

Factors affecting aerobic capacity

Sex difference in VO_2 max is attributed to a lower blood Hb concentration and low lean body mass in females after the onset of puberty. At full maturity, average North American female is approximately 13 cm shorter, 15-18 kg lighter with 25% body fat as compared to 15% body fat in male.

The relationship of aerobic capacity and chronological age is evident. A positive relationship with age exists in the first 18 years of life in both male and female sedentary group and reaches a peak at the age of 25 yrs (40-50 ml/kg/min) and then decline to 20-30 ml/kg/min at the age of 60 yrs. This is due to reduction of absolute aerobic power and partly for an increase in body weight after 30 yrs of age. Training can improve VO_2 max from 0-44%. Effect of training on VO_2 max depends on (a) Initial level of fitness (b) Type of training (duration, intensity and volume) (c) Physical characteristics of the person.

Environmental factors viz. altitude, hot, cold, pollution etc. affect VO_2 max. About 70% of VO_2 max is determined by the genetic endowment of the individual. Dietary manipulation/supplementation affect VO_2 max. Lack of optimal diet reduces max O_2 uptake by affecting the growth of the individual.

Training and aerobic capacity

No change or slight decrease in oxygen consumption at sub-maximal exercise. The decrease is due to an increase in mechanical efficiency. A decrease in O_2 consumption is most pronounced in comparisons of highly trained athletes and untrained individuals. The difference is also evident between good and average runners. At maximal effort, VO_2 max is increased. The increment is due to an increased oxygen delivery to the working muscles through an increased cardiac output and by an increased oxygen extraction from the blood by the skeletal muscles. The average improvement of 5-20% can be anticipated for college male and female student following 8-12 weeks of methodical training.

TRAINING AND ANAEROBIC THRESHOLD

Several studies have shown that even when the VO_2 max is not much increased significant improvement in anaerobic threshold (ATh) level is possible, provided the training schedule is administered at anaerobic threshold. Significant improvement in VO_2 max may not be possible when the runners reaches a plateau. It is ,therefore, suggested that more emphasis should be given to improve the anaerobic threshold (a) level of athletes.

During steady state exercise, sufficient oxygen is supplied to and utilized by the working muscles. In this condition lactic acid does not exceed resting values. However, if aerobic metabolism is insufficient, anaerobic glycolysis contributes to the energy requirements and lactic acid is formed. The onset of this anaerobiosis normally occurs between 65% and 75% of the max VO_2 in healthy untrained subjects. Almost all of the lactic acid generated during anaerobic metabolism is buffered in the blood by sodium bicarbonate in the following reaction

$$\text{Lactic acid} + NaHCO_3 \longrightarrow \text{Na Lactate} + H_2CO_3 \longrightarrow H_2O + CO_2$$

The CO_2 released in the buffering reaction is exhaled into the atmosphere as the venous blood entering the lungs.

The onset of metabolic Acidosis can be detected in one of several ways (i) an increase in blood lactic acid; (ii) a corresponding decrease in blood

pH and bicarbonate (iii) an increase in respiratory exchange ratio (R) due to the release of excess CO_2 in the buffering process (iv) a deviation from linearity in the relationship between oxygen consumption and ventilation due to strong ventilatory stimulus provided by both increased acidity and the release of CO_2 through buffering.

REFERENCE

Bachman, J. C., and Harvath, S. M. (1968) : Pulmonary function changes which accompany athletic training programs, ***Research Quarterly*** 39 : 235-242.

Carey, C. R. et al, (1955) : Effect of skin diving on lung volumes, ***Journal of Applied Physiology*** 8 : 519-527.

Dejours, P. : Control of respiration in muscular exercise. (1964) : In (W. Fenn, ed) Handbook of physiology, section 3. Washington : ***American Physiological Society.***

Dempsey, J. and Fregosy, R. (1985) : Adaptability of the pulmonary system to changing metabolic requirements, ***American Journal of Cardiology*** 55 : 59D-67D.

Duffin, J. (1994) : Neural drives to breathing during exercise, ***Canadian Journal of Applied Physiology*** 19 : 289-304.

Favier, R. et al : Ventilatory and circulatory transients during exercise (1983) : New arguments for a neurohumoral theory, ***Journal of Applied Physiology*** 54 : 647-653.

Green, J. and Schmidt, N. (1984) : Mechanism of hyperpnea induced by changes in pulmonary blood flow, ***Journal of Applied Physiology*** 56 : 1418-1422.

Green, J. and Sheldon, M. (1983) : Ventilatory changes associated with changes in pulmonary blood flow in dogs, ***Journal of Applied Physiology*** 54 : 997-1002.

Hagberg, J. et al (1982) : Exercise hyperventilation in patients with McArdle's disease, ***Journal of Applied Physiology*** 52 : 991-994.

Hammond, M. et al (1986) : Pulmonary gas exchange in humans during exercise at sea level, ***Journal of Applied Physiology*** 60 : 1590-98.

Kaufmann, D. A. et al (1974) : Pulmonary function of marathon runners, ***Medicine and Science in Sports*** 6 : 114-118.

Levitzky M. (1991) : ***Pulmonary Physiology***, New York, McGraw-Hill.

Newman, F. et al (1961) : A comparison between body size and lung function of swimmers and normal school children, ***Journal of Physiology*** 156 : 9-16.

Power, S. et al (1983) : Ventilatory threshold, running economy and distance running performance, ***Research Quarterly*** 54 : 179-182.

Reynolds, H. (1991) : Immunologic system in the respiratory tract, ***Physiological Review*** 71 : 1117-33.

Richter, D. (1982) : Generation and maintenance of the respiratory rhythm, ***Journal of Experimental Biology*** 100 : 93-107.

Richter, D., Ballantyne, D. and Remmers, J. (1986) : How is the respiratory rhythm generated? ***A model news in Physiological Sciences*** 1 : 109-11.

Wilmore, J. H. and Haskell, W. L. (1972) : Body composition and endurance capacity of professional football players, ***Journal of Applied Physiology*** 33 : 564-570.

6

MUSCULAR SYSTEM

MUSCULAR SYSTEM

THE STRUCTURE AND FUNCTION OF SKELETAL MUSCLE

A total of 217 pairs of skeletal muscles (striated and under voluntary control) constitutes 45% of the body weight in a man and 25% of the body weight in a woman (**Fox, S. 1987; Hole, 1987; Johnson, L. 1983**). Muscles, working in harmony with the nervous and skeletal systems, function as the focal point in movement.

Skeletal muscles perform three important functions (a) force generation for movement (b) force generation for postural support, and (c) heat production during period of cold stress.

Muscle tissue provides the necessary contractile force acting against the skeletal form to produce body movement. Shape of skeletal muscles vary greatly, each is designed by four basic attributes : (a) Connective and tendon tissue (b) Blood supply (c) Nerve supply (d) Varied muscle tissue design.

A muscle fiber is enclosed by a plasma membrane called the Sarcolemma. At the end of each muscle fiber, its sarcolemma fuses with the tendon which inserts into the bone. So typically each individual muscle fiber is ultimately attached to bone via the tendon. The cytoplasm of a muscle fiber is called the sarcoplasma. The sarcoplasm mainly contains dissolved proteins, mineral, glycogen, fat and necessary organelles, along with myoglobin, O_2 binding compound.

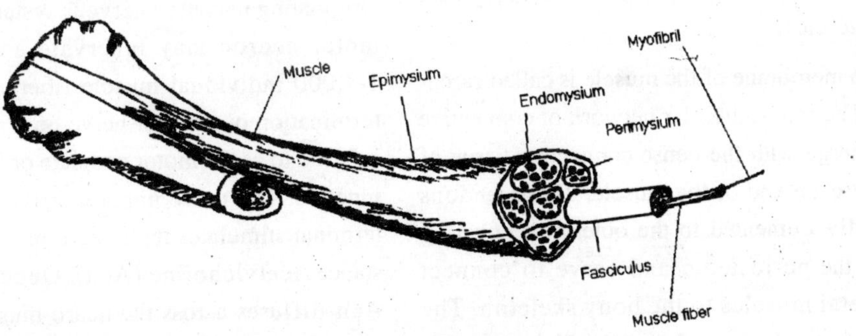

Fig. 6.1 : The basic structure of the skeletal muscle

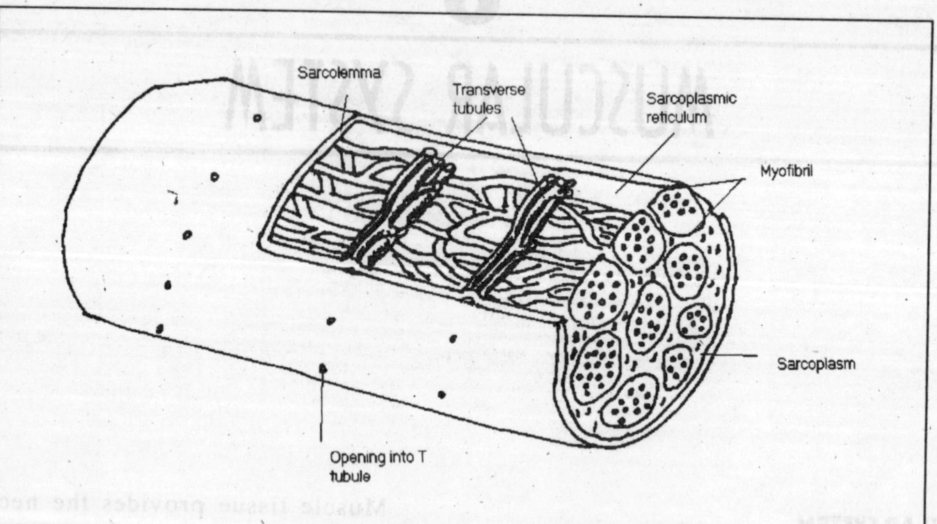

Fig. 6.2 : The cross-section of skeletal muscle

If we dissect a muscle, we first cut through an outer connective tissue covering. This is the Epimysium. Once we cut through the epimysium, we would see small bundles of fibers wrapped in a connective tissue sheath — these bundles are called Fasciculi. The connective tissue sheath surrounded by each fasciculus is the Perimysium. Finally, by cutting through the perimysium and using a magnifier, we could see the muscle fiber. Each muscle fiber is also covered by a sheath of connective tissue, called the Endomysium. The connective tissues of muscles are the Endomysium (fibers), Perimysium (bundles) and Epimysium (whole muscles).

The membrane of the muscle is called sarcolemma. The intra-muscular network of connective tissues merge with the dense connective tissue of tendon at each end of the muscle. These tendons are rigidly cemented to the outermost covering of bone, the periosteum and serve to connect the skeletal muscles to the bony skeleton. The design of attachment of muscle fibers to their tendon determines their muscle function. Muscles which have fibers running parallel throughout their length and taper into one tendon at each end (unicep) favour rapid contraction at the expense of power (Biceps). Muscles possessing fibers inserting from all directions (multipennate) favour power rather than the development of speed. (Deltoid) Tendons are non-living fibers and stronger than muscle. Small tendon can withstand the tension developed by a relatively large muscle.

Nerve supply

The nerves supplying a muscle contain both motor (efferent) fibers and sensory (afferent) fibers. Originating in central nervous system (CNS), each motor neuron may innervate anywhere from 1-1,000 individual muscle fibers. The point of termination of a motor nerve on a muscle fiber is referred to as the motor endplate or neuromuscular junction. The nerve impulse arriving at the nerve terminal stimulates the release of transmitter substance Acetylcholine (Ach). Once released, the Ach diffuses across the neuro-muscular junction where it acts on special receptor sites. This interaction changes the permeability of the motor endplate to Na^+ and K^+. So the membrane potential is lowered towards the threshold of depolarization.

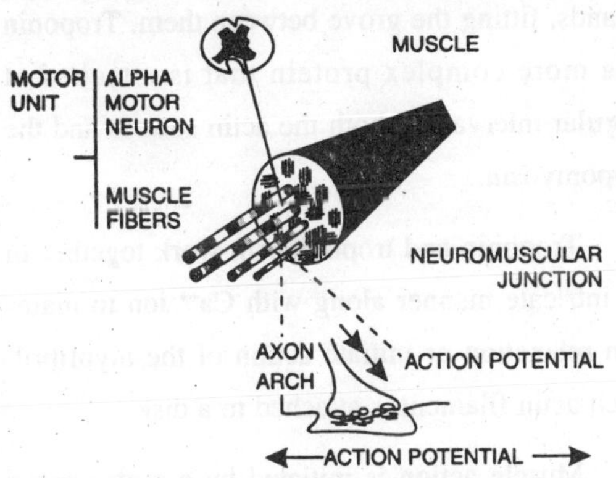

Fig. 6.3 : Sequence of events in the neuromuscular junction

This altered potential is referred to as the endplate potential (EPP). When E.P.P. reaches threshold it initiates an action potential across the entire sarcolemma, ultimately reaching the myofibril by way of transverse tubules.

Blood supply

Each muscle fiber receives a continuous supply of oxygenated blood through one or more small arteries that enter the epimysium and run parallel between fasciculus, eventually subdividing into capillaries. From the capillaries, the deoxygenated blood and other waste products (including lactate) drain into venule, regrouping to form veins. During exercise, a muscle group may require 60 times more blood than when at rest. Venous return is enhanced by the periodic compression of the blood vessels which results in increment of cardiac output.

The extensive tubule network found in the sarcoplasm includes T-tubules, which is the extension of sarcolemma that pass laterally through the muscle fiber. These tubules are interconnected as they pass along the myofibril, allowing nerve impulses received by the sarcolemma to be transmitted rapidly to individual myofibril. Tubules also provide pathways into the inner parts of the muscle fiber for substances carried in the ECF such as glucose, oxygen and ions. A longitudinal network of tubules known as sarcoplasmic reticulum (SR) is also found within the muscle fiber. These membranous channels parallel the myofibril and loop around them. The SR serves as a storage site for Ca^{++} which is essential for contraction. Each individual muscle fiber contains several hundred to several thousand myofibril. These are contractile elements of skeletal muscle. Myofibril appear as long strands of still smaller subunit sarcomere, the smallest functional unit of a muscle.

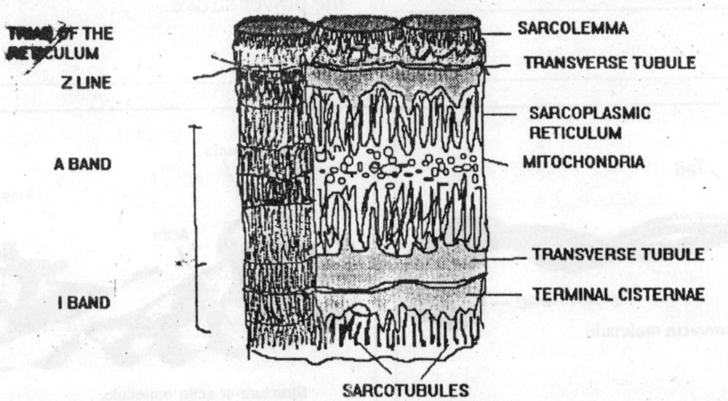

Fig. 6.4 : The alignment of sarcoplasmic reticulum and T-tubule system within the muscle fibre

A sarcomere is composed of filaments of two proteins which are responsible for muscular contraction. Myosin is a thick filament. Each myosin filament typically is formed by about 200 myosin molecules lined up end to end and side by side. Each myosin molecule is composed of two protein strands twisted together, one of each strand is folded into a globular head, called myosin head. Each filament contains several such heads that protrude from the myosin filament to form cross-bridges that interact during muscle action with specialized active sites on the actin filaments.

An actin filament is composed of 3 proteins. Actin molecules are globular and join together to form a strand of actin molecules. Tropomyosin is a tube-shaped protein that twists around the actin strands, fitting the grove between them. Troponin is a more complex protein that is attached at regular intervals to both the actin strands and the tropomyosin.

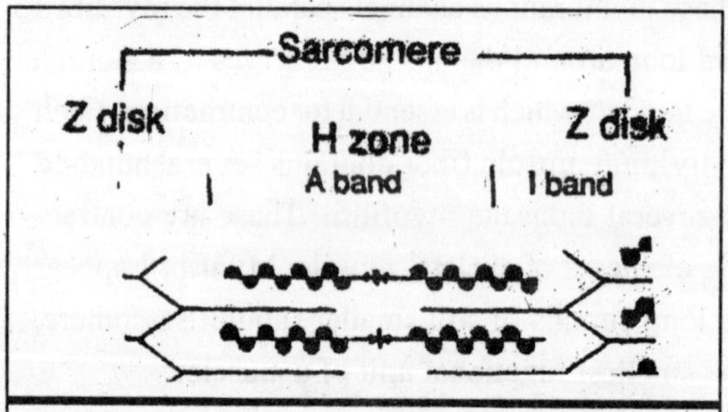

Fig. 6.5 : Muscle structure (microscopic)

Troponin and tropomyosin work together in an intricate manner along with Ca^{++} ion to maintain relaxation or initiate action of the myofibril. Each actin filament is attached to a disk.

Muscle action is initiated by a motor nerve impulse. The motor nerve releases Ach that opens ion gates in the muscle cell membrane, allowing sodium to enter the muscle (depolarization) if the cell is sufficiently depolarized, an action potential is fired and muscle action occurs. The action potential travels along the sarcolemma, even through the tubule system and eventually causes stored calcium to be released from the sarcoplasmic reticulum. Calcium binds which troponin and then troponin lifts the tropomyosin molecules off the active site on the actin filament, opening these sites for binding with the myosin head. Once it binds with actin active site, the myosin head tilts, pulling the actin filament so that the two slide across each other. The tilting of the myosin head is the power stroke.

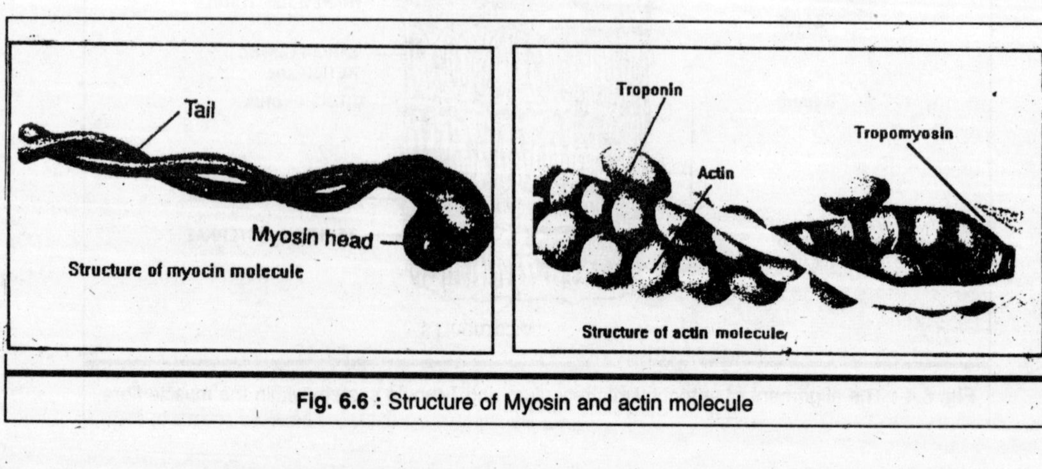

Fig. 6.6 : Structure of Myosin and actin molecule

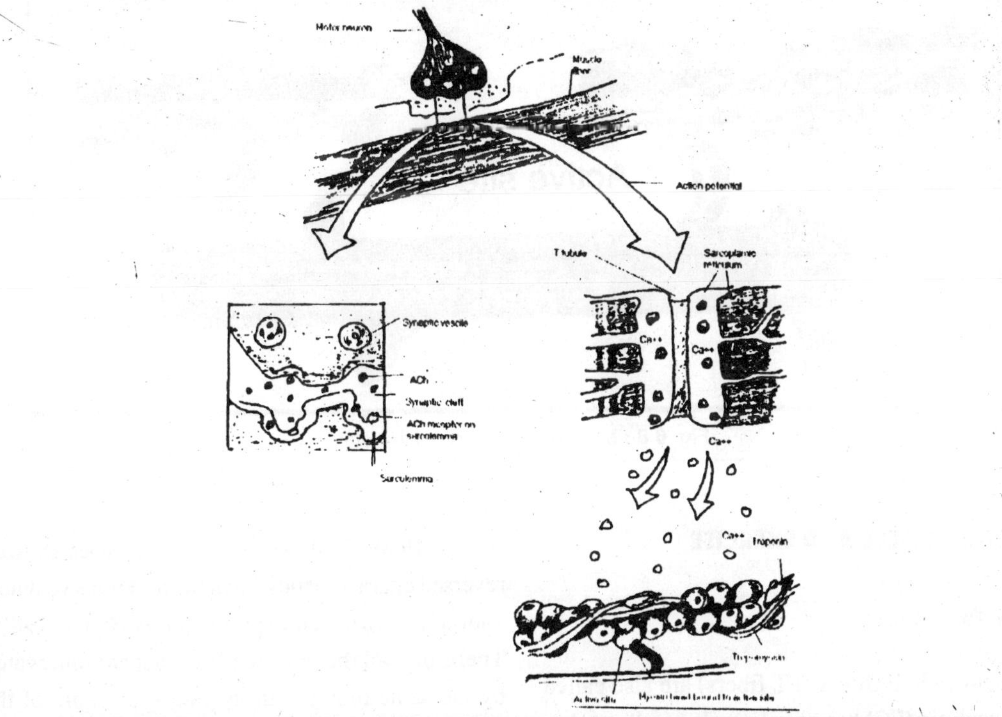

Fig. 6.7 : The sequence of events leading to muscle action : (a) A motor neuron releases acetylcholine (Ach), which binds to receptors on the sarcolemma. If enough Ach binds, an action potential is generated in the muscle fibre. (b) The action potential triggers Ca ++ release from the sarcoplasmic reticulum into the sarcoplasm. (c) The Ca ++ bind to troponin on the actin filament, and the troponin pulls the tropomyosin on the active sites, allowing myosin leads to attach to the actin filament

SUMMARY OF EVENTS OCCURRING DURING MUSCULAR CONTRACTION

Sliding Filament Theory (Ebahi S. 1976; Kodama 1985)

Rest

(a) Uncharged ATP cross-bridges extended, (b) Actin and myosin uncoupled (c) Ca^{++} stored in sarcoplasmic reticulum.

Excitation-coupling

(a) Nerve impulses generated, (b) Ca^{++} released from terminal cisternae, expanded position of sarcoplasmic reticulum vesicles, (c) Ca^{++} saturates troponin, turning on actin, (d) ATP cross-bridge 'charged', (e) Actin and myosin coupled ⟶ Actomyosin.

Contraction

$$\text{(a) ATP} \xrightarrow{\text{ATP ase}} \text{ADP + Pi + Energy,}$$

(b) Energy swivels cross-bridges. (c) Muscle shortens ⟶ Actin slides over myosin, (d) Tension developed.

Recharging

(a) ATP re-synthesized, (b) Actomyosin dissociates ⟶ Actin + Myosin (c) Actin and myosin recycled.

Relaxation

(a) Nerve impulse ceases, (b) Ca^{++} removed by calcium pump, (c) Muscle return to resting state.

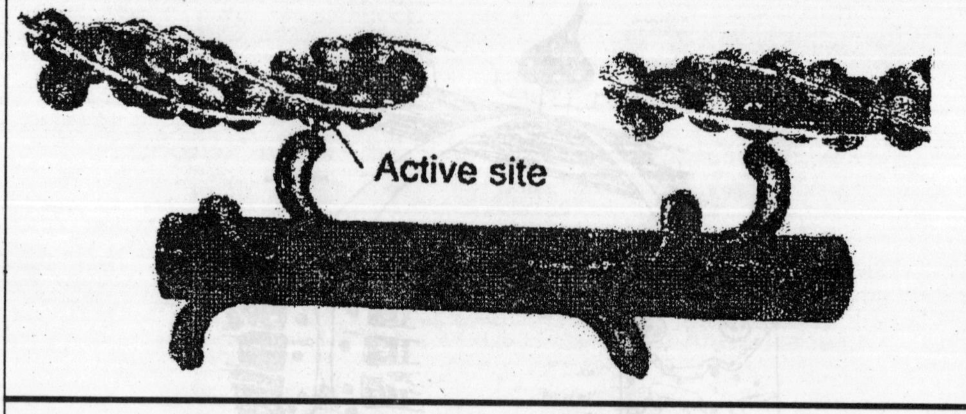

Fig. 6.8 : Muscle fibre in contractile state

SKELETAL MUSCLE AND EXERCISE

Muscle Fiber Types

Fast twitch fibers (FT fibers) are also called fast glycolytic (FG) have a relatively small number of mitochondria and a limited capacity for aerobic metabolism, hence less resistant to fatigue than slow twitch fibers (**Green, 1986; Pette and Spamer 1986**). FT fibers are rich in glycogen storage and glycolytic enzymes which provide large anaerobic capacity (**Pette, 1980**), FT fibers contain more myofibrils and ATP which results more force generation during rapid contraction.

Slow twitch fibers are also called (ST fibers) slow oxidative fibers; contain more number of mitochondria and are surrounded by more capillaries than FT fibers. Myoglobin content in ST fibers are more which increases O_2 binding capacity and acts as a "Shuttle" mechanism for O_2 between the cell and the mitochondria. All these characteristics provide slow twitch fibers with a high capacity for aerobic metabolism and a high resistance to fatigue.

The rate of conduction for fast twitch fibers is 80-90 meters/second, while the conduction rate for slow twitch fibers is only 60-70 meters/second (**Pette, 1980**). The two muscle fiber types showed reversed characteristics when the motor nerve innervation was switched experimentally (**Pette, 1980**). Therefore, all the muscle fibers that are innervated by the same motor neuron (motor unit) are of the same type.

Fiber type and Athletic success

Most skeletal muscles contain both Slow Twitch (ST) and Fast Twitch (FT) fibers. Fast twitch fiber can be subdivided into FTa, FTb and FTc. The differences among these fibers are still obscure but FTa fibers are believed to be the most frequently recruited. Only ST fibers are recruited more frequently than FTa fibers. FTc fibers are the least often used. On the average, most muscles are composed of roughly 50% ST fibers and 25% FTa fibers. The remaining 25% are mostly FTb, with FTc fibers making up only 1% to 3% of the muscle. The different fiber types have different ATPases. The ATP ase in the FT fiber acts faster, providing energy for muscle action more quickly than the ATP ase in ST fibers. FT fibers have a more highly developed sarcoplasmic reticulum, enhancing the delivery of Ca^{++} needed for muscle action. Motor neurons supplying FT motor units are larger and supply more fibers than do neurons for ST motor units. Thus FT motor units have more fibers to contract and can produce more force than ST motor units. The proportion of ST and FT fibers in an individual's arm and leg muscles are quite similar. There are some exceptions, however. The Soleus muscle (deep to gastrocnemius in the calf) for example, is almost completely composed of ST fibers in everyone. ST fibers have high aerobic endurance and are well-suited to low intensity endurance activities. Such as Marathon running or Channel swimming. FT fibers are better for anaerobic activity. FTa fibers are well-utilized in explosive bouts of exercise. FTb fibers are not well understood, but it is known that they are not easily recruited into activity.

Motor units give all or none responses, for a unit to be recruited into activity, the motor nerve impulse must meet or exceed the threshold. When this occur all threshold is not met, no fibers in that unit act. More is produced by activating more motor units and thus more muscle fibers. In the early 1970s **Gollnick et al** demonstrated that, indeed, this selective requirement is determined not by the speed of action but by the level of force demanded of the muscle. In low intensity activity, most muscle force is generated by ST fibers. As the resistance increases, FTa fibers are recruited, and if maximal strength is needed the FTb fibers are activated. The same pattern of recruitment is followed during events of long duration (**Gollnick & Hodgson, 1986**).

Sex difference in % slow & fast twitch muscle fiber

There are no apparent sex and age differences in fiber distribution (**Pette, 1980**). The average sedentary man or woman possesses approximately 45% to 55% ST fibers. It is reported that successful power athletes (sprinters, full-backs etc.) possess a large percentage of ST fibers (**Jesch et al, 1987**).

Table 1 : Sex difference in (%) slow & fast twitch muscle fiber

Athlete	Gender	Muscle	%ST	%FT	Cross-sectional area mm ST	FT
Sprinter	M	Gastrocnemius	24	76	5,878	6,034
	F	-do-	27	73	3,752	3,930
Distance	M	-do-	79	21	8,342	6,485
runner	F	-do-	69	31	4,441	4,128
Swimmer	M	Posterior Deltoid	67	33	—	—
Weight-lifter	M	Gastrocnemius	44	56	5,060	8,910
	M	Deltoid	53	47	5,010	8,450
Canoeists	M	Posterior Deltoid	71	29	4,920	7,040
Shot Putters	M	Gastrocnemius	38	62	6,367	6,441
Non Ath.	M	Vastus lateralis	47	53	4,722	4,709
	F	Gastrocnemius	52	48	3,501	3,141

(Costill & Wilmore, 94)

Table 2 : Classification of muscle fiber types

System 1	Slow twitch	Fast twitch a	Fast twitch b
System 2	Type I	Type II a	Type II b
System 3	SO	FOG	FG
Characteristic			
Oxidative Capacity	High	Moderately high	Low
Glycolytic Capacity	Low	High	Highest
Contractile speed	Slow	Fast	Fast
Fatigue resistance	High	Moderate	Low
Motor unit strength	Low	High	High

Table 3 : Structural and functional characteristics of muscle fiber type

CHARACTERISTICS	FIBER TYPE ST	FTa	FTb
Fibers/motor neuron	10-180	300-800	300-800
Motor neuron size	Small	Large	Large
Nerve conduction velocity	Small	Fast	Fast
Contraction Speed (ms)	50	100	100
Type of Myosin ATP Ase	Slow	Fast	Fast
SR development	Low	High	High
Motor unit force	Low	High	High
Aerobic Capacity (Oxidative)	High	Moderate	Low
Anaerobic Capacity (Glycolytic)	Low	High	High

Elite distance runners in 10,000 mts might differ in percentage of slow twitch fibers. For example, runner A might be found to possess 70% slow twitch fibers while runner B might contain 85% slow twitch fibers. This observation demonstrates that an individual's muscle fiber composition is not the only variable that determines success in athletic events. Success however depends on complex interaction of psychological, biochemical, neurological, cardiopulmonary and biomechanical factors (**Brooks and Fahey, 1984; Brooks and Fahey, 1987; McArdle, Katch and Katch, 1986**).

Numerous researchers have studied whether specific types of training changes a fast twitch fiber to a slow twitch fiber. The answer to this question is apparently no. Researchers concluded that endurance training does not result in a complete conversion of fast twitch fibers to slow twitch fibers (**Bagby et al, 1972; Baldwin et al, 1972 Edstrom and Grimby, 1986; Gollnick and Saltin, 1983; Hoppeler, 1986; Larsson, 1982; McArdle & Katch, 1986**). Endurance training results in a marked improvement of the oxidative capacity of the fiber types (**Pette, 1984; Pette and Spamer, 1986**).

Conversely, training for increased strength and power results in an improvement of the anerobic capacity of fast twitch and intermediate fibers (**Tesch et al, 1987**). Research continues in this area to determine the extent that training can alter the biochemical properties of skeletal muscle.

The leg muscle of distance runners, who rely on endurance, have a predominance of ST fibers. Studies of elite male and female distance runners revealed that, in many athletes, the gastrocnemius muscle contains more than 90% ST fiber. Although muscle fiber cross-sectional area varies markedly among elite distance runners, ST fibers in their leg muscles average about 22% more cross-sectional area than FT fibers. In contrast the gastrocnemius muscles are composed principally of FT fibers in sprinters who rely on speed and strength. Though swimmers have higher percentage of ST fibers (60% to 65%) in their muscles than untrained subjects (45-55%) fiber type differences between good and elite swimmers are not apparent (**Costill et al, 1976**).

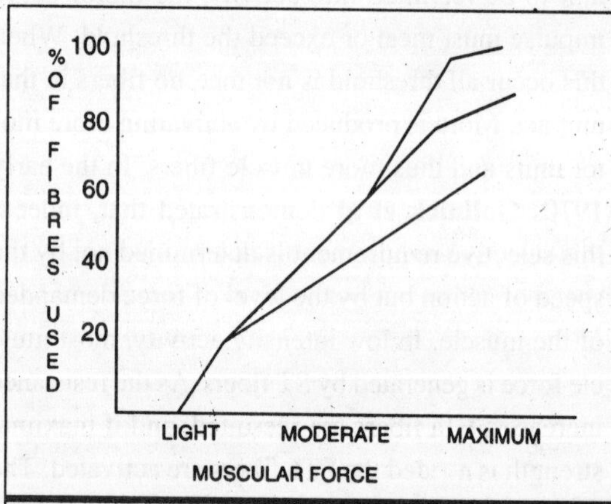

Fig. 6.9 : Percentage of fibers used in light, moderate and maximum muscular force

CLASSIFICATION OF MUSCLE MOVEMENTS

Muscles involved in a movement can be classified as Agonist (Prime movers); Antagonists (Opponent), Synergists (Assistants). Smooth flexion of elbow requires shortening of the brachialis and biceps brachii muscles (Agonist) and relaxation of the biceps brachii (Antagonist). The Brachioradialis muslce (Synergist) assist the brachialis and biceps brachii in their flexion of the joint. The three main types of muscle actions are — Concentric, in which the muscle shortens; Static, in which the muscle acts but joint angle is unchanged; Eccentric, in which the muscle lengthens.

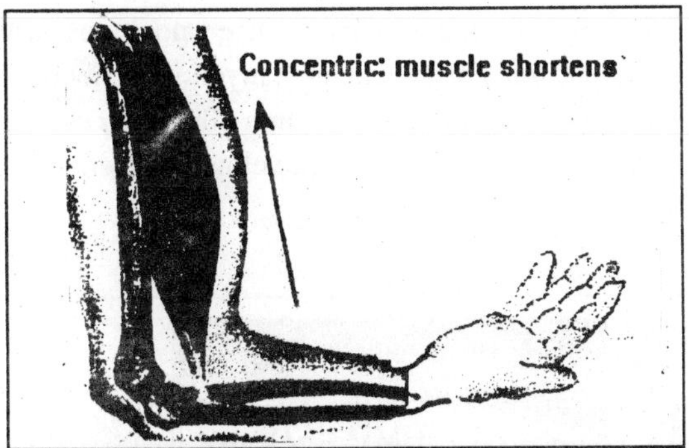

Fig. 6.10 : The action of synergistic muscle, during concentric muscle actions, the actin are pulled closer together increasing their overlap with myosin

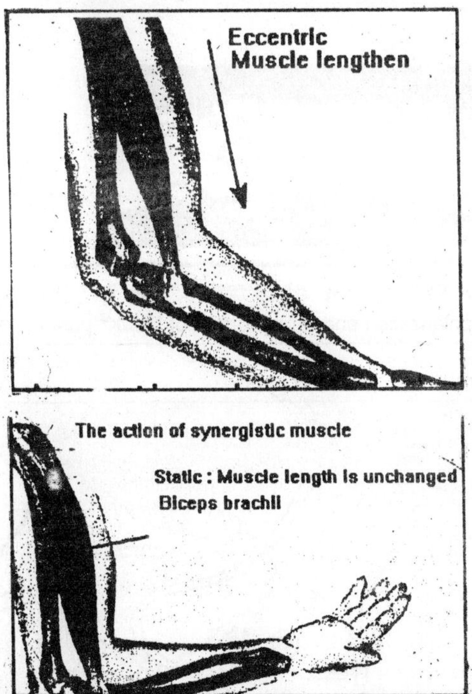

Fig. 6.11a : The action of synergistic muscle (Eccentric muscle lengthens), During eccentric muscle action the actin filaments move further apart. (b) During static contraction myosin cross bridges form and recycle, but the force is too great for the actin filament to move

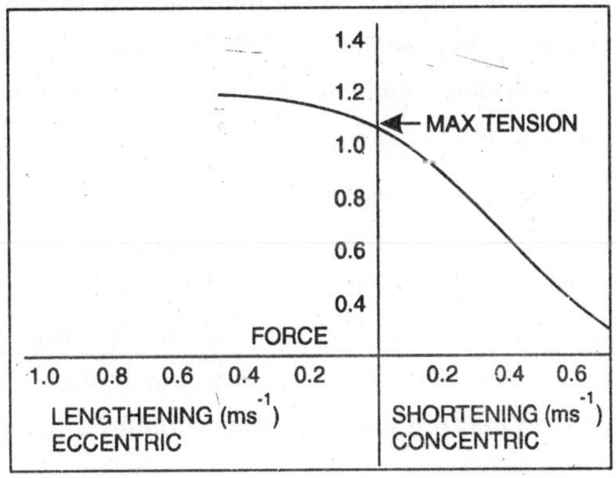

Fig. 6.12 : Relationship between muscle length and force production (Astrand & Rodhal, 1985 adopted)

The development of muscle force depends on the number of motor units activated; the type of motor unit activated; the size of the muscle; the muscle's initial length when activated; the angle of joint; the muscle's speed of action. Force production can be increased by recruiting more motor units. Force production can be maximized if the muscle is stretched 20% prior to action. At this point, the amount of energy stored and the number of linked actin-myosin cross bridges are optimum. All joints have an optimal angle at which the joint function which the muscles crossing the joint function to produce maximum force. This angle varies with the relative position of the muscle's insertion on the bone and load placed on the muscle. Speed of action also affect the amount of force produced. For concentric action maximum force can be achieved with slower contraction. The closer we get to the O velocity (Static), the more force can be generated. With eccentric actions however, faster movement allows more force production.

NEUROLOGICAL CONTROL OF MOVEMENT

All physiological activity in the human body can be influenced by the nervous system. Nerves provide the wiring through which the electrical impulse are received from and sent to virtually all parts of the body. A nerve impulse is an electrical charge or the signal that passes from one neuron to the next and finally to the end organ, such as a group of muscle fiber or back to the CNS.

A neuron's resting membrane potential (RMP) of – 70 mv results from the separation of Na^+ and K^+ ion maintained primarily by Na^+ and K^+ pump, coupled with low Na^+ permeability and high K^+ permeability (3 : 2) of the neuron's membrane. Any change making the membrane potential more

In myelinated neurons, the impulse travels through the axon by jumping between the nodes of Ranvier (gap between the cells that form the myelin sheath). This process, saltatory conduction is 5 to 50 times faster than in unmyelinated fibers of the same size. Impulse also travels faster in neurons of larger diameters. The velocity of nerve impulse transmission in large myelinated fibers can approach 120 ms $^{-1}$ (>250 mph 400 km/hr) — 5 to 50 times faster than in unmyelinated fibers of the same size.

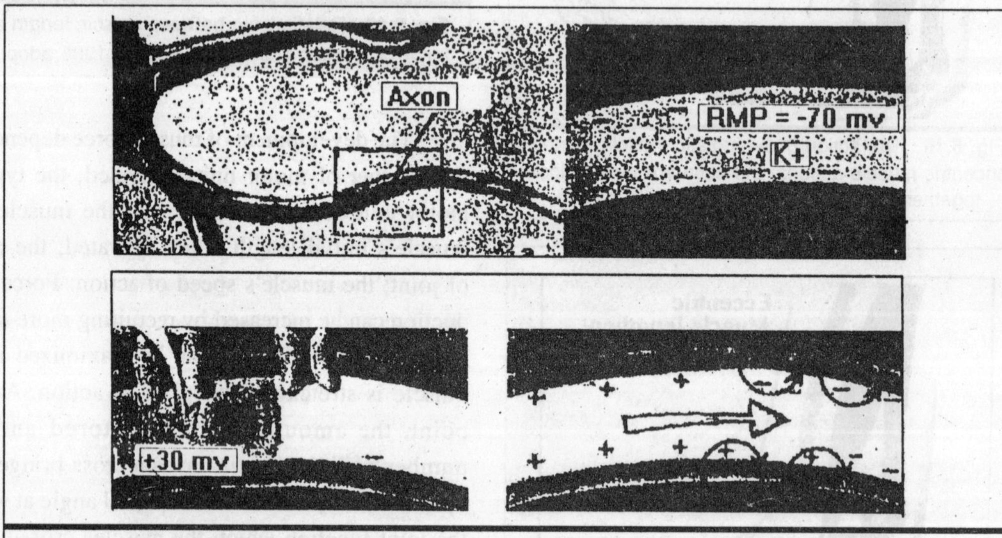

Fig. 6.13 : The sequence of events during an action potential, showing (a) the resting state, (b) depolarization, (c) propagation of an action potential, (d) repolarization and (e) the action of Na^+/K^+ pump

positive is the depolarization. Any change making this potential more negative is hyperpolarization. These changes occur when ion gates in the membrane open, permitting ions to move from one side to the other. If the membrane is depolarized by 15 to 20 mv, threshold is reached and an action potential results. Action potentials are not generated if threshold is not net.

The chain of events for an Action Potential are increased Na^+ permeability through opening of the Na^+ gate (– 70 mv to + 30 mv), decreased Na^+ permeability as the gate close(0 mv), Opening of K^+ gate and repolarization (– 70 mv).

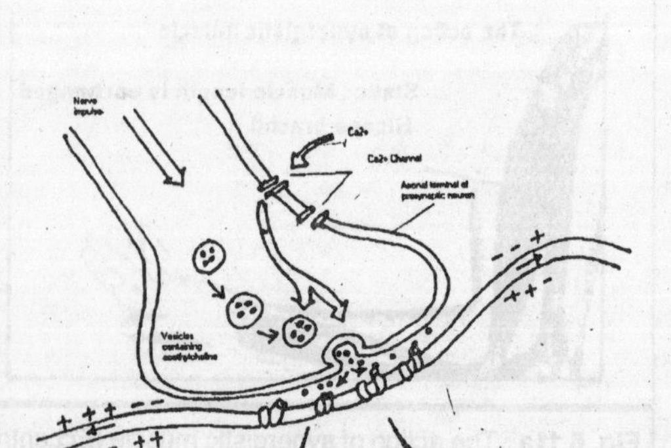

Fig. 6.14 : A chemical synapse between neurones

Nerves communicate with each other across synapses. A synapse involves : The action terminals of the presynaptic neuron. The post synaptic receptors, on the dendrite or cell body of the next neuron. The space between the two neurons (synaptic cleft). A nerve impulse causes chemicals called neurotransmitters to be released from pre-synaptic axon terminals into the synaptic cleft.

Peptides that act on the gut and the brain (eg. cholecystokinin neurotensin and leucine enkephalin). Peptides from other tissues (eg. Angiotensin II, bradykinin and calcitonin), Acetyl choline and norepinephrine are the two major neurotransmitters — chemical substances that transmit nerve impulses across synapses and synaptic clefts. Both can be either excitatory or inhibitory depending on the receptors involved. Neurotransmitters diffuse across the cleft and are bound to post synaptic receptors. Once neurotransmitters are bound the impulse has been successfully transmitted and the neurotransmitter is then either destroyed by enzymes or actively returned to pre-synaptic neuron for future use. Neurotransmitters binding at the post synaptic receptors open ion gates in the membrane and can cause depolarization (Excitation) or Hyperpolarization (Inhibition), depending on the specific neurotransmitter and receptor to which it binds. Neurons communicate with muscle cells at neuromuscular junctions. These involve pre-synaptic action terminals (motor and plates), synaptic cleft and the receptors on the sarcolemma of the muscle fiber. The neuromuscular junction functions much like a neural synapse.

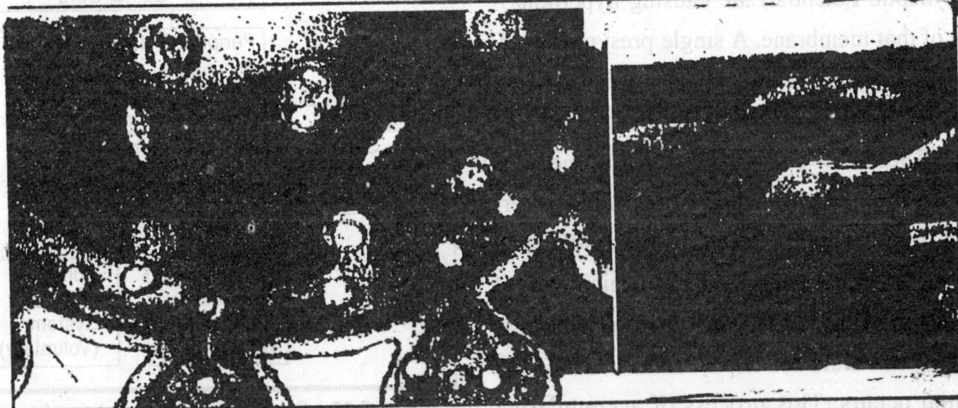

Fig. 6.15 : The neuromuscular junction showing the synaptic vesicles

CLASSIFICATION OF NEUROTRANSMITTERS

Small molecule, rapid acting transmitters :

Class I — Acetylcholine

Class II — Amines : norepinephrine, epinephrine, dopamine, serotonin and histamine.

Class III — Amino acid : GABA, glycine, glutamate and aspartate.

Neuropeptide, slow-acting transmitters.

Hypothalamic releasing hormones (eg. thyrotrophin-releasing-hormone somatostatin.

Pituitary peptide (eg, endropnin, thyrotropin and vasopressin).

The Post-Synaptic Response

After the neurotransmitter binds with the post synaptic receptors, the chemical signal that traversed the synaptic cleft, once again becames an electrical signal. The binding causes a graded potential in the post synaptic membrane. Excitatory post synaptic potential (EPSP) are depolarization of the post synaptic membrane. IPSP (Inhibitory Post Synaptic Potential) are causing hyperpolarization of that membrane. A single presynaptic terminal cannot generate enough of a depolarization to fire an action potential. Multiple signals are needed. These may come from numerous neurons or from a single neuron when numerous axon terminals release neurotransmitter rapidly and readily. The axon hillock keeps a running total of all EPSP and IPSPS when their sum meets or exceeds the threshold for depolarization, an action potential occurs. This process of accumulating incoming signals is known as summation.

CENTRAL NERVOUS SYSTEM

Central nervous system is composed of the brain and spinal cord. The four major divisions of the brain are the cerebrum, the diencephalon, the cerebellum and the brain stem.

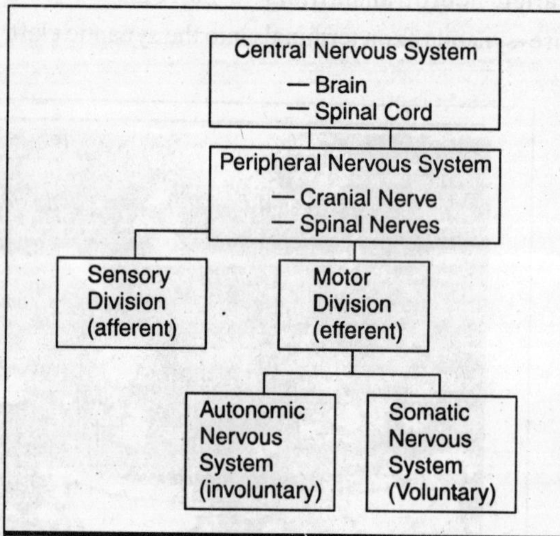

Fig. 6.16 : Schematic representation of central nervous system

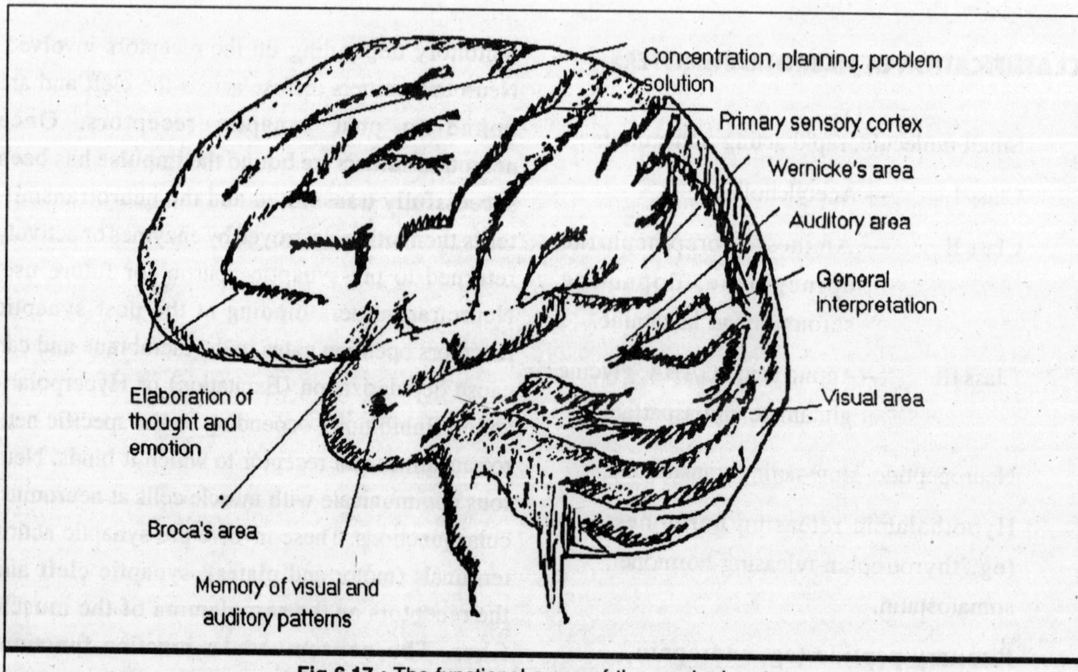

Fig 6.17 : The functional areas of the cerebral cortex

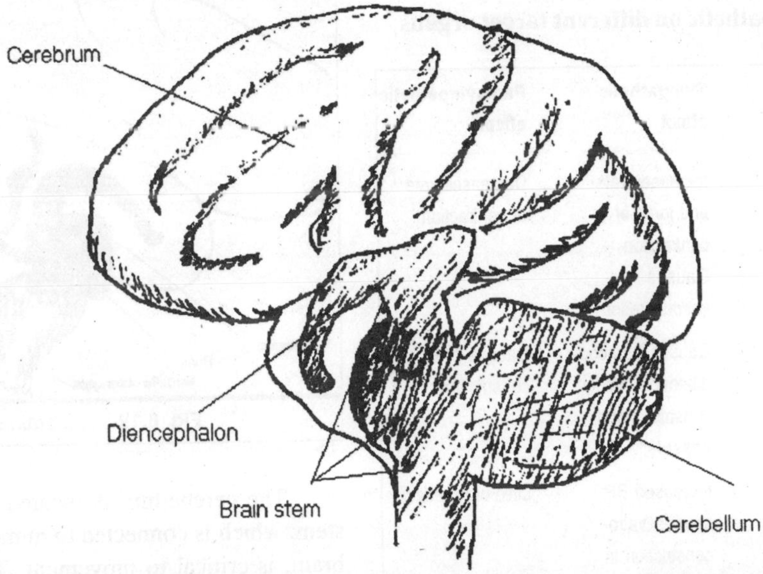

Fig. 6.18 : The four major regions of the brain

Cerebral cortex is our conscious brain, it allows is to think, to be aware of sensory stimuli and to voluntarily control our movement. The cerebrum consists of five lobes — four outer lobes and central insula.

The major lobes have the following general function : The frontal lobe is responsible for general intellect and motor control. The temporal lobe performs the function of auditory input and its interpretation. The parietal lobe controls general sensory input and its interpretation. Occipital lobe is functional for visual input and its interpretation. Three areas are in primary concern : (1) Primary motor cortex — in the frontal lobe (2) The basal ganglia, in the cerebral white matter (3) The primary sensory cortex. In the parietal lobe. The diencephalon includes the thalamus — which receives all sensory inputs entering the brain — and the hypothalamus — which is a major control center for homeostasis.

THE AUTONOMIC NERVOUS SYSTEM

The Autonomic Nervous System controls blood pressure, heart rate, respiration, digestion etc. Regulation of internal environment i.e., body temp.; fluid balance; neuroendocrine control; emotion; thirst; food intake; sleep-wake cycles. The autonomic nervous system includes the sympathetic nervous system which is our fight-or-flight system and the parasympathetic system, which is our house- keeping system. Though these systems often oppose each other, they always function together. Effect of sympathetic and parasympathetic nervous system on various organs are given next.

Table 4 : Effect of sympathetic and parasympathetic on different target organs

Target organ/ system	Sympathetic effect	Parasympathetic effect
Heart muscle	Increases rate and force of contraction	Decreases rate of contraction
Heart, coronary blood vessels	Causes vasodilatation	
Lungs	Causes broncho-dilatation, mildly constrict blood vessels	Causes broncho-constriction
Blood vessels	Increased BP, causes vaso-constriction in abdominal viscera and skin to deliver blood when necessary; causes vasodilatation in the skeletal muscle and heart during exercise	Little or no effect
Liver	Stimulate glucose release	No effect
Cellular metabolism	Increases metabolic rate	-do-
Adipose tissue	Stimulate lipolysis	-do-
Sweat gland	Increase sweating	-do-
Adrenal medulla	Stimulate secretion of epinephrine and norepinephrine	-do-
Digestive system	Decreases activity of gland and muscles; constrict sphincters	Increases peristalsis and glandular secretion; relaxes sphincters
Kidney	Causes vasoconstriction; decreases urine formation	No effect

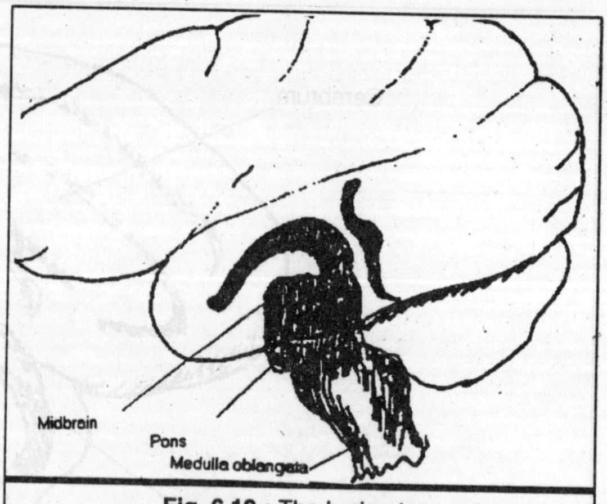

Fig. 6.19 : The brain stem

The cerebellum is located behind the brain stem, which is connected to numerous parts of the brain, is critical to movement. The brain stem is composed of the midbrain, the pons and medulla oblongata. Connecting the brain and the spinal cord. All sensory and motor nerves pass through the brain stem as they relay information between the brain and the spinal cord.

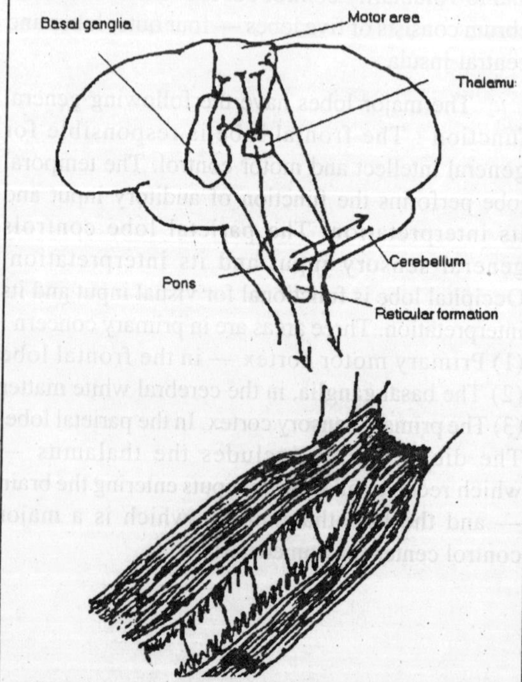

Fig. 6.20 : Motor pathway of the nervous system

This is the site of origin of 10 of the 12 pairs of cranial nerves. The brain stem also contains the major autonomic regulatory centers that exert control over the respiratory and cardiovascular system. A specialized collection of neuron running in the entire length of the brain stem, known as reticular formation. These neurons help to coordinate skeletal muscle function, maintain muscle tone, control cardiovascular and respiratory function, determine our state of consciousness (both arousal and sleep). The spinal cord carries both sensory and motor fibers between brain and the periphery.

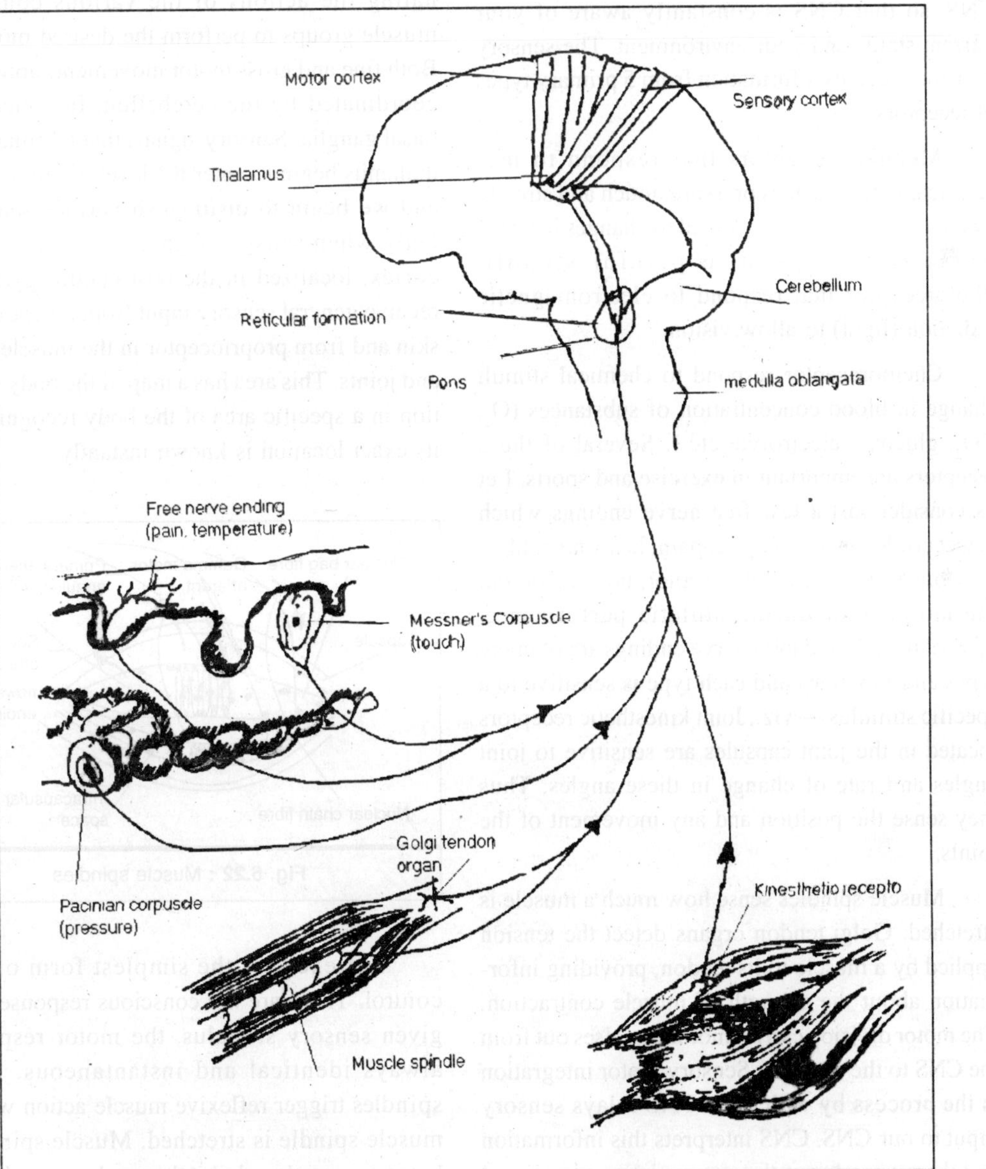

Fig. 6.21 : The sensory receptor and their pathways back to the Spinal Cord and brain

THE PERIPHERAL NERVOUS SYSTEM

The peripheral nervous system (PNS) contains 43 pairs of nerves — 12 cranial and 31 spinal. PNS can be subdivided into sensory and motor divisions. The motor division also includes the autonomic nervous system. The sensory division carries information from sensory receptors to the CNS, so that CNS is constantly aware of your current status and your environment. The sensory division receives information from 5 primary types of receptors :

Mechanoreceptors that respond to mechanical forces such as pressure, touch and stretch. Thermoreceptor which respond to changes in temp. Nociceptor respond to painful stimuli. Photoreceptor that respond to electromagnetic radiation (light) to allow vision.

Chemoreceptor respond to chemical stimuli change in blood concentration of substances (O_2, CO_2, glucose, electrolyte etc.). Several of these receptors are important in exercise and sports. Let us consider just a few free nerve endings which detect crude touch, pressure, pain, heat and cold — they function as mechanoreceptor, nociceptor and thermoreceptor during athletic performance. Special muscle and joint nerve endings are of many types and functions and each type is sensitive to a specific stimulus — viz., Joint kinesthetic receptors located in the joint capsules are sensitive to joint angles and rate of change in these angles. Thus they sense the position and any movement of the joints.

Muscle spindles sense how much a muscle is stretched. Golgi tendon organs detect the tension applied by a muscle to its tendon, providing information about the strength of muscle contraction. The motor division carries motor impulses out from the CNS to the muscles. Sensory motor integration is the process by which our PNS relays sensory input to our CNS. CNS interprets this information and then it sends out the appropriate motor signal to elicit the desired motor response. Sensory impulse that terminate in the spinal cord and integrated there (motor reflex) sensory signals that terminate in the lower brain stem in subconscious motor reactions of a higher and more complex nature than simple spinal cord reflexes. Eg, postural control when sitting or standing.

Sensory signals that terminate in the cerebellum results in subconscious control of movement, smoothing out movements by coordinating the actions of the various contracting muscle groups to perform the desired movement. Both fine and gross motor movements appear to be coordinated by the cerebellum in concert with basal ganglia. Sensory signals that terminate at the thalamus begin to enter the level of consciousness and we begin to distinguish various sensations. Only when sensory signals enter the cerebral cortex, localized in the post central gyrus, they receive general sensory input from receptors in the skin and from proprioceptor in the muscle, tendon and joints. This area has a map of the body stimulation in a specific area of the body recognized and its exact location is known instantly.

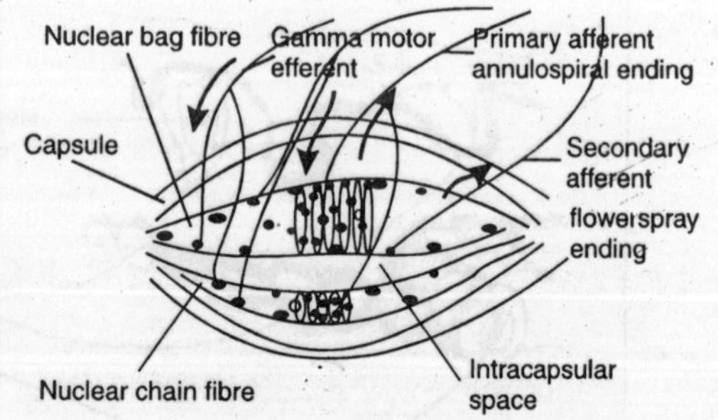

Fig. 6.22 : Muscle spindles

Reflexes are the simplest form of motor control. These are not conscious responses. For a given sensory stimulus, the motor response is always identical and instantaneous. Muscle spindles trigger reflexive muscle action when the muscle spindle is stretched. Muscle spindles lie between regular skeletal muscle, muscle fibers referred to as extrafusal fiber. A muscle spindle is composed of 4 to 20 small specialized muscle fibers called intrafusal fibers and the nerve endings sensory and motor associated with these fibers. A connective tissue sheath surrounds the muscle spindle and attached to the endomysium of the extrafusal fibers. The intrafusal fibers are controlled by specialized motor neurons, referred to as gamma motor neurons. In contrast, extrafusal fibers are controlled by alpha motor neurons. The central region of the intrafusal fiber cannot contract due to paucity of actin and myosin filament. Thus central region can only stretch. Because the muscle spindle is attached to extrafusal fiber, any time those fibers are stretched they transmit stretching to central intrafusal fiber. Sensory nerve ending wrapped around this central region of the muscle spindle transmit information to spinal cord when this region is stretched, they inform the CNS of the muscle length. In the spinal cord sensory neuron synapses with the alpha motor neuron, which triggers reflexive muscle contraction (in the extrafusal fibers) to resist further stretching.

Gamma motor neurons excite the intrafusal fibers, prestretching them slightly. Though the mid-section of the intrafusal fibers cannot contract, the ends can. The gamma motor neurons cause slight contraction of the end of these fibers, which stretches the central region slightly. This pre-stretch makes the muscle spindle highly sensitive to even small degree of stretch. When the α motor ncurons are stimulated to contract the extrafusal fibers, the gamma motor neurons are also activated, contracting the end of the intrafusal fibers. This stretches the central region of the muscle spindle, giving rise to secondary impulses that travel to the spinal cord and then to the motor neurons. In response, the muscle contracts. Thus neural muscle contraction is enhanced through this function of the muscle spindles.

Golgi tendon organs are encapsulated sensory receptors through which a small bundle of muscle tendon fibers pass. These organs are located just proximal to tendon fibers attachment to the muscle fibers. Approximately 5-25 muscle fibers are usually connected with each Golgi tendon organ. Golgi tendon organs trigger a reflex sensing changes in tension that inhibits contraction if the tendon fibers are overstretched.

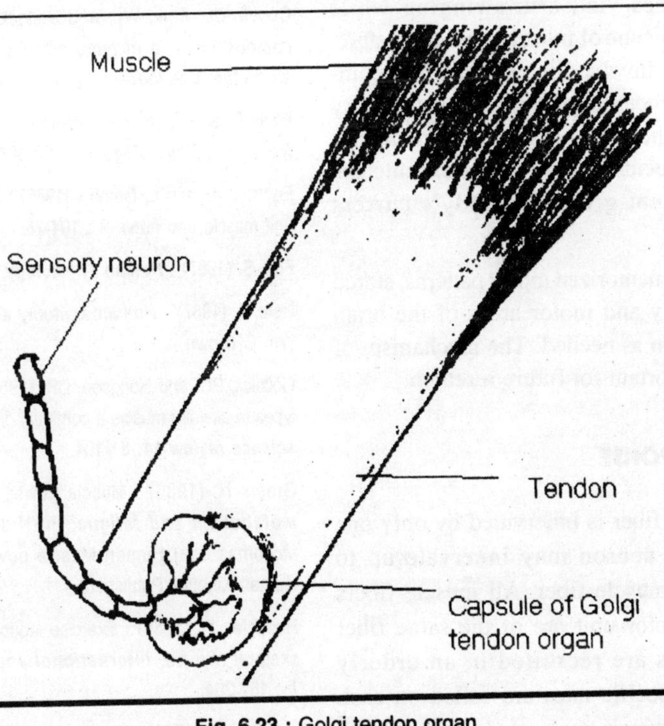

Fig. 6.23 : Golgi tendon organ

These sensory receptors perform a protective function by reducing the potential for injury. When stimulated, these receptors inhibit the contracting muscle (agonist) and excite the antagonist muscle. Some researchers speculate that reducing the influence of Golgi tendon results in disinhibition of the active muscles, allowing a more forceful action. The mechanism may explain at least part of the gains in muscular strength that accompany strength training.

THE HIGHER BRAIN CENTER

The primary motor cortex, located in the frontal lobe within the precentral gyrus is the center of conscious motor control, neurons here known as pyramidal cell. The cell bodies of the pyramidal cells are housed in the primary motor cortex and their axons form the extra-pyramidal tract. These are known as corticospinal tract — these tracts provide the major voluntary control of our skeletal muscles. The basal ganglia is the cerebral white matter, it helps initiate some movements (sustained and repetitive ones viz., arm swinging while walking) and help control muscle tone or posture. The cerebellum is involved in all rapid and complex movement processes and assists the primary motor cortex and the basal ganglia. It is an integration center that decides how to best execute the designed movement given our body's current status.

Engrams are memorized motor patterns, stored in both the sensory and motor areas of the brain that are called upon as needed. The mechanism of their action is important for future research.

THE MOTOR RESPONSE

Each muscle fiber is innervated by only one neuron, but each neuron may innervate up to several thousand muscle fiber. All muscle fibers within a single motor unit are of the same fiber type. Motor units are recruited in an orderly manner, so that specific ones are called on each time a specific activity is performed.

Motor units with smaller neurons (ST) are called on before those with larger neurons (FT). Neuromuscular activity is graded on the basis of a fixed order of recruitment from the available pool of motor units. The more force that is needed to execute a certain movement, the more motor units are recruited.

REFERENCES

Bagbay, G., W, Sembrowich. and P, Gollnick. (1972) : Myosin ATP are and fiber type composition from trained and untrained rat skeletal muscle, ***Journal of Applied Physiology*** 223 : 1415-17.

Baldwin, K. et al, (1972) : Respiratory capacity of white, red and intermediate muscle : Adaptive response to exercise, ***Journal of Applied Physiology*** 222 : 373-78.

Brooks, G. and Fahey, T. (1987) : ***Fundamentals of human performance***, New York : John Wiley and Sons.

Brooks, G. and Fahey, T. (1987) : ***Exercise Physiology*** : Human Bioenergetics and its applications. New York : John Wiely and Sons.

Costill, DL. Fink. WL. and Pollock, ML. (1976) : Muscle fiber composition and enzyme activities of elite distance runners, ***Medicine & Science in sport*** 8, 96-100.

Ebashi, S. (1976) : Excitation-contraction coupling, ***Annual Review of Physiology*** 38, 293-309.

Edstrom, L. and L, Grimby. (1986) : Effect of exercise on a motor unit muscle and nerve 9 : 104-26.

Fox, S. (1987) : ***Human Physiology***. Dubuque, la : Wm C Brown.

Hole, J. (1987) : ***Human anatomy and physiology***, Dubuque, la Wm C Brown.

Gollnick, PD. and Hodgson, DR. (1986) : The identification of fiber types in skeletal muscle a continual dilemma, ***Exercise and sports science review*** 14, 81-104.

Green, H. (1986) : Muscle power : ***Fiber type recruitment, metabolism and fatigue***. In (N Jones, N Mccartney and A Mccomas eds) Human Muscle power, 65-79. Champaign III. Human Kinetics Publishers.

Hoppeler, H. (1986) : Exercise induced ultrastructure changes in skeletal muscle. ***International Journal of Sports Medicine*** 7 : 187-204.

Johnson, L. (1983) : Biology : Dubuque, la : Wm C. Brown.

Kodama, T. (1985) : Thermodynamic analysis of muscle ATP mechanisms, ***Physiological reviews*** 65 : 468-540.

Larsson, L. (1982) : Physical training effect on muscle morphology in sedentary males at different ages, ***Medicine and Science in Sports Exercise*** 14 : 203.

McArdle, WF. Katch and V, Katch. (1986) ***: Exercise Physiology***, Energy, Nutrition and human performance, Philadelphia Lae and Febiger.

Pette, D. (1987) : Activity induced fast to slow transition in mammalian muscle, ***Medicine and Science in Sports and Exercise*** 16 : 517-28.

Pette, D. and Spamer, C. (1986) : Metabolic properties of muscle fibers, ***Federation proceedings*** 45 : 2910-14.

Pette, D. and C, Spamer. (1986) : ***Metabolic properties of muscle fibers***. Federation proceedings 45 : 2910-14.

Pette, D. (1980) ***: Plasticity of muscle***, New York : Walter de Gruyter

Tesch, PA. Thorsson and P, Kaiser. (1984) : Muscle capillary supply and fiber type characteristics in weight and power fibers, ***Journal of Applied Physiology*** 56 : 35-38

Tesch, PA. Thorsson and P, Kaiser (1984) : Muscle capillary supply and fiber type characteristics in weight and power fibers, ***Journal of Applied Physiology*** 56 : 35-38.

Willmore, JH. and Costill, DL. (1994) ***: Physiology of Sports and Exercise***, Human Kinetics. Gollnick, P. and Saltin, B. (1983) Hypothesis significance of skeletal muscle oxidative capacity with endurance training, ***Clinical Physiology*** 2 : 1-12.

7

ENERGY SYSTEM

Energy is defined as the capacity of doing work. The SI unit to measure heat energy is the Joule. However, a common unit employed to measure heat energy is the calorie. A calorie is defined as the amount of heat required to raise the temperature of one gram of water through one degree Celsius. Since calorie is very small, the term Kilocalorie (on C) is generally used to express energy expenditure and the energy value of foods. One Kcal is equal to, 1000 calories. In converting Kcal's to SI unit one Kcal is equal to 4.186 joules or 4.186 Kilojoules (Kj). Work is the product of a force acting through a distance. Common units — kg. Mt, ft. lb. Kcal. Power is the time rate of performing work. Common units — Kg. Mt/sec, ft lb/sec, Kcal/sec, Watt.

Basic energy system

About 60% to 70% of energy in the human body is degraded to heat. The remainder is used for mechanical work and cellular activities. Human machine requires energy for various activities. Energy produced in the body is in the form of chemical energy which is converted to mechanical energy. It is stored in the body as glycogen and fatty acids — mainly in liver, muscle and adipose tissue. Energy is stored intracellularly in the form of ATP and CP. We derive our energy from food sources — carbohydrate, protein and fats. Carbohydrate stores in the liver and skeletal muscle are limited to less than 2,000 Kcal of energy or the equivalent of the energy needed for about 32 km of running. Fat stores however, generally exceed 70,000 Kcal of stored energy. Protein can supply 5%-10% of energy needed to sustain prolonged exercise.

Body stores of fuels and energy

Carbohydrate	Gms	Kcal
Liver Glycogen	110	451
Muscle Glycogen	250	1,025
Glucose in body fluids	15	62
	375	1,538
Fat		
Subcutaneous	7,800	70,980
Intramuscular	161	1,465
	7,961	72,445

These estimations are based on an average body weight with 12% body fat. The energy we derive from food is stored in a high energy phosphate compound, ATP. Carbohydrate provides about 4 Kc of energy per gram, compared to about 9 Kc g^{-1} for fat. But CHO energy is more accessible. Protein can also provide energy.

METABOLISM

In some reactions in the human body energy is released and are known as catabolic reaction — catabolism. In some reactions small molecules are built up into large molecule known as anabolism. Energy required for these reactions is supplied by catabolic reaction. In the body, energy is released in two ways —

Anaerobic mechanism

Aerobic mechanism

ENERGY RELEASE IN MUSCULAR ACTIVITY

ATP-PC System

The initial energy required for muscular contraction and the energy for reabsorption of Ca^{++} into the Sarcoplasmic reticulum are provided by the synthesis of ATP. This energy released during the breakdown of ATP represents the immediate source of energy that can be used by the muscle cell to perform its work. ATP-PC system is the first active bioenergetics pathway followed by glycolysis and finally aerobic energy production **(Astrand and Rodahl, 1986, Brooks and Fahey, 1984, Essen and Kaijser, 1978; Hultman, 1973; Riley et al, 1981)**

$$ATP \xrightarrow{\text{ATP ase}} ADP + Pi + \text{energy (Utilised to perform work)}$$

During the breakdown of ATP, one of these phosphate bonds is spilt or removed from the rest of the molecule, and approximately 8 K per mole of energy are set free, free phosphate (Pi) and Adenosine Di-Phosphate (ADP) are formed. Creatine phosphate or phosphoryl creatine provides stored energy. It is used to resynthesize ATP from ADP. In the ATP-PCr system, Pi is separated from phospho-creatine through the action of creatine kinase. The Pi can then combine with ADP to form ATP. Through the process of phosphorylation of ADP and creatine are continually recycled into ATP and CP, respectively. This system is anaerobic and its main function is to maintain ATP levels. The energy yield is 1 mole of ATP per 1 mole of PCr. The PC store in the muscle is much higher than ATP store. The quantity of PC governs the duration capacity of the system. Through training, the system can provide energy for power type activities (up to 20 seconds duration for trained individuals), typical to those demonstrated by the explosive starts of sprinters and football players.

Cellular oxidation involves the transfer of electrons from hydrogen to molecular oxygen. The electrons (energy) from hydrogen are picked up in pairs by Nicotinamide Adenine Dinucleotide and NAD^+ while the substrate is being oxidized and loosing hydrogen (electron). NAD^+ is gaining a hydrogen and two electrons are being reduced to NADH, the other hydrogen appears in the cell fluid as H^+. The other important electron acceptor is Flavin Adenine Dinucleotide (FAD). FAD accepts both hydrogen to become $FADH_2$ on the inner membrane of the mitochondria. The electrons carried by NADH and $FADH_2$ are then passed in "bucket brigade" fashion by a series of iron protein electron carriers (in oxidized Fe^{3+} or reduced Fe^{2+}) — the cytochrome. By accepting an electron, the ferric portion of a specific cytochrome becomes reduced to its ferrous form. By shuttling between these iron forms, the cytochrome transfers electron. The transport of electron by specific carrier molecules constitutes the respiratory chain. Finally in the common pathway in which the electrons extracted from H^+ are passed to oxygen. For each pair of hydrogen atoms, the electrons flow down the chain and reduce one atom of oxygen to form water of the five specific cytochromes, only the last cytochrome oxidase (Cytochrome A^3) discharges its electron directly to molecular oxygen.

The energy in NADH is transferred to ADP at 3 distinct coupling sites during electron transport. This oxidation of hydrogen and subsequent phosphroylation can be summarized as follows :

$$NADH + H^+ + 3ADP + 3P + \tfrac{1}{2}O_2 \longrightarrow NAD^+ + H_2O + 3ATP$$

If hydrogen is donated by $FADH_2$, only two molecules of ATP are formed for each hydrogen pair oxidized. This occurs because $FADH_2$ enters the respiratory chain at lower energy level at a point beyond the site of the first ATP synthesis. Since O_2 is not directly involved in glycolysis the pathway is considered anaerobic. However, the presence of oxygen in the mitochondria, pyruvate can participate in the aerobic production of ATP. Thus in addition to being an anaerobic pathway capable of producing ATP without oxygen (O_2), glycolysis can be considered the first step in the aerobic degradation of carbohydrates.

Anaerobic pathway (lactic acid system)

The second major process involved in the production of ATP is commonly referred to as anaerobic glycolysis. Anaerobic glycolysis functions in the absence of oxygen. The system uses only carbohydrate in its simplest form in its food stuff. The pyruvic acid is converted to lactic acid — one mole of glucose yield 2 moles of ATP, but 1 mole of glycogen yields 3 moles of ATP. This yield represents only 5% of the total yield possible when the same amount of glucose is completely broken down to CO_2 and H_2O. Anaerobic glycolysis is extremely important as it provides a very rapid supply of ATP required during maximum intensities of 2-3 min. In absence of O_2, the end product of glycolysis i.e., pyryvic acid, is converted to lactic acid. Muscle can tolerate 2.0-2.3 gms of lactic acid per kg of muscle or 60 gms for the total muscle mass. Maximal amount of ATP manufactured 1.0-1.2 moles. This is twice as much ATP as that which is obtainable from ATP-PC system. In order to manufacture the equivalent ATP via the consumption of O_2, it would take about 15 minute of rest.

The ATP-PCr and glycolytic systems are major contributors of energy during the early minutes of high intensity exercise. Major limitation of anaerobic glycolysis is that it causes an accumulation of lactic acid in the muscle and body fluid. In all out sprint events lasting 1 or 2 min, the demands on the glycolytic system are high and muscle lactic acid levels can increase up to 20 to 25 m M/L. This acidification of muscle fibers inhibits glycolytic enzymes impairs glycogen breakdown. The acid also decreases Ca^{++} binding capacity and thus may impede muscle contraction.

The aerobic pathway (oxygen system)

The first series of reactions (in presence of oxygen) involved in the aerobic breakdown of glycogen/glucose to produce CO_2 and H_2O is aerobic glycolysis. Then, in the second series of reactions, the end product of glycolysis is pyruvic acid which entered into Kreb's cycle for further oxidation. In the presence of oxygen, a glucose molecule is metabolized to CO_2 and H_2O as a result of chemical reactions occurring in the Kreb's cycle and the electron transfer series (ETC). Energy production and subsequent replenishment are extremely time consuming (20-25 hrs). System functions primarily during long term activities (12 min minimum durations) which performed at a submaximal level. The system yields more energy than the ATP-PCr or glycolytic system.

Table 1 : Schematic representation of aerobic metabolism

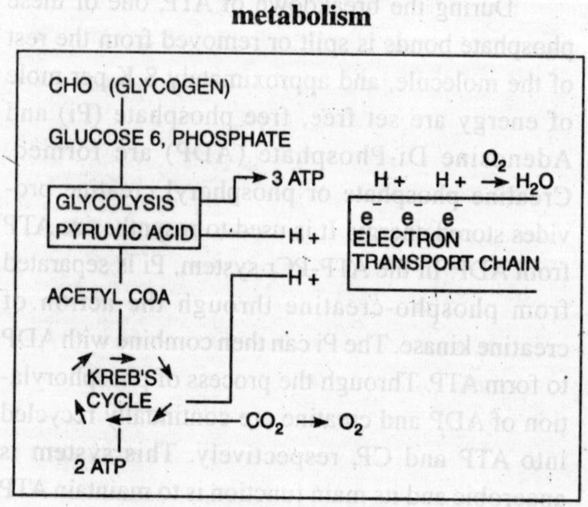

Oxidation of carbohydrate

Oxidation of carbohydrate (CHO) involves glycolysis, the Kreb's cycle and electron transport chain. The end result is H_2O, CO_2 and 38 or 39 ATP molecules per CHO molecule. Fat oxidation begins with β oxidation of FFA, then follows the same path as CHO oxidation; the Kreb's cycle and ETC. The energy yield for fat oxidation is much higher than for CHO oxidation. Although, fat provides more Kcal of energy per gram than CHO. Fat oxidation require more oxygen than CHO oxidation. The energy yield from fat is 5.6 ATP molecule per O_2. Oxygen delivery is limited by oxygen transport system, so CHO is the preferred fuel during high intensity exercise. Fat requires 2.01 L of O_2 for β-oxidation. Producing 147 molecules of ATP during breakdown of 18 carbon fatty acid molecule and during this course 26 O_2 molecules are required. Carbohydrate needs only 0.75 1 of O_2, producing 38 molecules of ATP of a 6 carbon glucose molecule. During this course 6 oxygen molecules needed.

Table 2 : Energy production from the oxidation of liver glycogen, ATP produced from 1 mole of liver glycogen

Stage of process	Direct	By oxidative phosphorylation
Glycolysis (Glucose to pyruvic acid)	3	6
Pyruvic acid to acetyl coA	0	6
Kreb's Cycle	2	22
Subtotal	5	34
	Total	39

Table 2(a) : Refers to ATP produced by transforming H⁺ and electrons to ETC. Energy production from oxidation of palmitic acid ($C_{16}H_{32}O_2$)

Stage of process	Direct	By oxidative phosphorylation
Fatty acid activation		–2
β oxidation		35
Kreb's cycle	8	88
Sub total	8	121
	Total	129

Protein oxidation is more complex because protein (amino acid) contains nitrogen, which cannot be oxidized. Protein contributes relatively little to energy production. So its metabolism is often overlooked. Oxidative capacity of the muscle depends on oxidative enzyme level (viz., SDH, citrate synthetase, mitochondrial enzyme involved in Kreb's cycle). Endurance athlete's muscles have oxidative enzyme activities nearly 2-4 times greater than those of untrained men and women **(Gollnick et al, 1972)**.

EXERCISE METABOLISM

In the transition from rest to light or moderate exercise oxygen uptake increases rapidly, generally reaching a steady state within one to four minutes. **(Bautellier et al, 1984, Cerretelli P et al, 1977, Powers et al, 1985)**. There is much evidence to suggest that at the onset of exercise the ATP-PC system is the first active bioenergetic pathway, followed by glycolysis and, finally, aerobic energy production. **(Astrand and Rodahl, 1986; Brooks, 1986; Essen and Kayser, 1978; Riley et al, 1981)**.

The term oxygen deficit is applied to the lag in oxygen uptake at the beginning of exercise. Specifically, the oxygen deficit is defined as the difference between oxygen uptake in the first few minutes of exercise and an equal time period after steady state has been obtained, **(Medbo et al, 1988; Power et al, 1987)**. Trained subjects have a lower oxygen deficit when compared to the untrained. It seems likely that the trained subjects have better developed aerobic bioenergetic capacity, resulting from either cardiovascular or muscular adaptations induced by endurance training which also means that aerobic ATP **(Dodd et al, 1988; Hickson et al, 1978; Power et al, 1985)**. Production is active earlier at the beginning of exercise and results in less production of lactic acid in the trained individual when compared to untrained individual.

Recovery from exercise : Metabolic responses

Metabolism remains elevated for several minutes immediately following exercise. The magnitude and duration of this elevated metabolism is influenced by the intensity of the exercise. (**Barnard and Foss, 1969; Gore and Wither, 1990; Powers et al, 1987**). The oxygen debt (also called excess post-exercise oxygen consumption EPOC) is the oxygen consumption above rest following exercise (**Hill A. V.; 1914**). Several factors contribute to the EPOC. First, some of the oxygen consumed early in the recovery period is used to resynthesise stored ATP and PC and replace tissue stores of O_2 in both muscle and blood. Other factors that contribute to the slow portion of the EPOC include an elevated body temperature (**Brooks G. et al, 1971; Hagberg et al, Power et al, 1982**). O_2 is required to convert lactic acid to glucose (gluconegenesis) (**Brooks, 1986**) and elevated blood levels of epinephrine and norepinephrine (**Gladder, et al, 1982**). EPOC was greater following high intensity exercise when compared to the EPOC following light to moderate work. This difference in EPOC is due to differences in the amount of body heat gained, the total PC depleted and the blood levels of epinephrine and nor-epinephrine (**Gore and Withers, 1990**) **Metabolic** responses to exercise : Influence of duration and intensity. The energy to perform short term exercise of high intensity cones primarily from anerobic metabolic pathways. Whether the ATP production is dominated by the ATP-PC system or glycolysis depends primarily on the length of the acitivity (**Armstrong R. 1979; Hultman, E 1973; Kmuttgen and Saltin, 1972**). During high intensity short term exercise (i.e., two to twenty seconds) the muscles ATP production is dominated by the ATP-PC system. Intense exercise lasting more than twenty seconds relies more on anaerobic glycolysis to produce much of the needed ATP. Finally, high intensity events lasting longer than fortyfive seconds use a combination of the ATP-PC system, glycolysis and the aerobic system to produce the needed ATP for muscular contraction.

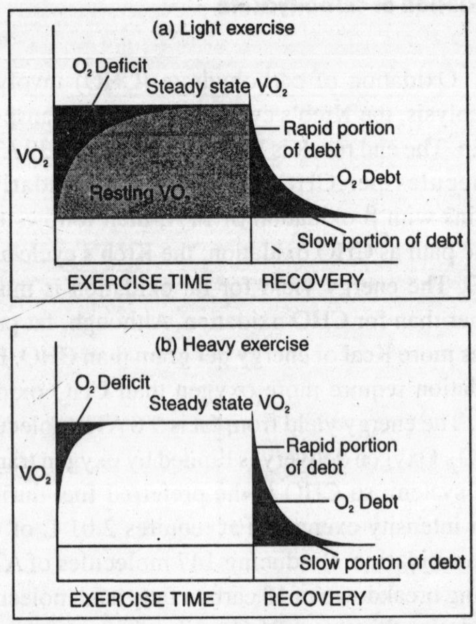

Fig. 7.1 : (a) Oxygen deficit and debt during light/ moderate exercise (b) and during heavy exercise

The energy to perform prolonged exercise (ie., > ten minutes) comes primarily from aerobic metabolism. A steady state oxygen uptake can generally be maintained during prolonged low intensity exercise. However, exercise in hot/humid environment or exercise in high relative work load (ie., 75% VO_2 max) results in a upward drift in oxygen consumption over time (**Hagberg et al, 1978**). Therefore steady state is not obtained in these types of exercise. This condition is influenced by increasing body temperature and to a lesser degree to rising blood level of the hormone epinephrine and norepinephrine. (**Gaesser and Brooks, 1984; Gladden et al, 1982**). Oxygen uptake increases in a linear fashion during incremental exercise until VO_2 max is reached. The physiological factors that influence VO_2 max include the following (1) the maximum ability of the cardiorespiratory system to deliver oxygen to the contracting muscle, and (2) the muscles' ability to take up the oxygen and produce ATP aerobically. Both genetics and exercise training are known to influence VO_2 max.

The point at which blood lactic acid rises systematically during graded exercise is termed the lactate threshold or anaerobic threshold. Controversy exists over the mechanism to explain the sudden rise in blood lactic acid concentrations during incremental exercise. It is possible that any one or the combination of the following factors might provide an explanation for the lactate threshold (a) low muscle oxygen, (**Wasserman and Mclroy 1964; Wasserman et al, 1973**). (b) accelerated glycolysis, NADH production may exceed (**Stainsby, 1986; Stryer, 1988**). The transport capacity of the shuttle mechanisms move hydrogen from sarcoplasm into the mitochondria. Blood levels of epinephrine and norepinephrine begin to rise at 50% - 65% of VO_2 max during incremental exercise and have shown to stimulate the glycolytic rate. This increase in glycolysis increases the rate of NADH production (**Stryer 1988**). Failure of the shuttle system to keep up with the rate of NADH production by glycolysis would result in pyruvic acid accepting some "unshuttled" hydrogen, and the formation of lactic acid could occur independent of whether the muscle cell had sufficient oxygen for aerobic ATP production.

A second explanation for the formation of lactic acid in exercising muscle is related to the enzy (LDH) that catalyses the conversion of pyruvic acid and lactic acid.

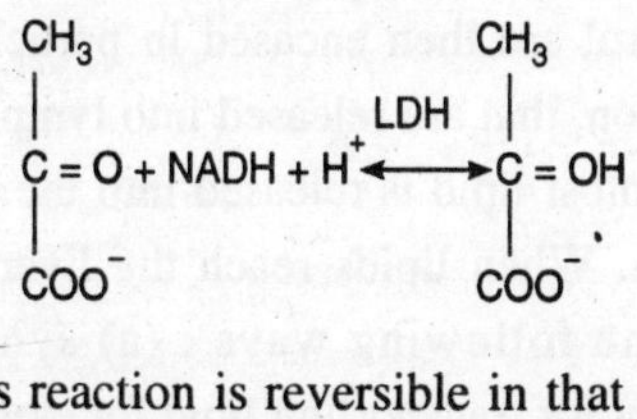

This reaction is reversible in that lactic acid can be converted back to pyruvic acid under appropriate condition. The LDH isoenzyme found in fast fibers has a greater affinity for attaching to pyruvic acid, promoting the formation of lactic acid (**Holloszy J., 1982, Skinner and Mclellan, 1980**). In contrast, slow fiber contain an LDH form that promotes the conversion of lactic acid to pyruvic acid. Therefore lactic acid formation might occur in fast fibers during exercise simply because of the type of LDH present. Thus lactic acid production would again be independent of oxygen availability in the muscle cell. Early in an incremental exercise test it is likely that slow fibers are the first called into action. However, as the exercise intensity increases, the amount of muscular force developed must be increased. This increased muscular force is supplied by recruiting more and more fast fibers. Therefore, the involvement of more fast fibers may result in increased lactic acid production and thus be responsible for the lactate threshold. A final explanation for the lactate threshold may be related to the rate of removal of lactic acid from the blood during incremental exercise. Thus a rise in the blood lactate concentration can occur due to either an increase in lactic acid production or a decrease in lactate removal. Recent evidence suggests that the rise in blood lactic acid levels in animals during incremental exercise may be the result of both an increase in lactic acid production and decrease in the rate of lactic acid removal (**Brooks, 1986; Donovan & Brooks, 1983**). The point of exponential rise in lactic acid during graded exercise has important implications for predicting sports performance and perhaps in planning training programs for endurance athletes. For example, several studies have demonstrated that the lactate threshold used in combinations with other physiological measurements (e.g., VO_2 max) is a useful predictor for success in distance running.

FIBER TYPE COMPOSITION

Training that places demands on oxidative phosphorylation stimulate the muscle fiber to develop more mitochondria that are also larger and contain more oxidative enzymes. By increasing the fibers enzymes for β oxidation, this training also enables the muscle to rely more heavily on fat for ATP production. Thus endurance training enhances the oxidative capacity to all fibers, especially FT fiber.

Oxygen availability

Oxidative capacity is determined by the no. of mitochondria and the amount of oxidative enzymes present, oxidative metabolism ultimately depends on an adequate supply of oxygen. To satisfy the O_2 need, the rate and depth of respiration increases improving gas exchange in the lungs and heart frequently also increases, pumping more oxygenated blood in the muscle.

Control of ATP-CP System

Creatine phosphate breakdown is regulated by creatine kinase activity. Creatine kinase is activated when sarcoplasmic concentration of ADP increase and is inhibited by high level of ATP.

Control of Glycolysis

The most important rate limiting enzyme is glycolysis is phosphofructokinase (PFK). When exercise begins ADP/Pi levels rise and enhance PFK activity, which serves to increase the rate of glycolysis. In contrast, at rest, when cellular ATP levels are high, PFK activity is inhibited and glycolytic activity is slowed further high cellular levels of free fatty acids or citrate (produced via Krebs cycle) also inhibit PFK activity via negative feedback. Another enzyme which regulate glycolysis is phosphorylase, responsible for degrading glycogen to glucose. At the beginning of exercise, calcium (Ca^{++}) is released from sarcoplasmic reticulum in muscle. This rise in sarcoplasmic Ca^{++} concentration indirectly activates phosphorylase which immediately begins to breakdown glycogen to glucose for entry into glycolysis. Additionally, phosphorylase activity may be stimulated by high level of hormone, epinephrine. Epinephrine released at a faster rate during heavy exercise, results in the formation of the compound, cyclic AMP which in turn activates phosphorylase.

Control of Kreb's cycle/Electron Transport Chain

The rate limiting enzyme in Kreb's cycle is isocitrate dehydrogenase which is inhibited by ATP and stimulated by increasing level of ADP/Pi (**Stryer, 1981; Suttice, 1977**). Electron transport chain is also regulated by the amount of ATP and ADP/Pi present (**Brazy and Mandel, 1986; Suttice, 1977**).

AEROBIC AND ANAEROBIC PATHWAYS DURING REST AND EXERCISE

During rest, the major fuel for energy production is lipid. Consumed fat in the diet must be further digested in the small intestine so that lipid can be absorbed into the blood stream. This is accomplished by the enzyme lipase, secreted by the pancreas, and by bile acids, lipase hydrolyses lipid producing monoglycerides, glycerol and fatty acids. These substances enter the epithelial lining of the small intestine and are reconstituted to from tryglycerides. Triglyceride along with cholesterol and glycerol are then encased in particles called chylomicron, that are released into lymphatic system. The most lipid is released into the blood via the lymph. When lipids reach the liver they are used in the following ways : (a) synthesis of lipoprotein for transporting lipid for storage in fat cell. (b) degradation of acetyl COA to produce ATP in TCA cycle or for conversion to ketone bodies (produced from the breakdown of fats) that can be used as fuel for the TCA cycle in other tissues, and (c) degradation to fatty acid and bound to serum albumin to pass to peripheral tissue. Most fuel stored in the human body is accomplished by fat storage, 98% is stored in adipose tissue and 2% in the muscle cells. Muscle cells can use lipid as a fuel by receiving either free fatty acid or ketone bodies from the liver, by receiving free fatty acid stored as fat or by using fat stored in muscle tissue. During light and moderate exercise that can be carried out over a long duration (up to 50% of VO_2 max) the predominate fuel is lipid. In contrast, during heavy exercise, exceeding 90% of VO_2 max, the predominate fuel is glycogen stored in the muscle and liver, liberates energy through the process of glycogenolysis.

Resting state

O_2 consumption = 0.3 l/min
Blood lactic acid = 1.5-2.0 mM/L of blood
O_2 Deficit + O_2 Consumed $\longrightarrow$ O_2 required

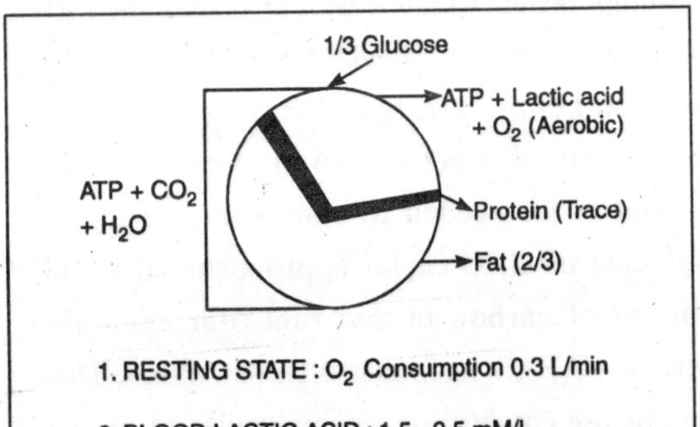

Fig. 7.2 : Metabolic contribution at resting rest

Short duration high intensity exercise

O_2 Consumption = 2.5 - 3.5 L/min

Blood Lactic Acid = 15-20 mM/L of Blood

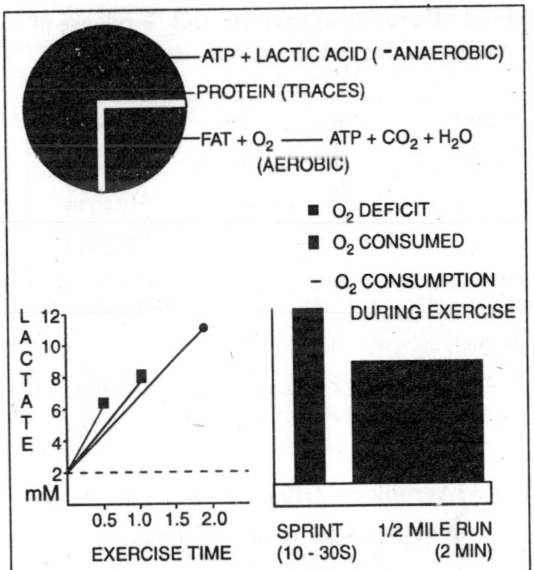

Fig. 7.3 : Metabolic contribution at short duration high intensity activity

Prolonged submaximal exercise

O_2 consumed = 3.5 - 5.6 l/min
Blood lactic acid level = 3 - 4mM/L blood

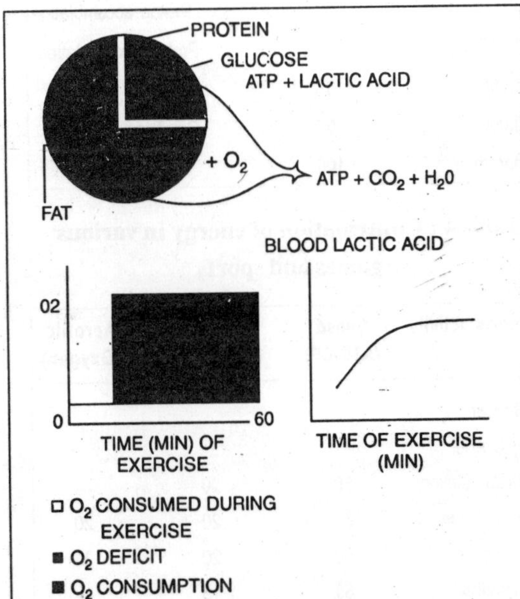

Fig. 7.4 : Metabolic contribution at prolonged submaximal exercise

Table 2 : Duration of exercise and % release of energy during maximal exercise Athletics

10 Sec.	99	1	ATP-PC
30 Sec.	80	20	ATP-PC
1 min.	70	30	Glycolysis
2 min.	40	60	Glycolysis
5 min.	20	80	Glycolysis & Oxidation
10 min.	9	91	Oxidation
60 min.	2	98	Oxidation
120 min	1	99	Oxidation

Table 3 : Aerobic contribution of various events and the major cause of fatigue

Is your run aerobic?

Event	ATP derived from Aerobic-metabolism (%)	Major causes of Fatigue
100 mt	0	Phosphocreatine
200 mt	10	Depletion
400 mt	25	Phosphocreatine
800 mt	50	Depletion and Proton accumulation
1,500 mt	65	Proton accumulation
5,000 mt	87	
10,000 mt	97	Glycogen depletion
Marathon	100	

Table 4 : Contribution of energy in various games and sports

Sports activity	Speed (ATP-CP)	Anaerobic (Lactic acid)	Aerobic (Oxygen)
Soccer			
(a) Goalie,			
Wings, Strikers	80	20	—
(b) Linkmen	60	20	20
Hockey	60	20	20
Basketball	85	15	—
Gymnastics	90	10	—
Volleyball	90	10	—

MEASURING ENERGY USE DURING EXERCISE

Direct calorimetry involves using a calorimeter to directly measure heat production of the body. It was developed by **Zuntz and Hagemanm in 1800s**, which is an insulated air tight chamber, the wall of the chamber contains copper tubing through which water is passed. The heat produced by the body radiates to the walls and warms the water. The waters temp. change is recorded, as are temperature changes in the air entering and leaving the chamber as an individual breathe. The air (out) entered the chamber contain CO_2 absorber which absorb CO_2 and pass through cooling circuit and, in turn, oxygenated air enters the chamber. These changes are due to the heat your body generates. By using the resting values, it is possible to calculate metabolism.

Indirect calorimetry involves measuring O_2 consumption and CO_2 release, calculating the RER value comparing it to standard values to determine the food being oxidized, then calculating the energy expended per liter of O_2 consumed. The amount of O_2 needed to completely oxidize a molecule of CHO or fat is proportional to the amount of carbon in that fuel. For example, glucose ($C_6H_{12}O_6$) contains 6 carbon atoms. During glucose combustion, six molecules of oxygen are used to produce 6 O_2 molecules and 6 H_2O molecules and 38 mol of ATP.

$$6O_2 + C_6H_{12}O_6 \longrightarrow 6CO_2 + 6H_2O + 38\ ATP$$

By evaluating how much CO_2 is released compared to the amount of O_2 consumed we find the RER is 1.0 :

$$RER = VCO_2/VO_2.\ \ 6CO_2/6O_2 = 1$$

RER varies with the type of food being used for energy.

RER varies with the type of food being used for energy

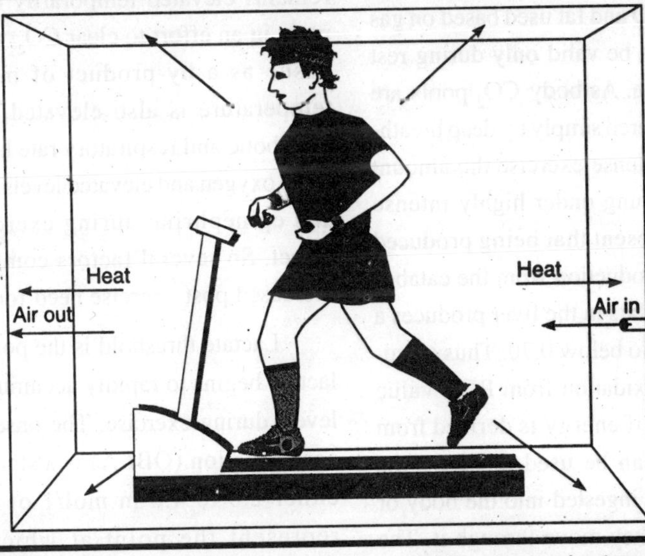

Fig. 7.5 : Direct calorimetry involves using a calorimeter to directly measure heat production of the body

FFA have considerably more carbon and hydrogen but less oxygen than glucose. Consider palmitic acid ($C_{16}H_{32}O_2$). To completely oxidize this molecule to CO_2 and H_2O require 23 molecules of oxygen.

$$16C + 16O_2 \rightarrow 16CO_2$$
$$32H + 8O_2 \rightarrow 16H_2O$$

Total = $24O_2$ needed

$-1O_2$ provided by the palmitic acid

$23O_2$ must be added

The oxidation results in 16 molecules of H_2O and 16 molecules of CO_2 and 129 molecules of ATP. During CHO oxidation, approximately 6.3 mol. of ATP are produced for each mol of O_2 used (38 ATP per $6O_2$) compared to 5.6 mol of ATP per mol of O_2 during palmitic acid metabolism (129 ATP per 23 O_2). Although fat provides more energy than carbohydrate, more O_2 is needed to oxidize fat than CHO. RER value of fat is substantially lower than for CHO, RER = VCO_2/VO_2 = 16/23 = 0.70. Once the RER value is determined from measurement of respiratory gases, the values can be compared to a table furnished below to determine the food mixture being oxidized.

Table 5 : Calorie equivalent of the respiratory exchange ratio and % K cal from CHO and fat

Respiratory exchange ratio	Energy K cal L^{-1} O_2	% K cal CHO	% K cal Fats
0.71	4.69	0	100
0.75	4.74	15.6	84.4
0.80	4.80	33.4	66.6
0.85	4.86	50.7	49.3
0.90	4.92	67.5	32.5
0.95	4.99	84.0	16.0
1.00	5.05	100.0	0

If, for example, RER value is 1, the cells are only glycogen/glucose and each liter of oxygen consumed would generate 5.05 K.cal. The oxidation of fat would yield 4.69 K cal. 1^{-1-02} and oxidation of protein would yield 4.46 K cal^{1-02} consumed.. Thus if the muscles were using only glucose and the body were consuming 2L of O_2 min than the rate of heat energy production would be 10.1 K cal min^{-1} (2L min^{-1} x 5.05 K cal).

Limitation

Calculation of CHO and fat used based on gas measurements appear to be valid only during rest and steady state exercise. As body CO_2 pools are quite large and can be altered simply by deep breathing or by performing intense exercise the amount of CO_2 released in the lung under highly intense condition may not represent that being produced in the tissue. Glucose production from the catabolism of amino acids and fats in the liver produces a respiratory exchange ratio below 0.70. Thus calculation of carbohydrate oxidation from RER value will be underestimated if energy is derived from this process. Isotopes can be used to determine metabolic rate. They are ingested into the body or ingested than traced as they move through it. The rates at which they are cleared can be used to calculate CO_2 production and then calorie expenditure.

Estimation of anerobic effort

The excess post-exercise O_2 consumption (EPOC) is the elevation above resting O_2 consumption that occur after exercise. Traditionally, the EPOC was thought to reflect the anaerobic effort of exercise. By classical theory the first curve represents the O_2 required to rebuild the ATP & PCM used during exercise, during recovery these bonds would need to be reformed via oxidative process to replenish the energy stores. The slow component of the curve was thought to result from removal of accumulated lactic acid from the tissue, by either conversion of glycogen or oxidation to CO_2 and H_2O,— thus providing energy needed to restore glycogen stores.

Traditionally, the EPOC was thought to reflect the anaerobic of exercise, but this is too simplistic. During the initial phase of exercise, some oxygen is borrowed from the O_2 stores (hemoglobin and myoglobin). That O_2 must be replenished during recovery. Also respiration remains elevated temporarily following exercise party in an effort to clear CO_2, accumulated in the tissue as a by-product of metabolism. Body temperature is also elevated, which keeps the metabolic and respiratory rate high, thus requiring more oxygen and elevated levels of nor-epinephrine and epinephrine during exercise have similar effect. So several factors combine to cause this increased post-exercise need for oxygen.

Lactate threshold is the point at which blood lactate begins to rapidly accumulate above resting levels during exercise. The onset of blood lactate accumulation (OBLA) is a standard value set at either 2.0 to 4.0 m mol/1 of O_2 consumed to represent the point at which blood lactate accumulation begins and is used as a common reference point. Lactate threshold, when expressed as a percentage of VO_2 max, is one of the best determinants of an athlete's pace in endurance events such as distance running and cycling.

Energy expenditure at rest & during exercise

The rate at which our body use energy is our metabolic rate. At rest an average person consumes about 0.3 L O_2 min. This equals 18 or 432 L per day.

How to calculate daily caloric expenditure?

At rest, the body usually burns a mixture of CHO & Fat. A PER value of 0.80 when at rest is fairly common for most individuals on a mixed diet. The calorie equivalence of an PER value of 0.80 is 4.80 K cal L O_2 consumed. So K cal per day —

= L of O_2 consumed per day × K cal used per liter O_2

= 432 L O_2 day 4.80 K cal O_2

= 2,074 K cal day^{-1}

This value is in close agreement with the average measuring energy expenditure expected for 70 kg man. One standardised measure of energy expenditure is BMR. BMR is typically in a range of 1,200 to 2,400 K cal day. BMR is the rate of energy expenditure for an individual at rest in a supine position, measured immediately after the 8 hours of sleep and at least 12 hours of fasting. The value reflects the minimum amount of energy required to carry out the essential physiological function.

BMR is related to = Fat free-mass
= Body surface area.

Many factors affect BMR
= Age — BMR gradually decreases with increasing age.
= Body temp BMR increases.

Increasing body temp. = Stress of sympathetic nervous system and increases the BM Hormone = Thyroxine and epinephrine both increases BMR.

Average total metabolic rate of an individual engaged in normal daily activity ranges from 1,800 to 3,000 K cal. The energy expenditure for very large athlete engaged in intense daily training can exceed 10,000 K cal.

Maximum capacity for exercise

Metabolism increases with the direct proportion of increased work. When the energy demand is more, body enventually reaches a limit for O_2 consumption. The O_2 consumption peaks and remains constant or drop slightly even though work intensity continues to increase. The peak value is referred to as maximal O_2 uptake or VO_2 max. VO_2 max increases with physical training only for 8-12 weeks then reaches a plateau, despite continued higher intensity training. Although VO_2 max does not continue to increase, the participants continue to improve their endurance performance. Athlete may develop a greater ability to perform at a higher % of VO_2 max. Consider the case of Alberto Salazav, the former world record holder in the marathon. His measured VO_2 max was 70 ml/kg/min. This is below the VO_2 max when performing at his racing pace, a percentage considerably higher than other runners. This may partly explain his world class running ability. Aerobic capacities of 80-84 ml kg^{-1} min^{-1} have been observed among elite male long distance runners and cross-country skiers. The highest VO_2 max value recorded for a male is from a champion Norwegian cross-country skier who had a VO_2 max of 94 ml kg^{-1} min^{-1}. The highest value recorded for a female is 74 ml kg^{-1} min^{-1} in a Russian cross-country skier. In contrast, poorly conditioned adults may have values below 20 ml kg min. Normally active 18-22 yr. old college students have average VO_2 max value of 38-42 ml kg^{-1} min^{-1} for women and 44 to 50 ml kg^{-1} min^{-1} for men. After the age of 25 to 30 yrs inactive peoples' VO_2 max value decreases about 1% per year, this may due to biological ageing and sedentary life style.

Success in endurance activities depend largely on high VO_2 max value, high lactate threshold, high economy of effort or low VO_2 value for the same rate of work and high percentage of ST fibers.

Energy cost of various activity

The amount of energy expended for different activities varies with the intensity and type of exercise. The energy cost is determined by monitoring the O_2 consumption during the activity to determine the activity to determine the average O_2 uptake per unit of time. Kilo calories of energy used per minute (K cal min^{-1}) can then be calculated from this value. This value typically ignores the anaerobic aspects of exercise and the excess post-exercise oxygen consumption. This is important because an activity that cost a total 300 K cal during the actual exercise period may cost an additional 100 K cal during the recovery period. Thus the total cost of the activity would be 400 not 300 K cal. An average body requires 0.2 to 0.35 L of O_2

per minute to satisfy resting energy requirement. This would amount to 1 to 1.8 K cal min^{-1}, 60 to 108 K cal L^{-1} or 1,440 to 2592 K cal day^{-1}. Obviously any activity above resting levels will add to the projected daily expenditure. The range for total daily calorie expenditure is highly variable. It depends on many factors — (i) activity level, (ii) age, (iii) gender, (iv) size, (v) weight & body composition.

The energy costs of sports activities also differ such as archery or shooting require only slightly more energy than when at rest. Others such as sprinting require so much energy than can be maintained for seconds. In addition to exercise intensity, the duration of activity must be considered. For example, approximately 29 K cal min^{-1} are expanded while running at 25 kph but this pace can be endured only for brief periods. Jogging at an 11 kph pace expends only 14.5 K cal min^{-1}.

Table 6 : Energy expenditure during various physical activities is furnished here under

ACTIVITY	♂ (K cal min^{-1})	♀ (K cal min^{-1})	Relative to body mass (K cal Kg^{-1} min^{-1})
Basketball	8.6	6.8	0.123
Cycling			
7.0 mph	5.0	3.9	0.071
10.0 mph	7.5	5.9	0.107
Handball	11.0	8.6	0.157
Running			
7.0 mph	14.0	11.0	0.200
10.0 mph	8.2	14.3	0.260
Sitting	1.7	1.3	0.024
Sleeping	1.2	0.9	0.017
Standing	1.8	1.4	0.026
Swimming (3.0 mph)	20.0	15.7	0.285
Tennis	7.1	5.5	0.101
Walking (3.5 mph)	5.0	3.9	0.071
Weight lifting	8.2	6.4	0.117
Wrestling	13.1	10.3	0.187

Values presented are for a 70 kg man and 55 kg woman. These values will vary depending on individual differences.

REFERENCE

Armstrong, R. (1979) ***Biochemistry*** : Energy liberation and use in sports medicine and physiology, ed. R. Strauss, Philadelphia WB Saunders.

Astrand, P. and Rodahl, K. (1986) : ***Text Book of Work Physiology***, New York Mc Graw Hill.

Barnard, R. and Foss, M. (1969) oxygen debt : Effect of beta adrenagic blockade and on lactacid and alactacid components, ***Journal of Applied Physiology***, 27 : 813-16.

Bautellier, U. et al, (1984) : Aftereffect of chronic hypoxia on oxygen kinetics and on oxygen deficit and debt. ***European Journal of Applied Physiology***, 53 : 87-91.

Brazy, P. Mandel, L. (1986) : Does availability of inorganic phosphate regulate cellular oxidative metabolism? ***News in Physiological Sciences***, 1 : 100-2.

Brooks, G. and Fahey, T. (1984) : ***Exercise Physiology*** : Human bioenergetics and its application. New York : John Wiley & Sons.

Brooks, G. et al, (1971) : Termperature skeletal, muscle, mitochondrial functions and oxygen debt, ***American Journal of Physiology***, 220 : 1053-59.

Brooks, G. (1986) : Lactate production under fully aerobic conditions. The lactate shuttle during rest and exercise. ***Federation proceedings***, 45 : 2924-29.

Cerretelli, P. et al, (1977) : Oxygen uptake transients at the onset and offset of arm and leg work. ***Respiration Physiology***, 30 : 81-97.

Dodd, S. et al, (1988) : Effects of beta blockade on ventilation and gas exchange during the rest to work transition. ***Aviation space and environmental Medicine***, 59 : 255-58.

Donovan, C. and G, Brooks. (1983) : Endurance training affects lactate clearence not lactate production. ***American Journal of Physiology***, 244 : E83-E92.

Essen, B. and Kayser, L. (1978) : Regulation of glycolysis in intermittent exercise in man, ***Journal of Physiology***, 281 : 499-511.

Essen, B. and L. Kayser. (1978) : Regulation of glycolysis in intermittent exercise in man, ***Journal of Physiology***, (London) 231 56.

Gaesser, G. and Brooks, G. (1984) : Metabolic bases of excess post-exercise oxygen consumption : A review. ***Medicine and Science in Sport and Exercise***, 16 : 29-43.

Gladden, B.W. Stains by and B. Macintosh (1982) : Norepinephrine increases canine muscle O_2 during recovery, ***Medicine and Science in Sports and Exercise***, 14 : 471-76.

Gladder, B. Stainby, W. and Macintosh B. (1982) : Norepinephrine increases canine muscle O_2 during recovery, ***Medicine and Science in Sports and Exercise*** 14 : 471-76.

Gollnic, P.D., Armstrong, R., Sanbert, C., Piew, K. and Saltin, B. (1972) : Enzyme activity and fiber composition in skeletal muscle of untrained and trained men. ***Journal of Applied Physiology*** 33 : 312-319.

Gore, C. and R. Wither. (1990) : Effect of exercise intensity and duration on post-exercise metabolism, ***Journal of Applied Physiology*** 68 : 2362-68.

Gore, C. and Withers (1990) : Effect of exercise intensity and duration on post-exercise metabolism, ***Journal of Applied Physiology*** 68 : 2362-68.

(1978) : Oxygen consumption during constant load exercise, ***Journal of Applied Physiology***, 45 : 381-84.

(1978) : Oxygen consumption during constant load exercise, ***Journal of Applied Physiology*** 45 : 381-384.

Hickson, R., Bonze, M. and Hollaszy, J. (1978) : Faster adjustment of oxygen uptake to the energy requirement of exercise in the trained state, ***Journal of Applied Physiology*** 44 : 877-81.

Hill, A. V. (1914) : The oxidative removal of lactic acid, ***Journal of Physiology*** (London) 48 : X-XI.

Holloszy, J. (1982) : Muscle metabolism during exercise, ***Archives of Physical and Rehabilitation Medicine*** 63 : 231-34.

Hultman, E. (1973) : Energy metabolism in human muscle, ***Journal of Physiology*** (London) 231 : 56.

Kmuttgen, H. and Saltin, B. (1972) : Muscle metabolites and oxygen uptake in short-term submaximal exercise in man, ***Journal of Applied Physiology*** 32 : 690-94.

Mc Ardle, W. F. Katch and Katch V. (1986) : ***Exercise Physiology*** Philadelphia, Lae & Febiger.

Medbo, J. et al, (1988) : Anerobic capacity determined maximal accumulated O_2 deficit, ***Journal of Applied Physiology*** 64 : 50-60.

Mole, P. (1983) : "Exercise Metabolism" In ***Exercise Medicine : Physiological principles and clinical application***, New York; Academic press..

Power, S. E. Howky and R. Cox, (1982) : Ventilatory and metabolic reactions to heat stress during prolonged exercise, ***Journal of Sports Medicine and Physical fitness*** 22 : 32 36.

Power, S., Dodd S. and Beadle, R. (1985) : Oxygen uptake kinetics in trained athletes differing in O_2 max, ***European Journal of Applied Physiology*** 39 : 407-15.

Power, S. et al, (1987) : Oxygen deficit debt relationship in ponies during submaximal treadmill exercise. ***Respiratory Physiology*** 70 : 251-64.

Powers S., Dodd, S. and Beadle, R. (1985) : Oxygen uptake kinetics in trained athletes differing in O_2 max. ***European Journal of Applied Physiology 39 : 407-15.***

Riley, W. S., Power, S. and Welch, H. (1981) : The effect of two levels of muscular work on urinary creatine excretion, ***Research Quarterly For Exercise and Sports*** 52 : 339-47.

Skinner, J. and Mclellan, T. (1980) : The transition from aerobic to anaerobic exercise. ***Research Quarterly*** 51 : 234-48.

Stainsby, W. (1986) : Biochemical and physiological bases for lactate production, ***Medicine and Science in Sports and Exercise*** 18 : 341-43.

Stryer, L. (1988) : ***Biochemistry***, San Francisco, W. H. Freeman, Holloszy, J. (1982) : Muscle metabolism during exercise, archives of physical and rehabilitation medicine 63 : 231-234.

Stryer, L. (1981) : ***Biochemistry***, San Francisco, W. H. Freeman.

Suttie, J. (1977) : ***Introduction to Biochemistry***, New York; Holt Rinehart & Winston.

Wasserman, K. and M. Mclroy, (1964) : Detecting the threshold on anerobic metabolism. ***American Journal of Cardiology*** 14 : 844-52.

Wasserman, K. et al, (1973) : Anaerobic threshold and respiratory gas exchange during exercise, ***Journal of Applied Physiology*** 35 : 236-43.

8

FATIGUE AND EXHAUSTION

Edwards (1983) has defined fatigue as the failure to maintain the required or expected force or power output. In the early studies of muscular fatigue, the CNS. was considered the culprit, but at late 70s' scientists suggested that fatigue may be local in origin with the brain simply modifying local events (**Karlsson, 1979; Edwards, 1981**). The recruitment of muscle depends, in part, on conscious control. The psychological trauma or exhaustive exercise may consciously or subconsciously inhibit the athlete's willingness to tolerate further pain. The CNS may slow the exercise pace to a tolerance level to protect the athlete, many researchers agreed that perceived discomfort of fatigue precedes the onset of a physiological limitation within the muscle. Unless they are highly motivated, most individuals end exercise before their muscles are physiologically exhausted. To achieve peak performance, athletes train to learn proper pacing and tolerance for fatigue. Fig. 8.1 suggests that central fatigue can be influenced by motivation, pain, perceived severity of exercise, dyspnoea and the central effects of systemic metabolic changes. Whereas peripheral fatigue can be considered to comprise 3 main components — impaired activation/excitation of the motor units, impaired energy supply and impaired actin-myosin cross bridge coupling.

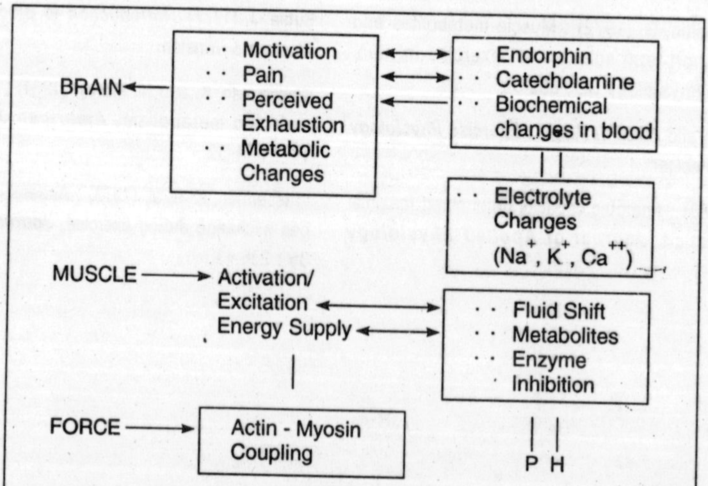

Fig. 8.1: Pathways to Fatigue (after Edwards, 1978)

FATIGUE DURING SHORT DURATION HIGH INTENSITY EXERCISE

Fatigue during short duration high intensity exercise could result from an impairment of the CNS, such that the optimal frequency of motor nerve activation is not maintained. **Bigland-Ritchie et al, (1979)** have shown that the frequency of motor nerve firing decreases during continuous contractile activity. From this finding two questions evolve (i) Whether this change precipitates muscle fatigue, or (ii) it results from neuronal feedback (muscle afferent) in an attempt to maintain optimal activation frequency as fatigue develops. Evidence suggests the latter, as the reduced motor neuron firing rate persisted during recovery when the fatigued muscle was kept ischemic (**Bigland-Ritchie et al, 1986**). The fatiguing muscle generally shows a prolonged force transient (primarily due to slower relaxation) in response to a single stimulus. Consequently a lower frequency of activation is required to elicit peak tension. From the above evidence it appears that primary sites of fatigue are located within the muscle and do not generally involve the CNS, peripheral nerves or the neuro-muscular junction (**Edwards, RTH, 1981**).

The action petential appears to reach the neuromuscular junction even when fatigue occurs, suggesting that the potential 'weak link' is the depletion of acetylcholine or a reduced excitability of the motor end-plate (**Merton, 1954**). However, evidence based on simultaneous measurements of electrical activity at the neuromuscular junction and in the individual muscle fibers suggests that the neuromuscular junction is not the site of fatigue (**Bigland-Ritchie, 1981**). The observation that fatigued muscles generate the same tension whether stimulated directly or via the motor nerve argues against NM junction fatigue (**Fitts et al, 1981**).

Fig. 8.2 Diagrammatic representation of the major components of a muscle cell involved in excitation-contraction coupling. The number indicate possible sites within the cell where alteration during short duration high intensity exercise could induce fatigue. (Fig. 8.2, No. 1) Fatigue during high frequency stimulation is in part due to an impaired surface membrane action potential transmission which result from an accumulation of extracellular K^+ and on reduction of Na^+ (**Edwards et al, 1977**), which would increase the excitation threshold of the membrane (**Jones, 1981**). With fatigue the shape of the sarcolemma Action Potential (AP) changes, showing a decreased amplitude and prolonged duration (**Metzger and Fitts, 1986**).

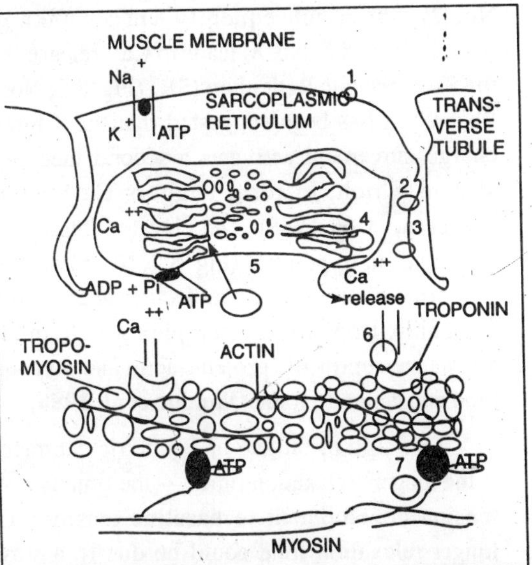

Fig. 8.2 : Diagrammatic representation of the major components of a muscle cell involved in excitation-contraction coupling

Failure to neutral transmission may be a cause of some fatigue. This failure may involve one or more of the following processes. The release or synthesis of Acetyl Choline (ACh), that relays the nerve impulse from the motor nerve to the muscle membrane, might be reduced. Cholinesterase, the enzyme that breaks down ACh once it has relayed the impulse, might become hyperactive, preventing sufficient concentration of ACh to initiate an AP. Cholinesterase activity might become hypoactive (inhibition), allowing ACh to accumulate excessively, paralyzing the fiber. The muscle fiber membrane might develop a higher threshold. Some substance might compete with ACh for receptors on the muscle membrane without activating the membrane.

The primary sites of muscular fatigue apparently involve process that occurs after depolarization of the sarcolemma and t-tubular membranes. It is likely that the general process of excitation-contraction coupling is disrupted. The t-tubular Action Potential (AP) produces a charge movement within the t-tubular membrane (Fig. 8.2, No. 2) which subsequently via an unknown process (Fig. 8.2, No. 3) leads to Ca^{++} release from the Sarcoplasmic Reticulum (SR) (Fig. 8.2, No. 4). Recently it has been suggested that the T-tubular charge movement activates a second messenger system which, in turn, triggers Ca^{++} release **(Vergera, et al, 1985**). The elevated intracellular Ca^{++} binds to troponin C (Fig. 8.2, No. 6) a regulatory protein, producing a molecular change in the troponin-c tropomyosin complex which, in turn, allows the contractile proteins actin and myosin to bind and generate force (**Vander et al, 1980**).

One sign of fatigue on isometric contraction is the longer 'relaxation time' — the time for peak tension development to baseline tension. This longer relaxation time could be due to a slower cycling of the crossbridge due to (1) Ca^{++} not being pumped back to the sarcoplasmic reticulum fast enough, and/or (2) inadequate ATP which is needed for dissociation of the cross-bridge as well as for Ca^{++} pumping (**Jones, 1981**). In fact, depletion of PCr and lactate build-up might simply increase the rate of Ca^{++} accumulation within T tubules. However, these theories of fatigue remain speculative. K^+ might leave the intracellular space of the contracting muscle, decreasing the membrane potential to half of its resting value.

To avoid fatigue, adequate tissue ATP levels must be maintained as this substrate supplies the immediate source of energy for force generation by the myosin cross-bridges. ATP is also needed in the functioning of Na/K pump, which is essential in the maintenance of a normal sarcolemma and t-tubular Action Potential. ATP is a substrate of the SR ATPase (Fig. 8.2, No. 5) and thus required in the process of Ca^{++} reuptake by the SR. The disturbance in any of these processes could lead to muscle fatigue. Phospho-creatine (PC) participates in the movement of ATP from the mitochondria to the cross-bridges — a process called the PC-ATP shuttle (**Savabi et al, 1984**). Critically low PC concentration may disrupt this shuttle system and slow the rate of ADP rephosphorylation to ATP. Thus PC could induce fatigue as the lowered ATP level hinder cross Bridge formation.

Dowson et al, (1986) have reported a strong linear relationship between the concentration of the acid form of Pi ($H_2PO_4^{-1}$) and the decline in force development in anaerobically stimulated frog Gastrocnemius muscle. They suggest that $H_2PO_4^{-1}$ reduces force by product inhibition, and that the effect of H^+ on force production can be attributed to an acidification of Pi.

Short duration high intensity exercise depends heavily on glycolysis and produce large amount of lactate and H^+ within the muscles. Cells and body fluid possess buffers such as **bicarbonate** (HCO_3^{-1}), that minimize the disrupting influence of H^+. Because of the body's buffering capacity the H^+ concentration remains low even during exhaustive workout allowing muscle pH to fall from resting value of 7.1 to no lower than 6.6 to 6.4 at exhaustion. An intracellular pH below 6.9 inhibits the action of phosphofructokinase (PFK), showing the rate of glycolysis and ATP production. (**Trevidi and Danfotgh, 1966**). At a pH of 6.4, the influence of H^+ stops any further glycogen breakdown, causing a rapid decrease in ATP and, ultimately, exhaustion. In addition, H^+ may displace calcium within the fiber, interfering with the coupling of the action myosin cross-bridges and decreasing the muscles contractile force (**Fuchs et al, 1970, Blanchard et al, 1984**). H^+ also inhibit the Sarcoplasmic-ATPase reducing Ca^{++} reuptake and subsequently Ca^{++} release from the terminal cisternae of the sarcoplasmic reticulum (**Fuchs, et al, 1970**) and the binding of Ca^{++} to troponin. (**Nakamura and Schwartz, 1972**). Most researchers agree that low muscle pH is the major limiter of performance and the primary cause of fatigue during maximal short term exercise. To delay fatigue, the athlete must control the rate of effort through proper pacing to ensure that PCr and ATP are not prematurely exhausted. Training and experience allow the athlete to judge the optimal pace that permits the most efficient use of ATP and PCr for the entire event. High intensity exercise involves an energy demand that exceeds the individual's max aerobic power and thus requires a high level of anaerobic metabolism. As fatigue develops the potential of metabolic agents increase/decrease as follows :

Increase	Decrease
Inorganic Phosphate (Pi)	High energy phosphate (ATP)
Lactate	
ADP	Phospho-creatine (PC)
H+	
Leads to Fatigue	Fatigue

Factors limiting All-out Anaerobic Performances

In events lasting less than ten seconds, optimal performance is dependent on the recruitment of appropriate Type II fibers to generate the great forces that are needed. Motivation or arousal is required, as well as the skill needed to direct the force. The primary sources of energy are anaerobic, with the focus on creatine phosphate. In short term performances lasting 10-180 seconds, there is a shift from 70% of the energy supplied anerobically at ten seconds to 60% being supplied aerobically at 180 seconds. As a result of this transition from anaerobic to aerobic energy production maximal running speeds slow as the length of the race increases. Anaerobic glycolysis provides a substantial portion of energy, resulting in an elevated H^+ ion and lactate level. The elevated H^+ concentration may actually interfere with the continued production of ATP via glycolysis (**Trevidi and Danforth, 1966**) or the contractile machinery itself, by interfering with troponin's ability to bind with Ca^{++} (**Fuchs, 1970**). In an effort to slow H^+ accumulation, some athletes have attempted to ingest buffer prior to the race.

FATIGUE DURING ENDURANCE ACTIVITY

Carbohydrates are important for contracting muscle during prolonged strenuous exercise, and fatigue is often associated with muscle glycogen depletion and or hypoglycemia (**Coggan and Coyle, 1987; Harmansen et al, 1967; Voltestad et al, 1984**). Recent studies have demonstrated that depletion of carbohydrate is associated with accumulation of ATP breakdown products (IMP and hypoxanthine, NH_3) in glycogen depleted muscle, (**Broberg and Saltin, 1989; Norman et al, 1987**) suggesting impaired ATP resynthesis. This appears to be due to a relative pyruvate deficiency, which results in reduced substrate for anaplerotic reactions that supply of TCA cycle intermediates necessary for the continued oxidation of acetyl units derived from other substances e.g., free fatty acid (FFA) and amino acids (**Saltin et al, 1990**). Increasing carbohydrate availability, by ingesting glucose during exercise, attenuates the rise in IMP, maintain TCA cycle intermediates and enhances endurance performance (**Spencer et al, 1991**). Thus the goal of carbohydrate in formulating nutritional strategies before, during, and after exercise are to optimize carbohydrate availability and oxidation during exercise.

Muscle glycogen depletion coincide with exhaustion during prolonged work bouts. Glycogen depletion/utilization was found to increase from 0.3 to 3.4 glucose units/kg/min as the relative work load increased from 25% to 100% of the VO_2 max. During heavy training, the carbohydrate requirement of the athletes may be as high as 8-10 gm per kg body weight or 60% to 70% of total energy intake (**Costill and Hargreaves, 1992**). The rate of body carbohydrate usage is dependent not only on the intensity of work but also on the individual's state of fitness (**Saltin and Karlsson 1971**). At a given work load, trained individuals have a lower RQ and deplete glycogen at a slower rate than untrained men (**Saltin and Karlsson 1971**).

Ingestion of diet high in carbohydrate should be encouraged in order to maintain carbohydrate reserves and ability to train intensely. Ingestion of high carbohydrate meal 3 to 4 hour prior to exercise ensures adequate carbohydrate availability and enhances exercise performance (**Coyle et al, 1985; Sherman et al, 1989**). Although hyperinsulinaemia associated with carbohydrate ingestion in the hour prior to exercise may result in some metabolic alterations during exercise, it may not necessarily impair exercise performance and may, in some cases, enhances performance (**Gleeson et al, 1986; Hargreaves et al, 1987; Levine et al, 1983**). Carbohydrate ingestion during prolonged strenuous exercise — where performance is often limited by carbohydrate availability — delays fatigue. This is due to maintenance of blood glucose levels and a high rate of carbohydrate oxidation, rather than slowing of muscle glycogen utilization, although liver glycogen reserves may be spared (**Costill and Hargreaves, 1992**). Recent studies have demonstrated that solutions containing 10% carbohydrate can be as effective as water in maintaining adequate hydration during prolonged exercise, while still providing sufficient carbohydrate to maintain blood glucose level and carbohydrate oxidation (**Kingwell et al, 1989; Owen et al, 1986**). There is little difference among maltodextrins, glucose and sucrose in their metabolic and performance effect during exercise, although 10% maltodextrin solution tend to be less sweet and, therefore, more palatable, than solutions of simple sugars. In contrast, fructose ingestion during prolonged exercise does not improve performance (**Bjorkman et al, 1984; Murray et al, 1989**).

During recovery from exercise, muscle glycogen resynthesis is critically dependent upon the ingestion of carbohydrate. The rate of postexercise muscle glycogen storage, when supplied with carbohydrate, is reported to be 5-8 mmol/kg/hr, which means at least 20-24 hrs is required for complete restoration of normal muscle glycogen levels. The rate of resynthesis is faster if carbohydrate is ingested immediately following exercise rather than delaying carbohydrate intake 2 hours (**Ivy et al, 1988[a]**). Thus athlete should be encouraged to ingest carbohydrate as soon after exercise as possible.

Furthermore, in the early post- exercise period the optimal carbohydrate intake appears to be 50 gm every 2 hours (**Blom et al, 1987[b], Ivy et al, 1988[b]**) aiming for a total carbohydrate intake in 24 hrs of 600 gms. Ingestion of simple, rather than complex carbohydrate results in a greater muscle glycogen storage in the first 6 hours post exercise (**Kien et al, 1990**), although after 24 hours glycogen repletion is similar regardless of the type of carbohydrate ingested (**Costill et al, 1981; Kiens et al, 1990**).

It was reported that ingestion of carbohydrate food with a high glycemic index in a 24 hours after prolonged submaximal exercise results in a greater glycogen resynthesis than that observed after ingestion of an equal amount of carbohydrate foods with a low glycemic index (**Burke et al, 1991**). Glucose and sucrose result in a faster muscle glycogen resynthesis than fructose (**Blom et al, 1987[b]**) although fructose may be of more benefit in the restoration of liver glycogen.

It was observed that muscle glycogen resynthesis is reduced or even absent, following activities such as eccentric exercise (**Costill et al, 1990; O Railly et al, 1987**) and exhaustive running (**Blom et al, 1987[a]; Sherman et al, 1983**) that produce muscle damage and soreness. The presence of inflammatory cells, which possess a large capacity for glucose oxidation within damage muscle probably results in less glucose being available for glycogen depleted muscle cells (**Costill et al, 1990**).

Furthermore, disruption of sarcolemma may interfere with the membrane structures involved in insulin binding and glucose transport. The effect of muscle damage can be partially overcome by the ingestion of increased amount of carbohydrate (**Costill et al, 1990**). Thus, one should be aware of the potential need of increased dietary carbohydrate following intense, prolonged exercise that produces muscle damage and soreness.

Glycogen depletion in different muscle groups

The comparative assessment of vastus lateralis (knee extensor), Gastrocnemius (ankle extensor) show that, the gastrocnemius uses more glycogen than the vastus lateralis or the soleus (uphill downhill or level). This suggests that ankle extensor muscles are worked more during distance running and are more likely to become depleted during distance running than are the thigh muscles.

Glycogen depletion in different fiber types

The pattern of glycogen depletion from ST and FT fibers depends on exercise intensity. ST fibers are the first fibers to be recruited during light exercise. As muscle tension requirement increases FTa fibers are added to the work force. In exercise approaching to maximum intensities the FTb fibers are added to the pool of recruited fibers. Glycogen depletion also follows the similar pattern. During relatively low intensity exercise (40%-60% of VO_2 max). ST fibers are most active and FTa and FTb fibers are relatively inactive. At higher intensities of effort (75% to 90%) FT fibers are recruited more frequently and are depleted of their glycogen at a greater rate than the ST fibers in the vastus lateralis muscle during cycling.

Muscle fibers are recruited in the following order with increasing intensities of exercise : Up to about 40% of VO_2 max, the Type I slow twitch oxidative muscle fibre which is recruited to provide tension development (**Sale, 1987**). This fibre type is dependent on a continuous supply of blood to provide the oxygen needed for the generation of ATP from carbohydrates and fats.

Any factor limiting the oxygen supply to the fibre type (e.g., altitude, dehydration, blood loss, or anemia) would cause a reduction in tension development in this fibers and necessitate the recruitment of Type IIa fibers to generate the needed tension. Type IIa fast twitch, fatigue resistant muscle fibers are recruited between 40%-75% VO_2 max (**Sale, 1987**). These fast twitch fibers are rich in mitochondria, as are the type I fibers, making them somewhat dependent on oxygen delivery for tension development. However, they also have a great capacity to produce ATP via anaerobic glycolysis. The mitochondrial content of Type IIa fibers is sensitive to endurance training, so that with detraining more of the ATP supply would be provided by glycolysis, leading to lactate production.

If oxygen delivery to this fiber type is decreased, or the ability of the fiber to use oxygen is decreased (due to low mitochondrial number), tension development will fall, requiring Type IIb fibers to came into play to maintain tension. Type IIb is the fast twitch muscle fiber with a low mitochondrial content. This fiber can generate great tension via anaerobic sources of energy, but fatigue quickly. It comes into play at about 75% VO_2 max, making heavy exercise dependent upon its ability to develop tension (**Sale, 1987**).

Apart from muscle glycogen, adequate level of free fatty acid (FFA) and blood glucose are available at exhaustion. Certain level of muscle glycogen metabolism is required for either the optimal production of NADH and the electron transport on the maintenance of fat oxidation. Perhaps intermediates of Krebs cycle become limiting without adequate glycogen metabolism leads to fatigue. Translocation of FFA into mitochondria may be rate limiting and/or high conc. of long chain FFA may inhibit ATP translocation across the mitochondrial membrane which also leads to fatigue and exhaustion.

Factors limiting aerobic performances

In moderate length performances lasting three to twenty minutes, aerobic metabolism provides 60%-90% of the ATP, respectively. These activities require an energy expenditure near VO_2 max, with Type II fiber being recruited. Any factor interfering with oxygen delivery (e.g., altitude or anemia) would decrease performance since it is so dependent on aerobic energy production. High level of lactate accompany these type of activities. Intermediate length activities lasting twentyone to sixty minutes are usually conducted at less than 90% VO_2 max, and are predominantly aerobic. Since races of this duration are not run at VO_2 max, a person who can run at a high percentage of VO_2 max would have an advantage. The ability to run at a high percentage of VO_2 max is related to the high concentration of lactate in the blood. One of the best predictor of race pace is the 'lactate threshold'. Given the length of the activity, environmental factors such as heat, humidity, and the state of hydration of the subject play a role in the outcome.

In long term performances of one to four hours duration, environmental factors play a more important role as the muscle and liver glycogen stores try to keep up with the rate at which carbohydrate is used. Diet fluid ingestion, and the ability of the athlete to deal with the heat and humidity all influence the final outcome.

Fatigue of ventilatory muscles and limitation of ventilation

Diaphragm and accessory ventilatory muscles can induce fatigue. When diaphragm muscle preparations isolated from experimental animals are electrically stimulated to contract at high rates, the muscle demonstrates distinct fatigue characteristics. Maximum voluntary ventilation tests repeated in rapid succession will also usually produce decreasing values.

The central question regarding ventilatory muscle fatigue during exercise, however, is whether or not ventilatory fatigue precedes or coincides with — and results in — decrements in body exercise performance. The answer to this question is, usually, no. As noted previously, VE max during exercise is usually less than MVV, even MVV determined after exercise. Further, most athlete scan volitionally increase VE above normally occurring volume at the end of exercise (**Brooks and Fahey, 1987**). The issue of adequacy of the ventilatory system during maximal exercise in very fit individuals has recently been raised (**Brooks and Fahey, 1987**).

Decreases in characteristics PaO_2 have been observed when some subjects were stressed to VO_2 max. Because the PaO_2 decreased even though V_E approached MVV, pulmonary system did not adequately oxygenate blood passing through it. Therefore, it was suspected that compliance in the ventilatory system prevented VE from rising sufficiently to maintain arterial O_2 concentration. Compliance is a measure of expansibility of the lungs and thorax. These structures do provide a resistance to ventilatory movements and ventilatory flow. Consequently, a limitation in the ventilatory flow is imposed by the internal resistance of the pulmonary tissues. It is, therefore, possible that in some individuals PaO_2 could be affected by pulmonary compliance during maximal exercise.

The failure to cope with lactate production during exercise results in blood acidosis. Acidosis of the blood also causes a fall in muscle pH because hydrogen ion accumulation in the blood inhibits the efflux of hydrogen ion from muscle.

Acidosis is another fatigue factor during exercise. Decrease in muscle force development has been shown to be linked to increases in muscle lactate in both frog muscle (**Fitts and Holloszy, 1976**) and human muscle (**Tesch P., 1978**). Finally, when **Adams and Welch (1980)** showed that performance time in heavy exercise (90% VO_2 max) could be altered by breathing 60% O_2 compared to 21% or 17% O_2, the point of exhaustion was associated with the same arterial H^+. The primary means by which H^+ are buffered during exercise is through its reaction with the plasma bicarbonate reserve to form carbonic acid, which subsequently yields CO_2 that is exhaled (respiratory compensation). As the bicarbonate buffer store decreases, the ability to buffer H^+ is reduced and the plasma H^+ will increase. Knowing this, scientists have explored ways of increasing plasma buffer store to slow down the rate of H^+ increase during strenuous exercise.

Dill (1932) induced alkalosis in a subject (means unknown) and showed that run time to exhaustion could be extended (5 : 22 to 6 : 04). **Jones et al (1977)** used 0.3 gm/kg body weight sodium bicarbonate and contrasted it with 0.3 gm/kg calcium carbonate, used as the control condition, and 0.3 gm/kg ammonium chloride, which caused a plasma acidosis. Subjects worked at 33% and 66% of VO_2 max for twenty minutes each, followed by work to exhaustion at 95% VO_2 max. The ammonium chloride condition decreased the duration of the ride to exhaustion (160 seconds) while the sodium bicarbonate treatment increased the ride time (438 seconds) over control (270 seconds).

Wilkes et al (1983) supported these findings in a study in which they used sodium bicarbonate to induce alkalosis and compared it with a calcium carbonate placebo condition, as well as control trial with no placebo. The subjects were six varsity track athletes and the test was an 800 mt run. The sodium bicarbonate resulted in a significantly faster time (2 : 02.9) compared to either the control (2 : 05.8) or placebo (2 : 05.1) run. **Robertson et al (1982)** supported these studies showing a lower perceived exertion during work at 80% VO_2 max with sodium bicarbonate.

The usefulness of the procedure may depend on the length of the anaerobic exercise bout. Studies in which the duration of the work task was thirty second (**Parry-Billing and Maclaren, 1986**), sixty second (**Kinderman et al, 1977**), and one hundred second (**Katz et al, 1984**) showed that the induced alkalosis did not result in significant improvement over a control condition. The reason may be that glycolysis is more important in these activities. It is logically assumed that some short-term anaerobic activities are more dependent on the plasma H^+ as a primary cause of fatigue than others. **Welch (1987)** indicates that while subjects may stop at the same H^+ within any exercise protocol, the difference that exists among studies in the 'terminal' H^+ suggest the other factors are more limiting as far as performance is concerned. The use of these agents to cause an alkalosis is not without risks. Large doses of sodium bicarbonate can cause diarrhea and vomiting, both of which are sure to affect performance (**Gledhill, 1985**).

CENTRAL FATIGUE

The central nervous system (CNS) would be implicated in fatigue if there was a reduction in the number of functioning motor units involved in activity, or a reduction in motor units' firing frequency (**Edwards, 1981**). There is evidence both for and against the concept of central fatigue. **Merton (1954)** demonstrated no difference in tension development when a voluntary contraction was compared to an electrically induced maximal contraction. In addition, when the muscle was fatigued by voluntary contractions, electrical stimulation could not restore tension. This suggested that the CNS was not limiting performance, and that the 'periphery' was the site of fatigue. **Ikai and Yabe (1969)** reported that electrical stimulation of a muscle fatigued by voluntary contractions resulted in an increase in tension development. It suggests that the upper limit of voluntary strength is 'psychologically' set, given that certain motivational or arousal factors are needed to achieve a physiological limit. In agreement with these result that CNS can limit performance are two studies by **Asmussen and Mazin, 1978[a]**. There subjects lifted weighs thirty times a minute, causing fatigue in two to three minutes. Following a two minute pause, the lifting continued. These investigators showed that when either a physical diversion, consisting of the contraction of non fatigued muscles, or mental diversion, consisting of doing mental arithmetic, was used between fatiguing bouts of exercise, work output was greater than when nothing was done during the pause. In addition, they found that if a person did a series of muscle contractions to the point of fatigue with the eye closed, simply opening the eye restored tension (**Asmussen and Mazin, 1978[b]**). These studies suggest that alteration in central nervous system 'arousal' can facilitate motor unit recruitment to increase strength, and alter the state of fatigue.

SYMPTOMS OF FATIGUE

Colour of face	-> Red
Sweating	-> Increased
Execution of movement	-> Crude, Staggering, Lack of Coordination.
Concentration	-> Lack of concentration, Nervousness, Negative learning
Continuity of training	-> Rest period prolonged
Behaviour changes	-> Aggressive, Depressed, irritated etc.
General health symptoms	-> Heaviness, Dizziness, Breathing difficulty

Nausea, Vomiting, Burning sensation, Restlessness, Insomnia
Pulse rate high
(low physical performance)

Training load and recovery

It depends upon level of fitness of sportsman ⟶ Functional capacity
+
Voluntary effort (it gives optimum performance) ⟶ Reserve capacity
It gives performance capacity ⟶ Maximum functional capacity

Performance

Adaptational changes (Physiological, Psychological, Bio-mechanical, Morphological etc.)

Laws

Adaptation processes are evident when training load reaches optimum intensity (Physical and physiological tolerance). Correct interplay of work and recovery. (Adaptation process taken place during recovery — super-compensation is the basis of improvement in performance).

Recovery is essential for re-establishment of full ability to function. Adaptation process leading to functional improvement in performance and Morphological reorganization of functional system under stress.

METHODS OF RECOVERY

Pedagogical method

Attitude of athlete to training session; Aims, objectives and tasks of all aspects of training should be clear; Correct organization of training cycle (active recovery); Recovery must start in the concluding part of training. Recovery in micro and meso cycle through change in activity; Recovery through recreation (low intensity physical exercise).

Medical-biological method

(a) Rest ⟶ Good living condition, Hygiene, Ventilated room, Proper rest.

(b) Diet ⟶ Well balanced dict (Qualitative and Quantitative).

(c) Physical therapy ⟶ Massage, Self-relaxation.

(d) Hydro-therapy ⟶ Stimulation of blood circulation.

Removal of metabolites	Hot bath (37°C - 39°C) Contrast bath (1 : 4) Shower bath at jet pressure

(e) Thermo therapy ⟶Wax bath (For connective tissue and joints), Steam packs (muscle).

Temperature 90°C to 95°C ⟵	Increase metabolism
Sweating Media to perspiration remove ⟵ waste	Eliminates waste products Toning of autonomic nervous system. Physical qualities of connective tissue increases. Tone up excretory system and skin.

(f) Electrotherapy ⟶ Ultrasound, short wave diathermy and microwave diathermy.

(g) Therapy by special movements ⟶ Music, Dancing, Stretching and bending with music, Limbering down, Special exercise for spine and joints; Stimulating climate, (Beaches, garden etc.).

(h) Psychological therapy : Psychotherapy : Psychoanalysis; Relaxation; Spiritual; Yoga; Meditation, Autogenic training; Elimination of psychic factors.

REFERENCE

Adams, R. P. and H. G. Welch. (1980) : Oxygen uptake, acid-base status, and performance with varied inspired oxygen fractions. ***Journal of Applied Physiology*** 49 : 863-868.

Asmussen and Mazin. (1978)[a] : A central nervous component in local muscle fatigue. ***European Journal of Applied Physiology*** 38 : 9-15.

Asmussen and Mazin. (1978)[b] : Recuperation after muscular fatigue by "diverting activities". ***European Journal of Applied Physiology*** 38 : 1-7.

Bigland-Ritchie B., Dawson, N. J., Johansson, R. S., Leppold OCJ., (1986) : Reflex origin for the slowing of motorneurone firing rates in fatigue of human voluntary contraction. ***Journal of Physiology.*** London 379 : 451-459.

Bigland-Ritchie. (1981) : EMG and fatigue of human voluntary and stimulated contractions. In ***Human Muscle Fatigue : Physiological Mechanisms*** 130-56. London : Pitman Medical.

Bigland-Ritchie B., Jones, D. A., Hoods, J. J. (1979) : Excitation frequency and muscle fatigue : Electrical responses during human voluntary and stimulated contractions.***Experimental Neurology*** 64 : 414-427.

Bjorkman, O., Sahlin, K., Hagenfeidf, L., Wahren, J. (1984) : Influence of glucose and fructose ingestion on the capacity for long term exercise in well trained men. ***Clinical Physiology*** 4 : 483-494.

Blom, PCS., Hostmark, AT., Voage, O., Kardel, K., Maehlum, S. (1987)[b] : Effect of different sugar diet on the rate of muscle glycogen synthesis. ***Medicine & Science in Sports and Exercise*** 19 : 491-496.

Blom, PCS., Costill, DL., Vpllestad, NK., (1987)[a] : Exhaustive running : inappropriate as a stimulus of muscle glycogen compensation, ***Medicine & Science in Sports and Exercise*** 19 : 398-403.

Broberg, S., Sahlin, K. (1989) : Adenine nucleotide degradation in human skeletal muscle during prolonged exercise. ***Journal of Applied Physiology*** 67 : 166-172.

Burke, L., Collier, G., Hargreaves, M., (1991) : Effect of glycemia index on muscle glycogen resynthesis following exhaustive exercise. Submitted for publication.

Coggan, A. R., Coyle, E. F. (1987) . Reversal of fatigue during prolonged exercise by carbohydrate infusion or ingestion, ***Journal of Applied Physiology*** 63 : 2388-2395.

Costill, DL., and Hargreaves, M. (1992) : Carbohydrate nutrition and fatigue. ***Sports Medicine*** 13(2) : 86-92.

Costill, DL., Pascoe, DD., Fink, WJ., Robergs, RA., Barr, SI. et al, (1990) : Impaired muscle glycogen resynthesis after eccentric exercise. ***Journal of Applied Physiology*** 69 : 46-50.

Coyle, EF., Coggan, AR., Hemmert, MK., Lowe, RC., Walters, TJ. (1985) : Substrate usage during prolonged exercise following a pre-exercise meal. ***Journal of Applied Physiology*** 59 : 429-433.

Dill, D. B., H. T. Edwards. and J. H. Talbot. (1932) : Alkalosis and the capacity for work. ***Journal of Biological Chemistry*** 97 : LVII-LIX.

Dowson, M. J., Smith, S. and Wilkie, D. R. (1986) : The ($H_2PO_4^{-1}$) may determine cross-bridge cycling rate and force production in living fatiguing muscle, ***Biophysics Journal*** 49 : 268a.

Edward, R. H. T., Hill, D. K., Jones, D. A., Merton, P. A. (1977) : Fatigue of long duration in human skeletal muscle after exercise. ***Journal of Physiology***. Lond 272 : 769-778.

Edwards, R. H. T. (1981) : Human muscle function and fatigue; in Porter (ed) : ***Human muscle fatigue : Physiological Mechanisms*** pp 1-18 (Pitman, London).

Fitts, R. H., Kim, D. H., Witzmann, F. A. (1976) : The development of fatigue during high intensity endurance exercise in Nagle (ed) : ***Exercise in health and disease*** pp 188-135 (Thomas Springfield).

Fitts, R. H. and J. O. Holloszy. (1976) : Lactate and contractile force in frog muscle during development of fatigue and recovery. ***American Journal of Physiology*** 231 : 430-33.

Fuchs, F., V. Reddy, and F. N. Briggs, (1970) : The interaction of cations with the calcium-binding site of troponin. ***Bi chemistry Biophysics***. Acta 221 : 407-9.

Gledhill, N. (1985) : The influence of altered blood volume and oxygen transport capacity on aerobic performance. In (R.L. Terjung. ed.), ***Exercise and Sport Sciences Reviews***, Vol. 13 : 75-94. New York, Macmillan Publishing Company.

Gleeson, M., Manghan, RJ., Greenhaft, PL. (1986) : Comparison of the effects of pre-exercise feeding on glucose, glycerol and placebo on endurance and fuel homeostasis in man. ***Eur. Journal Applied Physiology*** 55 : 645-653.

Hargreaves, M., Costill, DL., Fink, WJ., King, DS., Fielding, RA. (1987) : Effect of pre-exercise carbohydrate feeding on endurance cycling performance. ***Medicine & Science in Sports & Exercise*** 19 : 33-36.

Hermansen, I., Hultman, E., Saltin, B. (1967) : Muscle glycogen during prolonged severe exercise, ***Acta Physiologica Scandinavia*** 71 : 129-139.

Ikai, M., and Yabe, K. (1969) : Training effect of muscular endurance by means of voluntary and electrical stimulation. ***European Journal of Applied Physiology*** 28 : 55-60.

Jones, N. L. et al, (1977) : Effect of pH on cardiorespiratory and metabolic responses to exercise. ***Journal of Applied Physiology*** 43 : 959-64.

Ivy, JL., Katz, AL., Culler, CL., Sherman, WM., Coyle, EF. (1988) : Muscle glycogen synthesis after exercise, effect of time of carbohydrate ingestion. ***Journal of Applied Physiology*** 64 : 1480-1485.

Jones, D. A. (1981) : Muscle fatigue due to changes beyond the neuromuscular junction. In ***Human Muscle Fatigue : Physiological Mechanisms*** 178-96. London : Pitman Medical.

Karlsson, J., and Saltin, B. (1970) : Lactate, ATP and CI77 in working muscle during exhaustive exercise in man, ***Journal of Applied Physiology*** 29 : 598-602.

Katz, A. et al, (1984) : Maximal exercise tolerance after induced alkalosis. ***International Journal of Sports Medicine*** 5 : 107-10.

Kinderman, W., J. Keul. and G. Huber. (1977) : Physical exercise after induced alkalosis (bicarbonate or Tris-buffer). ***European Journal of Applied Physiology*** 37 : 197-204.

Kingwell, B., McKenna ,MJ., Sandstrom, ER., Hargreaves, M. (1989) : Effect of glucose polymer ingestion on energy and fluid balance during exercise. ***Journal of Sports Sciences*** 7 : 3-8.

Levine, L., Evans, WJ., Cararette, BS., Fisher, EC., Bullen, BA. (1983) : Fructose and glucose ingestion and muscle glycogen during submaximal exercise. ***Journal of Applied Physiology*** 55 : 1776-1771.

Merton, P. A. (1954) : Voluntary strength and fatigue. ***Journal of Physiology*** 123 : 553-64.

Metzger, J. M., Fitts, R. H. (1986) : Fatigue from high and low frequency muscle stimulation. Role of sarcolemma action potentials. ***Experimental Neurology*** 43 : 320-333.

Murray, R., Pau,l GL., Seifert, JG., Eddy, DE., Halaby, GA. (1989) : The effect of glucose, fructose and sucrose ingestion during exercise. ***Medicine & Science in Sports and Exercise*** 21 : 275-282.

Nakamura, Y. and S. Schwartz, (1972) : The influence of hydrogen ion concentration on calcium binding and release by skeletal muscle sarcoplasmic reticulum. ***Journal of General Physiology*** 59 : 22-32.

Norman, B., Sollevi, A., Kaijser, L., Jansson, E. (1987) : ATP breakdown products in human skeletal muscle during prolonged exercise to exhaustion. ***Clinical Physiology*** 7 : 503-509.

O. Reilly KP., Warhol, MJ., Fielding, RA., Frontera, W., Meredith, CN. et al, (1987) : Eccentric exercise induced muscle damage impairs muscle glycogen repletion. ***Journal of Applied Physiology*** 64 : 252-256.

Owen, MD., Kregel, KC., Wall, PT., Gislfi, CV. (1986) : Effects of ingesting carbohydrate beverages during exercise in the heat. ***Medicine & Science in Sports and Exercise*** 18 : 568-575.

Parry-Billings, M. and D. M. MacLaren. (1986) : The effect of sodium bicarbonate and sodium citrate ingestion on anaerobic power during intermittent exercise. ***European Journal of Applied Physiology*** 55 : 524-29.

Robertson, R. et al, (1982) : Effect of induced alkalosis on differentiated perceptions of exertion during arm and leg ergometry. ***Medicine and Science in Sports and Exercise*** 14 : 158.

Sahlin, K., Katz, A., Broberg, S. (1990) : Tricarboxitic acid cycle intermediates in human muscle during prolonged exercise. ***American Journal of Physiology*** 259 : C834-C841.

Sale, D. G. (1987) : Influence of exercise and training on motor unit activation. In (K.B. Pandolf. ed) ***Exercise and Sport Sciences Reviews***, Volume 15 : 95-151. New York : MacMillan Publishing Company.

Saltin, K., Kartz, A., Broborg, S. (1990) : Tricarboxylic acid cycle intermediate in human muscle during prolonged exercise; ***American Journal of Physiology*** 259 : C834-C841.

Saltin, B. and Karlsson, J. (1971) : Muscle glycogen utilization during work of different intensities, in pernow (ed) : ***Muscle metabolism during Exercise***, pp 289-299 (Pienum press, New York.).

Savabi, F., Geiger, P. J., Bessman, S. P. (1984) : Myofibrillar end of creatine phosphate energy shuttle. ***American Journal of Physiology*** 247 : C424-C432.

Sherman, WM., Brodowicz, G., Wright, DA., Allen, WK., Simonsen J. et al, (1989) : Effect of 4th pre-exercise carbohydrate feedings on cycling performance. ***Medicine and Science in Sports and Exercise*** 21 : 598-604.

Sherman, WM., Costill, DL., Fink, WJ., Hagerman, FC., Armstrong, LE. et al, (1983) : Effect of a 42.4 Km foot race and subsequent rest or exercise on muscle glycogen and enzymes. ***Journal of Applied Physiology*** 55 : 1219-1224.

Spencer, MK., Yan, Z., Katz, A. (1991) : Carbohydrate supplementation attenuate IMP accumulation in human muscle during prolonged exercise. ***American Journal of Physiology*** 261 : C71-C76.

Tesch, P. et al, (1978) : Muscle fatigue and its relation to lactate accumulation and LDH activity in man. ***Acta Physiologica Scandinavia*** 103 : 413-420.

Trevidi, B. and W.H. Danforth. (1966) : Effect of pH on the kinetics of frog muscle phosphofructokinase. ***Journal of Biological Chemistry*** 241 : 4110-4112.

Vander, A. J., Sherman, J. H., Luciano, D. S. (1980) : Chapter 10 Muscle, in ***Human Physiology : The mechanism of body function***, 3rd ed. pp 211-249 (Mc. Graw-Hill, New York).

Vergara, J., Tsien, R. Y., Delay, M. (1985) : Inositoll, 4, 5 triphosphate, A possible chemical link in excitation contraction coupling in muscle. ***Proceeding of National Academy of Sciences*** USA. 82 : 6352-6356.

Vollestad, NK., Vaage, O., Harmansen, L. (1984) : Muscle glycogen depletion pattern in type I and subgroups of type II fibers during prolonged severe exercise in man. ***Acta Physiologica Scandinavia*** 122 : 433-441.

Welch, H. G., (1987) ; Effects of hypoxia and hyperoxia on human performance. In (K.B. Pandolf. ed.) ***Exercise and Sports Sciences Reviews*** Vol. 15 : 191-222. New York : Macmillan Publishing Company.

Wilkes, D. N., N. Gledhill. and R. Smyth. (1983) : Effect of acute induced metabolic alkalosis on 800-m racing time. ***Medicine and Science in Sports and Exercise*** 15 : 277-80.

9

GROWTH & DEVELOPMENT OF YOUNG ATHLETES

Growth, development and maturation are terms that can be used to describe changes starting at conception and continuing through adulthood that occur in the body. Children gradually develop a readiness (learning capacity based on physiological maturation) for specific motor skills and type of exercise. This readiness depends on factors such as neurological, cardiovascular and psychological development. Training principles of the young group of sports persons have to be considered on the basis of physiological development of various organs and systems. Understanding the principle of growth and development helps in preparing their long term and short term training programs to achieve high level performance in the long run. The correct approach is required for better adaptation with training at the right time since it is not possible to reverse the process and remodify the training. The training of growing children has to be different then the adults and the children should not be taken as miniature adults.

Growth

Growth involves the transformation of nutrients into living tissue. Growth of an individual may be defined in terms of changes in its magnitude, gain in its mass or weight, increase in size of the individual as a whole i.e., it is the measurable change in the size of the various body systems for example, muscles grow in size towards maturity. Growth can be estimated by changes in physical and physiological characteristics with age.

Development

Development refers to differentiation along specialized lines of function, so it reflects the functional changes that occur with growth. The degree of competence in a variety of performance-related area, for example, development of strength/endurance with growth are :

Table 9.1

Change in body composition	Change in system
1. LBM	1. Skeletal
2. Physique	2. Circulatory
3. Height	3. Muscular
4. Weight	4. Respiratory and others
5. Body fat	
Development of	
1. Speed	
2. Strength	
3. Endurance and other performance-related qualities	

Maturation

Finally maturation refers to the process of taking on the adult form and becoming fully functional, and is defined by the system or function being considered. For example, skeletal maturity refers to having a fully developed skeletal system in which all bones have completed normal growth and ossification. Whereas, sexual maturity refers to having a fully functional reproductive system. The state of child's or adolescent's maturity can be defined by, Chronological age, Skeletal age and the State of sexual maturation.

Height

Growth in height is very rapid during the first two years of life, with a child reaching 50% of adult stature by age 2. After that the rate is slower throughout childhood until a marked increase occurs near puberty. During childhood, the period between about two years and onset of puberty, there is a steady but gradual increase in height and weight, with height increasing faster than weight. Males tend to be taller and heavier than females; however, females have relatively longer leg, which indicate greater level of maturity (the focus of growth progress from head to feet, so greater leg length indicate further progression on the growth curve). Although the growth rate is faster in males, the relative changes are similar in both sexes. The skeletal age of girls are more advanced throughout childhood. Between the age of six to ten years, the girls gain in pelvic width faster than boys, while boys tend to have larger thoraxes and forearms. Although there are some sex difference in growth during childhood, the anthropometric characteristics are almost the same until puberty. The gradual growth rate during the childhood is conducive for learning motor skill. The relatively constant ratio between height and lean body mass provides a stable environment for developing coordination and neuromuscular skill.

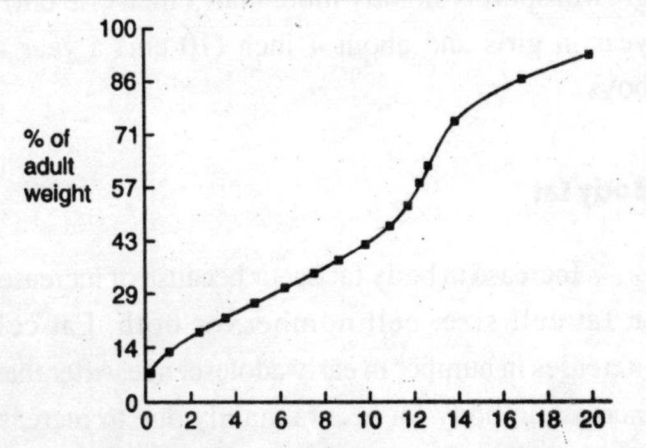

Fig. 9.1 : Growth in weight from age 2 to 20 years

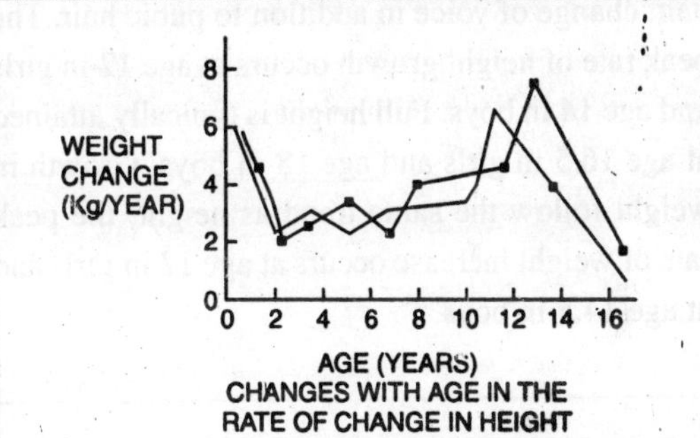

Fig. 9.2 : Rate of change of height with age

This is an important **period for the introduction and development of gross motor activities such as running, jumping, hopping and throwing. However, the limited muscle mass and the fragile skeletal epiphysial growth centers make vigorous strength training less appropriate and effective. Adolescence is the final period of growth process leading to maturity. The adolescence growth spurt generally begins at about 10.5 to 13 years in girls and 12.5 to 15 years in boys. Because puberty and growth spurt occur at the same time, the degree of sexual maturation is often used to assess the position of the growth curve (Larid, 1984).**

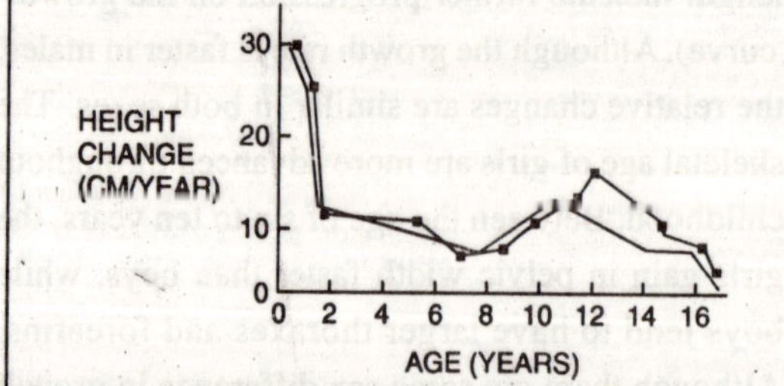

Fig. 9.3 : Rate of change of height with age

In girls, the growth spurt generally occurs when the breast and pubic hair first appear. This is followed by menarche, the first menstruation. Menarche provides a definite landmark for the assessment of maturation for girls. The indicators of maturity in boys are the appearance of facial hair, change of voice in addition to pubic hair. The peak rate of height growth occurs at age 12 in girls and age 14 in boys. Full height is typically attained at age 16.5 in girls and age 18 in boys. Growth in weight follow the same trend as height, the peak rate of weight increase occurs at age 12 in girls and at age 14.5 in boys.

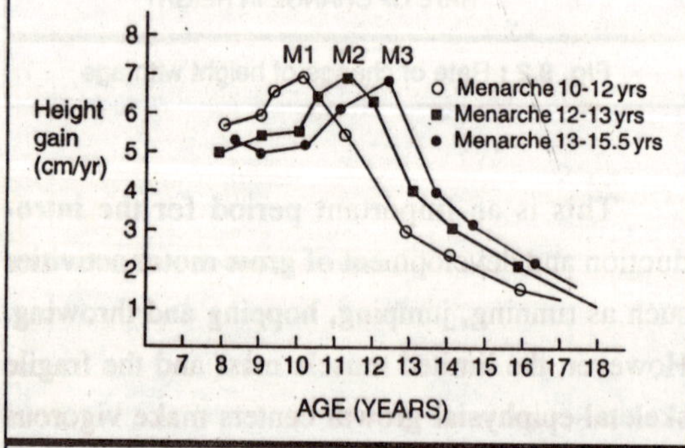

Fig. 9.4 : Peak velocities in height for early average and late maturing girls. M1, M2, M3 average time of menarche for each group

The general sequence of growth is to examine the change in stature with increasing chronological age. A linear increase in height and weight occurs with age. Development of height and weight in female children is in correspondence with the male children till pubertal age. The average increase from 7-13 year age is 40.6 cms in female and 43.1 cms in case of male. Peak highest velocity in male occurs at the age of 13-14 years. Whereas, in female, it occurs at the age of 11-12 years. In Indian talented male children of 10-16 years age, average gain in height was found to be 3.8 cms per year. The body weight of 10 years of trained children is 31.7 kgs. It increases to 53.3 kg at the age of 16 years.

Weight

The average gain of weight of 10-16 years boys is 3.1 kgs per year. Adolescent growth characteristics are different in late and early maturer. The rate of growth is more intense the earlier the growth spurt occurs (**Tanner, 1984**). Boys who mature earlier tend to be more muscular, with shorter leg and broader hips. Girls who mature earlier have shorter legs and narrower shoulders than those who mature late. Additionally, the late maturers tend to become slightly taller adults. Even though growth spurt is less in late maturers, they are growing over a longer period of time. The characteristic sexual differences in anthropometric measures arise during puberty. Males develop greater height and weight with larger musculature and broader shoulders, while females develop larger hips. The growth spurt is slightly more than 3 inch (7.5 cm) a year in girls and about 4 inch (10 cm) a year in boys.

Body fat

Increase in body fat occur because of increases in fat cell size, cell number, or both. Fat cell increases in number in early adolescence. After that, increase in body fat occurs mainly due to increasing cell size. During childhood females have slightly more fat than males. Typically body fat % are 16% for 8-year old boys and 18% for 8-year old girls.

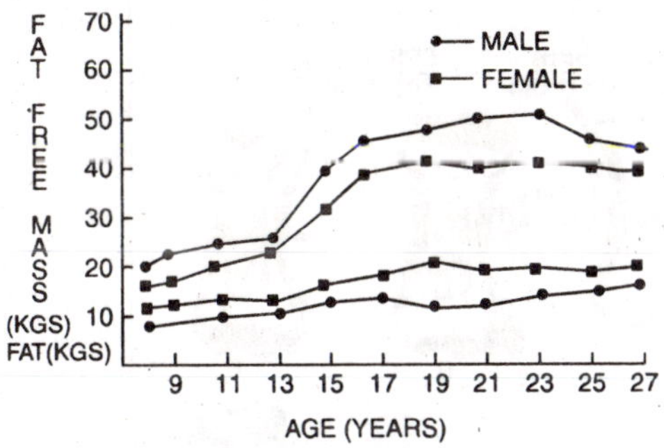

Fig. 9.5 : Fat content of male and female at various age group

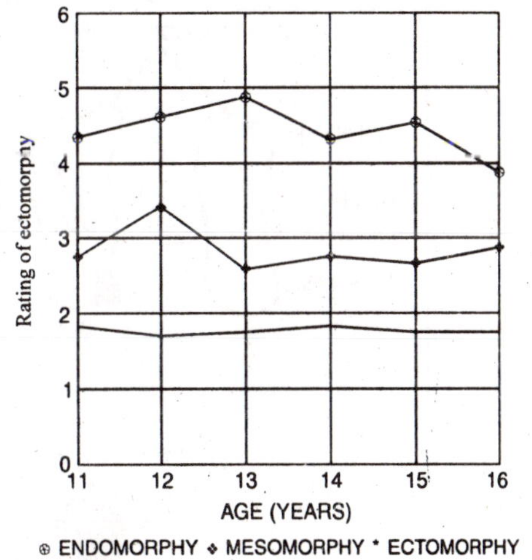

Fig. 9.6 : Variation of somatotype rating with age

At puberty marked change in body composition occurs. Boys make rapid increases in lean weight and decreases in percentage of fat. Percentage of fat typically drops 3% to 5% between ages 12 to 17.

Females also experience increase in lean mass, although less than boys, and increase in body fat. Body fat in case of growing male children does not significantly vary with age. Although, there is no general agreement on the ideal amount of body fat of children. However, it has been reported that children should not exceed 17% of body fat. Fat cells can increase in size and number throughout life (**Bjorntorp, 1986**). The amount of fat accumulation depends on diet, exercise habit and heredity. At physical maturity, the body fat content average 15% in males and 25% in females. The differences are primarily caused by higher testosterone level in males and higher estrogen levels in females.

Physique

Somatotype of the athlete does not significantly vary with growth and development in children under training. Although fluctuation in mean somatotype rating are reported with growth and development. Keeping in view this aspect the most desirable physique should be slected at the right age for making a champion.

Development of bone "Ossification"

Bones are formed through ossification, which spreads from primary (diaphysis) and secondary (epiphysis) ossification centers. The vast majority of bones develop from hyaline cartilage. During fetal development as well as during the initial 14-22 years of life, membrane and cartilage are transformed into bone through the process of ossification.

The central shaft of the long bone is referred to as the diaphysis and each end of the long bone is epiphysis. Ossification — through which cartilage is transformed into bone — begins at the diaphysis. The cartilage that will be transformed is covered by a fibrous membrane, the perichondrium. Ossification is initiated when this membrane is penetrated by blood vessels. Once perichondrium is vascularized, it is called the periosteum, and the chondrocyte-(çartilage forming cells) in it become osteoblasts (bone-forming cells). Osteoblast secretes substances that form a ring or collar of bone around the diaphysis. At the same time the cartilage cells in the central area of the diaphysis undergo a series of complex changes, which, eventually, result in calcification of the bone. This area of bone formation is known as primary ossification center.

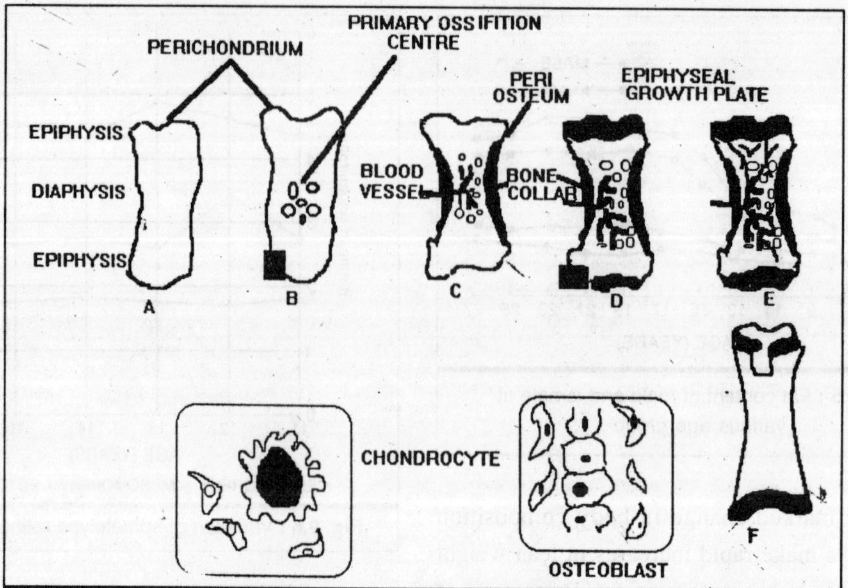

Fig. 9.7 : Process of bone ossification

The cartilage continues to grow in length and thickness, the periosteal development and bone formation from the primary ossification center continues towards the epiphysis.

At birth, each of our long bones has a body diaphysis and also cartilaginous epiphysis. Shortly after birth, secondary ossification center arise in the epiphysis. With the establishment of these secondary centers, the epiphysis begin to ossify. Bone formation then occurs in the diaphysis and epiphysis, leaving a plate of cartilage between the diaphysis and each epiphysis — that is known as epiphysial or growth plate. This epiphysial plate allow our bones to elongate as we grow. Cartilage growth continues on the epiphyseal border of these plates as cartilage is replaced on the diaphyseal border, so the growth plates remain approximately the same thickness.

Ossification is completed and bone growth ceases when the cartilage cells cease to grow and the epiphyseal plates are replaced by bone. This fuses the diaphysis with each epiphysis, and bone lengthening then is no longer possible. In the tibia (shin bones) of males, ossification is completed in the distal epiphysis (ankle) on the average age of 17 years, and the proximal epiphysis at the age of 20 years, although actual age varies considerably. In females, this fusion process is completed approximately 2 to 3 years earlier. With certain exception, bones typically begin to fuse pre-tens and all are fused by early twenties. On the average, girls achieve full bone maturity several years before boys.

Bone is a living tissue that requires essential nutrients, so it receives a rich blood supply. Bone consists of cells distributed throughout the matrix, and it is dense and hard due to deposit of lime salt, viz., calcium phosphate and calcium carbonate. Calcium is an essential nutrient, particularly during the periods of bone growth and in the latter years of life, when bone tends to become brittle due to aging. Bone store Ca^{++}, when our blood Ca^{++} level is high, excess Ca^{++} is deposited in our bone for storage, and when Ca^{++} level is too low, bone is reabsorbed or broken down to release Ca^{++} into blood. When injury occurs or when extra stress is placed on the bone, the more Ca^{++} is deposited. Thus throughout life our bone is constantly changing. Exercise, along with an adequate diet, is essential for proper bone growth. Exercise affects primarily bone width, density and strength but has little or no effect on length.

Bone injury

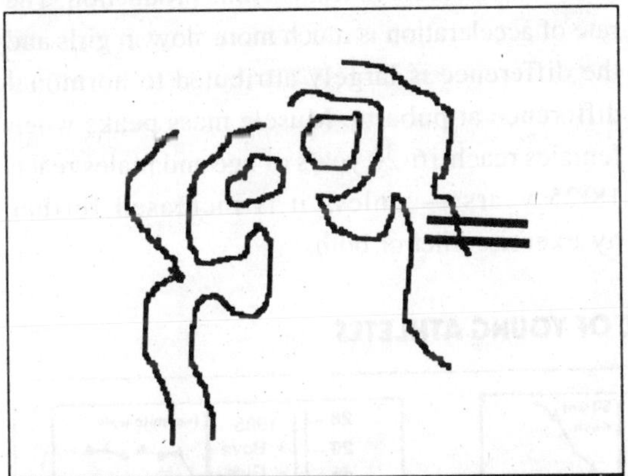

Fig. 9.8 : A slipped epiphysis on the head of the femur in an 8 - year old girl

In a study of 31 epiphyseal injuries, only 23% were sports induced. The remainder resulted from falls and vehicular accident (**Larson, 1974**). Fig. 9.8 illustrate a slipped epiphysis on the head of the femur in an 8 year old girl. The epiphysis of her femur was displaced or had slipped from its correct alignment with the diaphysis. The injury occur during a championship soccer match, and her symptoms were initially diagnosed as a groin pull.

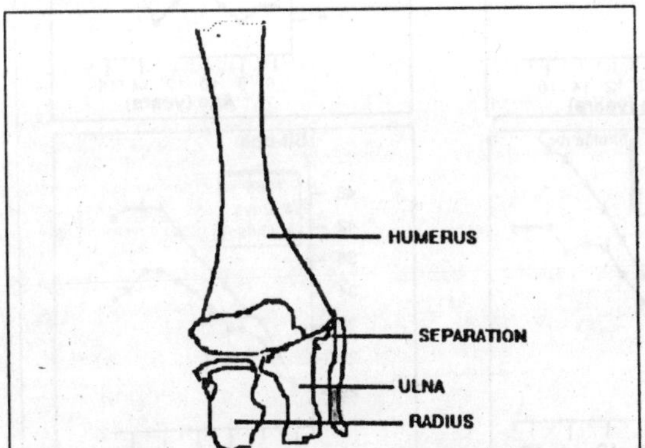

Fig. 9.9 : Inflammation of epiphysis

Traumatic epiphysis (inflammation of the epiphysis) is a type of epiphyseal injury that occurs in young athletes. One form of this little 'leaguer's elbow' is a condition that results from repetitive strains to the medial epicondylar epiphysis of the humerus (inner aspect of the elbow). A 12 year old boy can throw a baseball 129 kph, this causes a sudden pull on the epiphysis that anchors the tendons of the involved muscle, and can even result in its separation. Short of the total separation, the stress of repetitive throwing can produce an inflammatory response — epiphysitis. Another study reviewed 1,338 consecutive athletic injuries seen by 4 orthopedists in a major sports medicine practice. Of all those injuries, 28% occurred in young age of 15 years or younger (**Larson and McMahan, 1966**). Only 6% of the total injuries in those 15 year olds and youngers involved the epiphysis. The study also concluded that epiphyseal injuries do not always result in crippling or permanent trauma and that early recognition is important. Tennis (tennis elbow), Swimming (swimmer's shoulder) are two other sports which share an increased risk of epiphyseal injury.

Muscle

There is a steady growth of muscle tissue during the first seven years of life, followed by a slowing trend in the year immediately preceding puberty. During the pubertal growth spurt, muscle grows at a rapid rate, particularly in boys. The increase in muscle tissue typically occurs slightly after the greatest increase in height. Significant training induced muscle hypertrophy does not occur until adolescence in boys. This is because of low level of male hormones (principally testosterone) found in sexually immature children.

Male hormone, called androgens, are important regulators of protein synthesis. Adult males have about ten times the amount of androgens as pubertal children and adult women. Sex differences in strength may also be partially attributed to the higher number of muscle cell nuclei in males. Males probably have a greater capacity for muscle hypertrophy (and, thus, strength) because of the critical role that the muscle cell nuclei play in protein synthesis. The increased muscle mass with growth and development is accomplished primarily by hypertrophy of individual muscle fiber through increases in their myofilament and myofibril. Muscle length increases through the addition of sarcomere and by increases in the length of existing sarcomere. In males, total muscle mass increases from 25% of body weight at birth to 40% or more in the adult. Much of the gain occurs when the muscle development rate peaks at puberty due to 10-fold increase in testosterone production. The rate of acceleration is much more slow in girls and the difference is largely attributed to hormonal difference at puberty. Muscle mass peaks when females reach 16-20 years of age and males reach 18-25 years — unless it is increased further by exercise, diet or both.

PHYSICAL PERFORMANCE OF YOUNG ATHLETES

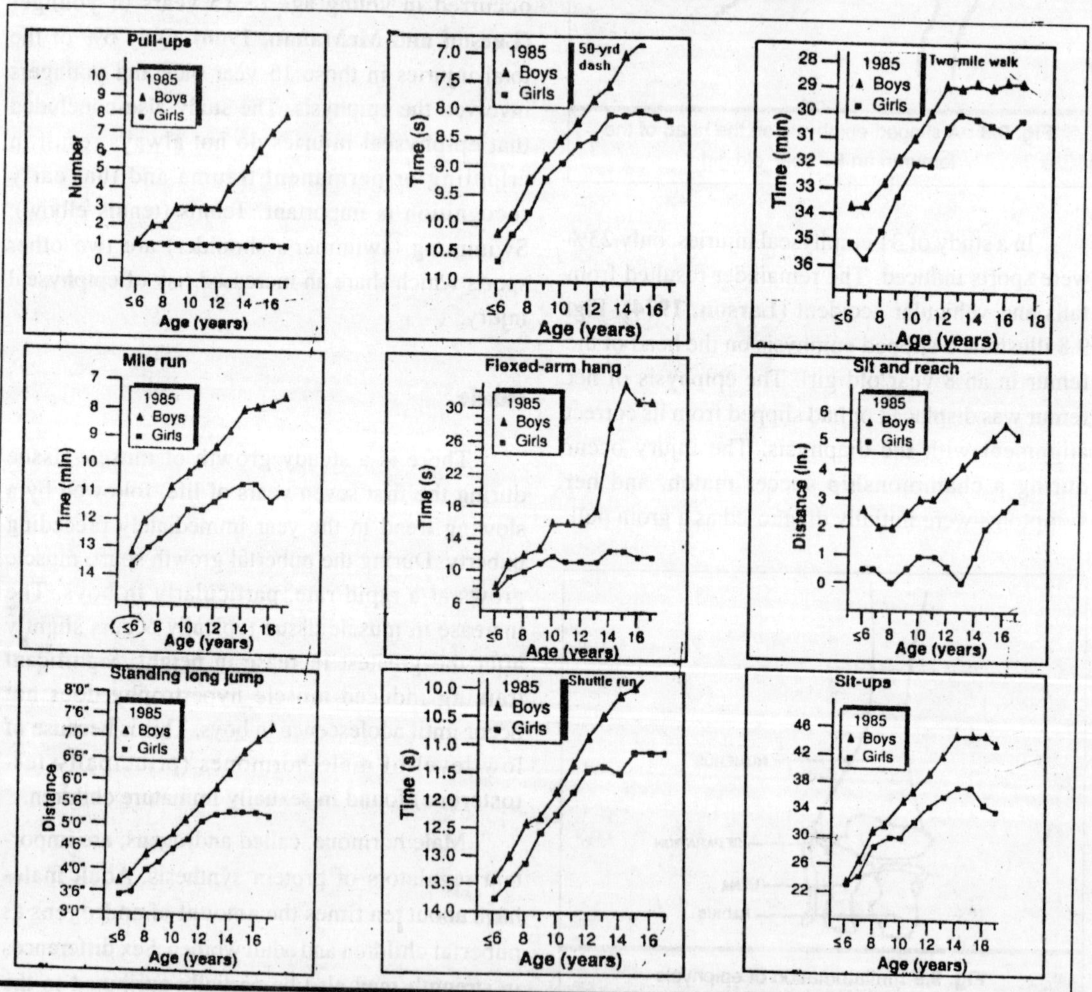

Fig. 9.10 : Graphical representation of motor abilities from age 7 to 18 years

Balance, agility and coordination improve as children's nervous system develop. Myelination of nerve fibers must be completed before fast reactions and skilled movements are fully developed because myelination speeds the transmission of electrical impulses.

Motor ability

Motor ability generally increases for the first 18 years of life, although in girls it tends to plateau around puberty. This plateau is probably due to increased estrogen level, which promotes greater fat deposition, as well as girls' typical assumption of more sedentary life style.

Strength

Strength improves as muscle mass increases with age. In Medford study the boys were followed longitudinally from age 7 to age 18 (**Clarke, 1971**). The rate of strength gain increases noticably around the age of 12, the typical age for onset of puberty. Cross-sectional study for girls indicate that girls experience a more gradual increase in strength and do not exhibit a marked change in their rate of strength gain with puberty. Gain in strength also depend on neural maturation (**Brooks and Fahey, 1984**) because neuromuscular control is limited until myelination has been completed, usually around sexual maturity. Muscular strength increases with age and peak highest gain is achieved one year after the maximum weight gain i.e., at the age of 14-15 years. Grip strength of boys begins to increase rapidly in 13th year and coincides with the rapid weight gain. Physiologically it is observed that strength spurt coincides with increased selection of male sex hormones. In case of physically active children grip strength in 8 years of age is 10 kg and it increases to 44 kg by 18 years.

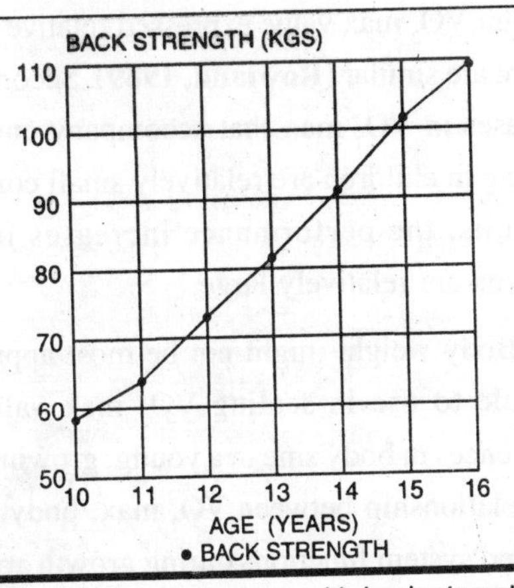

Fig. 9.11 : Age changes with back strength

The rate of growth in strength is slow. Back strength in the physically active children is 33 kg at the age of 8 years and increases to 126 kg at the age of 18 years. There is not much difference of muscle strength till the age of 12 years in male and female adolescent. The strength in boys increases at faster rate. The maximum strength is reached in between at the age of 20-30 years.

Pulmonary Function

Lung function changes are marked by with age. All lung volumes increase until physical maturity. For example, cross-sectional study show that V_E max average about 40 L min^{-1} for 4-6 year-old boys and increase to 110 L min^{-1} to 140 L min^{-1} at full maturity. Girls follow the same general pattern, but their absolute values remain considerably lower, primarily due to their smaller size. There is about 2.59 times increase in ventilation from 8-18 years of age. The increase is in proportion to the body size. Peak highest velocity is attained at the age of 13-14 years. This age corresponds with the peak highest velocity of the height and weight.

Cardiovascular Function

There is a progressive decline in resting and maximum heart rate during childhood and adolescence. Heart rate tend to be same in girls and boys during childhood, but are about three to four beats higher in females during and after adolescence. At puberty, in boys there is a tendency for submaximal and recovery heart rate even in absence of vigorous training. The decreased heart rate is accompanied and perhaps caused by a greater resting and exercise stroke volume resulting from an increased heart size and blood volume.

Resting and exercise systolic blood pressure rise progressively, particularly during puberty. Blood pressure assumes adult values shortly after adolescent growth spurt. The pubertal acceleration in blood pressure occurs in females before males, but the boys quickly catch-up and surpass the girls. Blood pressure is directly related to body size, it is lower in children than adult but increases to adult levels in the late ten years, because children have less peripheral resistance.

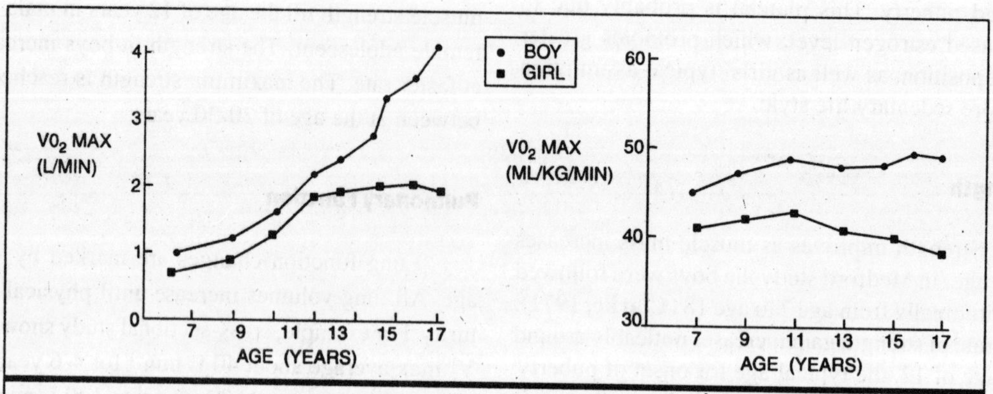

Fig. 9.12 : Age-related changes in aerobic capacity in boys and girls

During both submaximal and maximal exercise, the child's smaller heart and blood volume results in a lower stroke volume than in adult. In partial compensation child's heart rate is higher than an adult's. Maximum heart rate (MHR) of Indian children (8-18 years) varies from 202-184 bpm. Peak decline in MHR occurs at the age of 15 years. Smaller heart and blood volume results in a lower stroke volume than in adult. In partial compensation child's heart rate is higher than an adult's.

Even with increased heart rate, a child's cardiac output remains less than an adult's. In submaximal exercise, an increase in the a-VO_2 differences adequate O_2 delivery to the active muscles. But at maximal work rates oxygen deliver limit performance in activities, other than those in which the child merely needs to move his or her body mass. As pulmonary and cardio-vascular function improve with continued development, so does aerobic capacity. VO_2 max expressed in L/min peaks between ages 17 to 21 years in male and 12 to 15 years in female. (**Robinson, 1938**). However, expressing VO_2 relative to body weight might not provide an accurate estimate of aerobic capacity. Such VO_2 max values do not reflect the significant gains in endurance performance capacity that are noted with both maturation and training.

Although VO_2 max values expressed relative to body weight remain relatively stable or decline with age, endurance performance steadily improves. The average 14 year old boy can run a mile (i.6 Km) almost twice as fast as average 5 year old boy, yet their VO_2 max value expressed relative to body weight are similar (**Rowland, 1989**). Secondly, the increases in VO_2 max that accompany endurance training in children are relatively small compared to adults, the performance increases in these children are relatively large.

Body weight might not be most appropriate variable to use in scaling VO_2 max values for differences in body sine in a young, growing child. The relationship between VO_2 max, body dimension and system functions during growth are extra-ordinarily complex (**Rowland, 1991**).

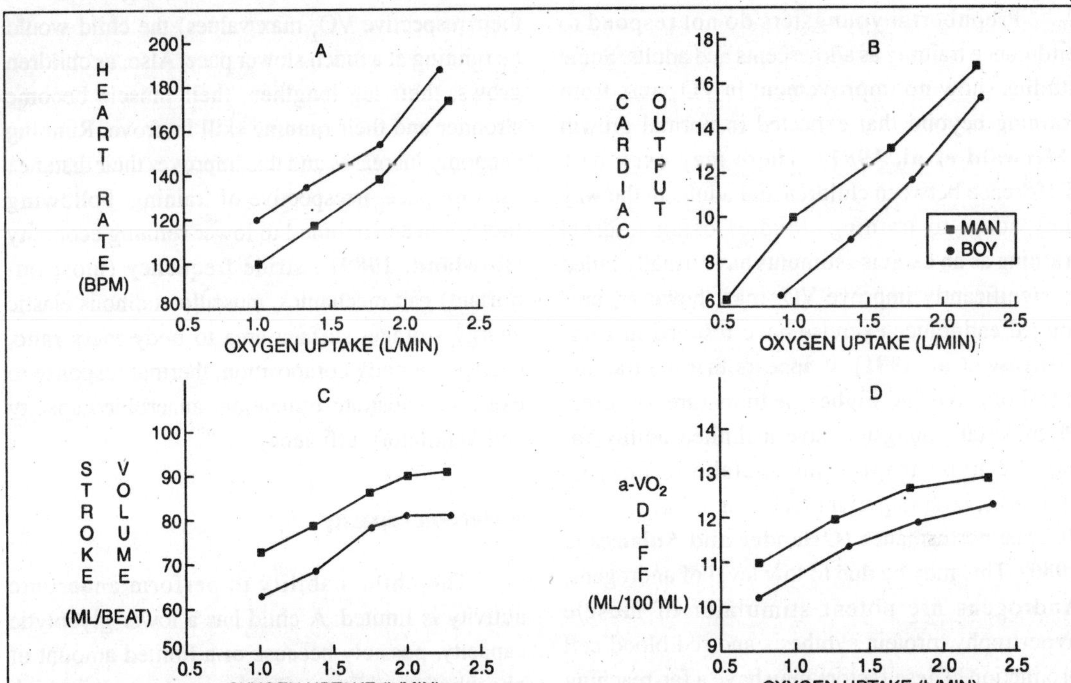

Fig. 9.13 : Relationship of heart rate, Cardiac output, stroke volume and a-VO_2 difference with oxygen uptake between men and boys

The total increase in VO_2 max is approximately 30% throughout the total growth period. The percentage increases in O_2 max corresponds with the increase in proportion to average weight. If the data are expressed per unit of body weight, results remain relatively constant. In girls the VO_2 max is almost similar till the age of 10 years, thereafter girls have relatively low VO_2 max as compared to boys. Along with increase in aerobic power during the growing years other variables are known to increase. When aerobic power increases by about 55%, pulmonary ventilation, pulmonary diffusion capacity and cardiac output increase proportionately — 49%, 45% and 50%, respectively. During this period RBC and hemoglobin concentration increase about 20% in boys. Girls experience less increase after the age of 12 years a sex difference can be observed with boys; having larger contour.

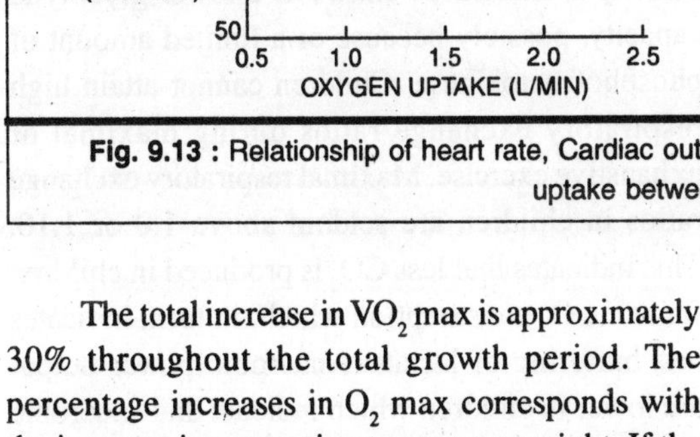

Fig. 9.14 : Relationship of relative VO_2 with age

Table 2 : VO_2 max of age group talented Indian sports children

Age group yrs	VO_2 max l/min	VO_2 max ml/kg/min
10	1.65 ± 0.29	51.83 ± 6.93
11	1.82 ± 0.33	52.22 ± 6.19
12	2.13 ± 0.38	55.16 ± 6.19
13	2.38 ± 0.44	56.60 ± 5.97
14	2.69 ± 0.49	59.12 ± 5.81
15	2.90 ± 0.45	58.42 ± 5.92
16	3.10 ± 0.07	58.86 ± 7.38

Prepubertal youngsters do not respond to endurance training as adolescents and adults. Some studies show no improvement in VO_2 max from training beyond that expected in normal growth (**Mirwald et al, 1981**). There may even be a difference between children and adults in the way they adapt to training. Studies using interval training as an exercise stimulus have usually failed to significantly improve VO_2 max, however, prolonged endurance exercise have resulted in gains (**Murase et al, 1981**). It appears that the training threshold may be higher in immature children. Prepubertal youngster have a limited ability for cardiac hypertrophy and metabolic enzyme synthesis, both important factors in improving endurance performance (**Orlander and Aniansson, 1980**). This may be due to low level of androgens. Androgens are potent stimulator of muscle hypertrophy, protein synthesis and red blood cell production. These factors may have a far-reaching effect on O_2 transport and ATP production. Some researchers (**Mirwald et al, 1981**) have called the adolescent growth period a critical time for development of maximal aerobic power. Adolescence provides the first opportunity for large increases in physical capacity. Those who take advantage of this may develop a superior capacity for exercise that may persist into adulthood.

Physical performance in children and adolescents must always be assessed in light of the growth process. Growth involves a series of developmental stages that are remarkably similar in all people. Individual differences in diet, exercise and health may affect those stages to a certain extent, but the basic pattern remains the same. Each of these stages has a profound influence on individual capability for physical performance.

How do growth related changes affect performance? Child cannot maintain as fast running pace as the adult in spite of having similar relative VO_2 max. This is due to the reason of differences in economy of effort. Even if the child's lactate threshold occurred at the same relative oxygen consumption as the adult (at the same percentage of their respective VO_2 max values) the child would be running at a much slower pace. Also, as children grows, their leg lengthen, their muscle become stronger and their running skill improve. Running economy increases and this improves their distance running pace, irrespective of training. Following factors are attributed to lower running economy (**Rowland, 1989**) : stride frequency (most important) gait mechanics, musculotendinous elastic energy storage, surface area to body mass ratio, changes in body composition, thermal response to exercise, substrate utilization, anaerobic capacity and ventilatory efficiency.

Anaerobic capacity

The child's ability to perform anaerobic activity is limited. A child has a lower glycolytic capacity, possibly because of a limited amount of phosphofructokinase. Children cannot attain high respiratory exchange ratios during maximal or exhaustive exercise. Maximal respiratory exchange ratios in children are seldom above 1.0 or 1.10. This indicates that less CO_2 is produced in children for same O_2 consumption which, in turn, indicates less buffering of lactate. Anaerobic power output are lower in children which indicate that anaerobic

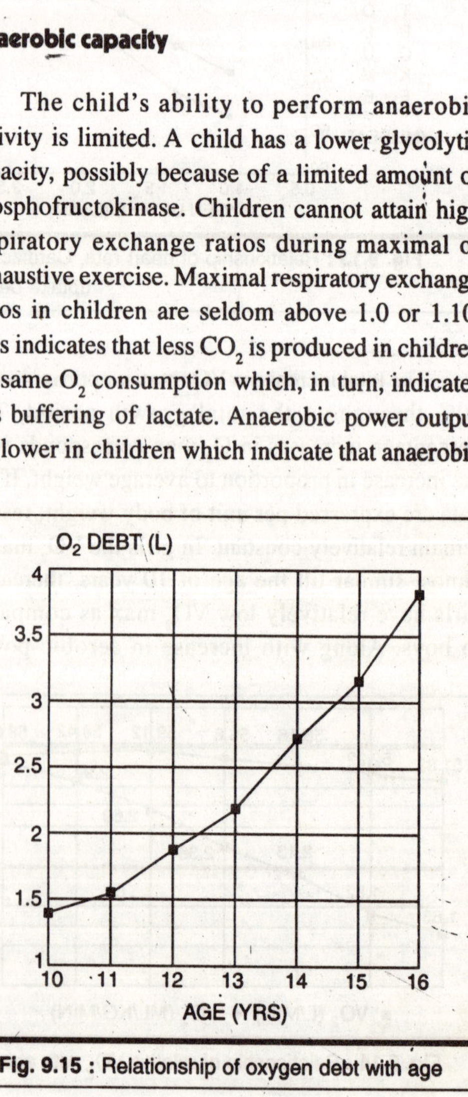

Fig. 9.15 : Relationship of oxygen debt with age

power increases with growth and development, even when the values are expressed relative to body weight (Watt kg^{-1}). It increases with growth due to increase in muscle mass, increase in enzymes and increase tolerance to blood lactate. Peak highest velocity corresponds with puberty. **Bar-or-O (1983)** has summarized the development of both the aerobic and anaerobic characteristics in boys and girls from age 9 through 16 using 18 years of age as the criteria for 100% of the adult value. Aerobic power is represented by a child's VO_2 max, whereas anaerobic power is represented by child's performance on the Margeria step running test. Maximum energy expenditure per kg represents the maximum energy generating capacities of the aerobic and anaerobic systems, scaled to body weight (kg) to account for body size differences with growth..

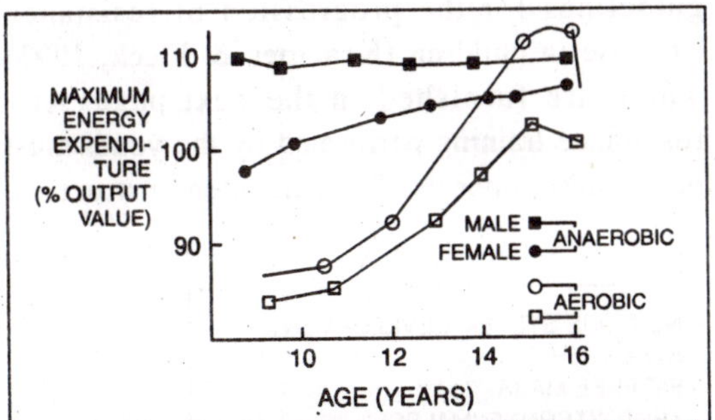

Fig. 9.16 : Relationship of maximum energy expenditure with reference to contribution in aerobic and anaerobic metabolism with age

Thermal Stress

Laboratory study indicate that children are more susceptible to injury or illness from thermal stress. A major concern is the child's apparently lower capacity when exercising in the heat to dissipate heat through evaporation. Children appear to rely much more on convection and radiation, which are exhausted through greater peripheral vasodilatation. **(Bar-Or-O, 1989)** Children are capable of less evaporative heat loss than adult because children sweat less (less sweat is produced by each active sweat gland). Young boys acclimatize to heat more slowly than adults do. Children appear to have greater conductive heat loss than adults, due to larger surface area to mass ratio. This should place them at higher risk for hypothermia in cold environment. Until more is known about children's susceptibility to thermal stress, a conservative approach should be used for children who exercise in temperature extremes.

TRAINING THE YOUNG ATHLETE

Training can improve the strength, aerobic capacity and anaerobic capacity of the young athletes. Generally the youngster will adapt well to the same type of training routine used by the mature athlete. But training programs for children and adolescents should be designed specifically for each age group, keeping in mind the developmental factors associated with that age. In these section we address the issue of most concern for young athletes who are involved in — Resistance training — Aerobic training — Anaerobic training.

Resistance Training

For many years, the use of resistance training to increase muscular strength and endurance in prepubescent and adolescent boys and girls was highly controversial. Boys and girls were discouraged from using free weight in fear that they might injure themselves and primarily stop the growth process. Animal studies suggest that resistance training can lead to stronger, broader, more compact bones **(Kraemer & Fleck, 1993)**. The risk of injury from resistance training in young athletes is relatively low — for example, by strengthening the muscle that cross joint.

Several studies conducted in mid 1980s demonstrated that prepubescent boys and girls can participate safely in resistance training and they can gain substantial strength. In one study, prepubescent boys and girls took part in a 9-week progressive resistance training program (**Sewall & Micheli, 1986**). They exercised 25-30 mins/day 3 days each week. The mean strength increase was 42.9% compared to a 9.5% increase in non-training control group. In another study, 16 prepubescent males between age 6 and 11 participated in a 14-week strength program using isokinetic technique i.e., hydraulic resistance, while another 10 boys served as non-training controls. Isokinetic strength increased between 18% and 37% in the training group, but little or no change was observed in the control group (**Weltman et al, 1986**).

Researchers hypothesized that prepubescent growth would experience the greater strength gains because testosterone levels increase dramatically during this period, but this was not the only case. Strength gain achieved from resistance training in prepubescent results primarily from (**Ramsay et al, 1990**) improved motor skill coordination, increased motor unit activation and other neurological adaptation.

Unlike in adults, prepubescents who resistance trained experience little change in muscle size. In this model strength was influenced by the amount of fat-free mass, testosterone concentration, the extent or nervous system development and the determination of FT-ST muscle fibers. The early gains in strength are up through puberty and largely the result of changes in neuromuscular pattern.

Specific guidelines were established at a workshop in 1985 by a group representing 8 different professional organizations : The Am. Orthopaedic Society for Sports Med., The Am. Academy of Paediatrics, The Am. Col. of Sports Med., National Athletic Trainers Association, The National Strength and Conditioning Association, The President's Council on Physical Fitness and Sports, The USOC and The Society of Pediatric Orthopaedics.

Kramer and Fieck have also established basic guidelines for the progression of resistance exercise in children (**Kraemer & Fleck, 1993**) which are furnished in the next page. Any resistance training performed by the youth must be carefully supervised by competent instructors.

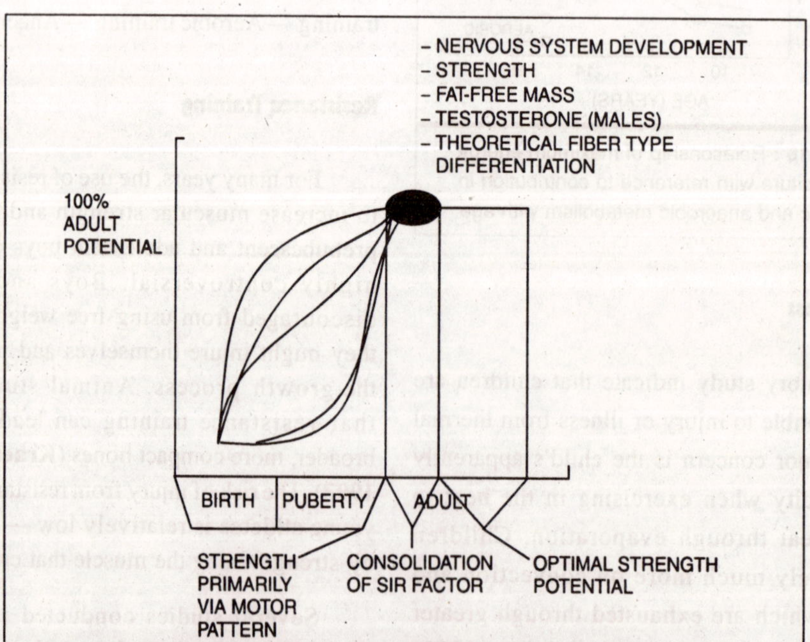

Fig. 9.17 : Model shows how strength is influenced by other factors

Strength training recommendation for the prepubescent children

Equipment

Strength training equipment should be of appropriate design to accommodate the size and degree of maturity of the prepubescent. It should be cost-effective. It should be safe and free of defect & inspected frequently. It should be located in an uncrowded area, free of obstruction, with adequate lighting and ventilation.

Program consideration

A preparticipation physical examination is mandatory. The child must have the emotional maturity to accept coaching and instruction. There must be adequate supervision by coaches who are knowledgeable and the strength training and special problem of prepubescent. Strength training should be a part of an overall comprehensive program designed to improve motor skill and level of fitness. Strength training should be preceded by a warm-up period and followed by a cool down. Emphasis should be on dynamic-concentric contraction. All exercise should be carried through a full range of motion; Competition is prohibited; No maximum lift should ever be attempted.

Prescribed program

Training is recommended 2 or 3 times a week for 20 to 30 mins period. No resistance should be applied until proper form is demonstrated — 6-15 rep. equal one set; one to three sets per exercise should be done. Weight or resistance is increased in 1-3 lb increments after the prepubescent does 15 rep. in good form.

Table 9.3 : Basic guidelines for resistance exercise program in children

Age	Consideration
7 or younger	Introduce child to basic exercises with little or no weight; develop the concept of a training session; teach exercise technique; progress from body weight calisthenics, partner exercises; and lightly resisted exercises, keep volume low.
8-10 years	Gradually increase the number of exercises; practice exercise technique in all lifts, start gradual progressive loading of exercise, keep exercise simple gradually increase training volume; carefully monitor toleration of exercise.
11-13 years	Teach all basic exercise techniques, continue progressive loading of each exercise, emphasize exercise technique, introduce more advanced exercises with little or no resistance.
14-15 years	Progress to more advanced youth prog. in resistance exercise, add sports-specific components, emphasize exercise technique, increase volume.
16 or older	Move child to entry level adult prog. after all background knowledge has been mastered and the basic level of training experience has been gained.

If a child of any age begins the prog. with no previous experience, start the child at previous levels and move him or her to more advanced levels as exercise toleration, skill, amount of training time and understanding permit (**Represented from kraemer & Fleck, 1992**).

Aerobic and anaerobic training

Aerobic training in preadolescents does not alter VO_2 max (**Rowland, 1985**) as much as would be expected for the training stimulus, possibly because VO_2 max is dependent on heart size. But endurance performance does increase with aerobic training. Anaerobic training appears to improve children's anaerobic capacity. Following training, children have (**Eriksson, 1972**) increased resting level of phosphocreatine, ATP and glycogen, increased phosphofructokinase activity and increased maximum blood lactate level. Ventilatory threshold has also been reported to increase with endurance training in 10-14 year old boys (**Mohon & Vaccaro, 1989**).

Regular training typically results in decreased total body fat, increased fat free mass and increased total body mass. As for maturation, the age at which peak height velocity occurs is generally not affected by regular training nor is the rate of skeletal maturation. Although some data suggest that menarche (initial onset of menstruation) is delayed in highly trained gilrs, this may due to multiple factors. Malina (1989) concludes his review with the following statements. Responses of the developing individual to the physical activity of regular training are probably not sufficient to alter genotypical programmed growth and maturation process. Thus training has no apparent effect on stature and on maturation as ordinarily assessed in growth studies.

REFERENCE

Bar-Or-O. (1989) : ***Temperature Regulation During Exercise in Children and Adolescents***. In V. V. Gosolfi and D. R. 1Lamb (Eds) perspective in exercise science and sports medicine : Youth exercise and sports (pp 335-362) Carmel In Benchmark Press.

Bar-Or-O. (1983) : ***Pediatric Sports Medicine for the Practitioner***. From physiological principles to clinical application, New York, Springer-Verlag.

Bjorntorp, P. (1986) : ***Fat Cells and Obesity***. In K. D. Brownell and J. P. Forey (Eds) Hand book of eating disorders. Physiology, psychology and treatment of obesity, anorexia and bulimia. New York. Basic books.

Brooks, G. A. and Fahey, T. D. (1984) : ***Exercise Physiology : Human Bioenergetics and its Applications***. New York, Wiley.

Clarke, H. H. (1971) :***Physical and Motor Tests in the Medford Boys Growth Study***. Englewood cliffs, N. J. : Prentice, Hall.

Eriksson, B. O. (1972) : Physical training, oxygen supply and muscle metabolism in 11-13 years old boys. ***Acta, Physiologica Scandinavia*** suppl. 384.

Kramer, W. J. and Fleck, S. J. (1993) :***Strength Training for Young Athletes***. Champaign IL, Human Kinetics.

Larid, A. K. (1967) : Evolution of the human growth curve. ***Growth*** 31 :.345-355.

G. A. Brooks and T. D. Fahey (1984) : ***Exercise Physiology, Human Bioenergetics and its Application***. New York. Macmillan.

Larson, R. L. & Mcmahan, R. O. (1966) : The epiphysis and the childhood athlete. ***Journal of American Medical Association*** 196 : 607-612.

Larson, R. L. (1974) : Physical activity and the growth and development of bone and joint structures. In G. L. Rarick (ed) Physical activity : ***Human Growth and Development*** (pp 32-59). Academic press.

Mahon, A. D. and Vaccaro, P. (1989) : Ventilatory threshold and VO_2 max changes in children following endurance training, ***Medicine and Science in Sports and Exercise*** 21 : 425-431.

Malina, R. M. (1989) : Growth and maturation : Normal variation and effect of training. In C. V. Gosofi and D. L. Lamb (Eds) ***Perspective in Exercise Science and Sports Medicine, Youth Exercise and Sports*** (pp 223-265) Carmel In, Benchmark Press.

Mirwald, R., Bailey, D. A., Cameron, N. and Rasmussen, R. L. (1981) : Longitudinal comparison of aerobic power in active and inactive boys aged 7 tc 17 years. ***Annals of Human Biology*** 8 :405-414.

Murase, Y., Kobayashi, K., Kamei, S. and Matsui, H. (1981) : Longitudinal study of aerobic power in superior junior athletes. ***Medicine and Science in Sports and Exercise*** 13 : 180-184.

Orlander, J. and Anniansson, A. (1980) : Effect of physical training on skeletal muscle metabolism and ultrastructure. ***Acta Physiologica Scandinavia*** 109 : 149-154.

Ramsay, J. A., Bilmkie, C. J. R., Smith, K., Garner, S., Macdougall, J. D. and Sale, D. G. (1990) : Strength training effects in prepubescent boys. ***Medicine and Science in Sports and Exercise*** 22 : 605-614.

Robinson, S. (1938) : Experimental studies of physical fitness in relation to age. ***Arbeitsphysiologie*** 10 : 251-253.

Rowland, T. W. (1991) : 'Normalizing' maximal oxygen uptake or the search for the holy grail (per kg), ***Pediatric Exercise Science*** 3 : 95-102.

Rowland, T. W. (1978) : Oxygen uptake & endurance fitness in children. A developmental perspective. ***Pediatric Exercise Science*** 1 : 313-328.

Rowland, T. W. (1985) : Aerobic response to endurance training in prepubescent children — a critical analysis, ***Medicine and Science in Sports and Exercise*** 17 : 493-497.

Sewall, L. and Michei, L. J. (1986) : Strength training for children the ***Journal of Pediatric Orthopaedia strabismus*** 6 : 143-146.

Tanner, J. M. (1984) : Growth at adolescence Oxford. Blackwell publication ltd. 1962 in : G. A. Brooks and T. D. Fahey. ***Exercise Physiology, Human Bioenergetics and its Application***, New York, Macmillan 667.

10

WOMEN IN SPORTS

BODY SIZE & COMPOSITION

Skeletal system

Female usually smaller, shorter	—	lower center of gravity, lighter body frame
Before adolescence	—	not much difference
During adolescence	—	gain in height — leg length increased.
Female wider pelvis	—	different running mechanics
Thighs slant inward toward knees,		Some believe more prone to injury.
Lower leg bones, less bowed	—	due to more knee instability than male.
Female has shorter limbs (rel tive to body length)	—	Shorter lever arms for movement, important for use of implements.
Female shoulders narrower and slope more	—	Different mechanics of upper limb musculature.
Upper arms do not hang vertically	—	Important in throwing pattern. Marked 'caring angle' of elbows

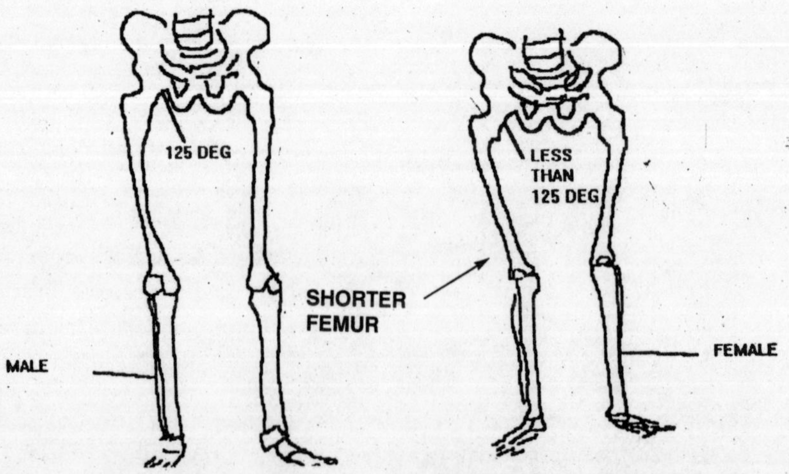

Fig. 10.1 : Sex difference in skeletal system (lower extremity)

Body Composition

Female contours more rounded, less angular.	— Female greater % body fat.
Female physique less mesomorphic and more endomorphic.	— Female less LBM (less bone, less muscle)
Female has greater concentration of subcutaneous adipose tissue, particularly in buttock.	— Female, less metabolically active tissue. Female more buoyant.
Smaller proportion of muscle in relation to body fat.	— Female lower ratio of strength

Until puberty females and males do not differ significantly in most measurements : viz. height; weight; girth; bone width; skinfolds thickness. A study of 609 normal boys and girls ages 7.5 to 20.5 found no gender differences in fat-free mass (FFM) prior to adolescence when FFM was expressed per unit of height (**Forbes, 1972**). At age 12-13, the fat-free mass to height ratio in female begins a plateau, but in males it continues to increase to age 20. The peak FFM attained by female is 72% of the FFM attained by males. Females typically have lower body density values at all ages, including pre-adolescence, which would normally indicate a higher relative body fat. But from age 7 to age 25, the density of fat-free mass in females is consistently lower than in male (**Lohman, 1986**).

The calculations used to determine relative body fat typically assume that these densities are

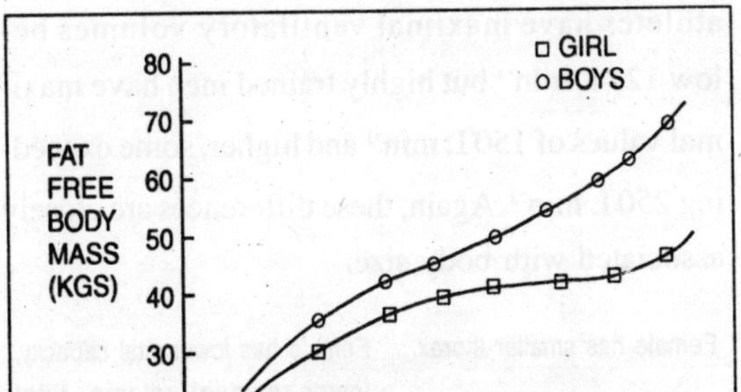

Fig.10.2 : Gender difference in fat-free body mass

the same in both sexes. As result, most existing data on females in this age range overestimate their true relative body fat. At puberty, the body composition of the sexes begin to differ markedly primarily because of endocrine changes. During puberty, the anterior pituitary begins to secrete FSH and LH. In female when sufficient quantities of FSH and LH are secreted, the ovaries develop and estrogen secretion begins. Estrogen has sufficient influence on body growth by broadening the pelvis, stimulating breast development, and increasing fat deposition, particularly in thighs and hips. The increased fat deposition (thigh and hips) is the result of increased lipoprotein lipase activity and low lipolytic activity. Lipoprotein lipase is considered the gatekeeper for storing fat in adipose tissue. Lipoprotein lipase is produced in the fat cells (adipocytes) but is bound to the wall of the capillaries where it exerts its influence on the chylomicron, which are the major transporters of triglycerides in blood. When lipoprotein lipase activity in any area of the body is high, chylomicron are trapped and their triglycerides are hydrolyzed and transported into the adipocytes in that area for storage. Estrogen also increases the growth rate of bone, allowing the final length to be reached within 2 to 4 years following the onset of puberty. As a result females grow very rapidly for the first few years following puberty, then cease to grow. In male, FSH and LH trigger development of testes and in turn testosterone secretion. Testosterone causes increased bone formation, which leads to longer bones as well as increased protein synthesis, which leads to increased muscle mass. As a result, adolescent males are larger and more muscular than females, and these characteristics continue into adulthood. Males have a much longer growth phase allowing them to attain a greater height.

Because of these differences, comparatively females are on average 13 cm (5 inch) shorter, 14 to 18 kg (30-40 Ib) lighter in total weight, 18 to 22 kg (40-50) lighter in FFM, 3 to 6 kg (T-13lb) heavier in fat mass, 6% to 10% higher in relative body fat.

Table 1 : Relative body fat values for women and men of various age

Age group	Relative body fat Women	Men
15 - 19	20 - 24	13 - 16
20 - 29	22 - 25	15 - 20
30 - 39	24 - 30	18 - 26
40 - 49	27 - 33	23 - 29
50 - 59	30 - 36	26 - 33
60 - 69	30 - 36	29 - 33

PHYSIOLOGICAL DIFFERENCES

Female lower Blood volume	— Total oxygen carrying capacity
Female fewer RBC (15%) Female has smaller heart	— Higher HR, smaller SV and lower oxygen pulse for a given Q and VO_2
Female has lower Q max	— Females have lower maximum aerobic capacity (20 - 25%)

Cardiovascular response

For the same rate of work, trained women generally have cardiac output similar to those of comparably trained men, but this is achieved by higher heart rates and lower stroke volume — which primarily results from at least 3 factors : Women have smaller hearts and, therefore, smaller left ventricles because of their smaller body size and possibly due to lower testosterone concentration. Women have a smaller blood volume which is also related to their size. Average woman is typically less active and, therefore, less well coordinated. Women also have a lower capacity to increase a VO_2 difference, probably because of their lower Hb content, which results in a lower arterial O_2 content and a reduced muscle oxidative potential. Girls achieve VO_2 max (ml/kg/min) between 8-9 yrs of age, after that it declines slowly up to age of 15 and reaches a plateau and remain constant through young adulthood. Boys reach their peak at about 15-16 yrs. and maintain the peak throughout adulthood. At the age 7 to 9 years the difference is small, at 12 to 13 yrs of age the observed difference noted as 13%-16% and at adulthood it is approximately 18%.

Table 2 : Gender difference on Aerobic capacity in various sports and events

Aerobic capacity

Events	VO_2 max (ml/kg/min) (male)	(female)
Long distance runners	70 - 75	58 - 72
Cyclists	55 - 70	45 - 60
Basketball players	45 - 55	35 - 45

Table 3 : Gender difference on heart size, stroke volume, cardiac output and hemoglobin

Parameters	Mean values in male	Mean values in female
Heart size	800 ml	580 ml
Stroke volume		
(Rest)	100 - 120 ml	70 - 90 ml
(Exercise)	150 - 170 ml	100 - 120 ml
Cardiac output	25 - 30 l/min	18 - 20 l/min
Hemoglobin	16 gm%	12 gm%

Respiratory responses

Tidal volume and ventilatory volume are generally smaller in women at the same relative and absolute power outputs, up to and including maximal levels. Most highly trained female athletes have maximal ventilatory volumes below 125 L min^{-1} but highly trained men have maximal values of 150 L min^{-1} and higher, some exceeding 250 L min^{-1}. Again, these differences are closely associated with body size.

Female has smaller thorax	Female has lower vital capacity, lower residual volume, tidal volume, low maximal breathing capacity.
Female has less lung tissue	Female has lower max ventilation.

Table 4 : Spirometric evaluation of lung function

	Men	Women
Minute Ventilation	160 l/min	120 l/min
Vital capacity	4 - 6 l	3 - 4 l
Residual Volume	1,200 ml	1,000 ml
Total Lung Capacity	6,000 ml	4,200 ml

Muscular response

No differences in distribution of ST/FT fibers, females are 40 - 60% weaker in upper body strength & 25% weaker in lower body strength. Females have smaller muscle mass (fewer fibers and smaller fibers), when strength is expressed relative to LBM. No sexual differences in some instances is observed. Females have less lactate tolerance. Performance of female in anaerobic type of activities is lower.

Strength

Up to the age of 10-12 yrs — boys are slightly stronger than girls. During adolescent years biological and structural difference becomes more pronounced — strength gap between the sexes widens. Generally the differences between males and females continue to increase from 12-18 yrs. The males continue to improve but females do not change. Physical changes are brought about by the greater hormonal secretions in the male of testosterone, which enhances muscle and bone size.

The innate qualities of muscle and the mechanism of motor control are similar for women and men. In lower body strength, when expressed relative to body weight or to fat-free mass, women and men do not differ — But women show less upper body strength — 43% to 63% and lower body by only 25-30%. Although differences in upper body strength are reduced somewhat when expressed relative to total body weight and FFM, substantial differences remain. There are at least 2 possible reasons for this. Women have a higher percentage of FFM below the waist, which implies that they have more muscle there as well. In addition and probably related to this FFM distribution, women use the muscle mass of their lower bodies much more than upper body muscle mass, particularly when compared to use pattern in man. This indicates the importance of neuromuscular recruitment and synchronization of strength. From the biopsy data, we have learnt that men and women in the same sports or events have similar fiber type distributions, although men in one study reached greater extremes (> 90% ST or > 90% FT). However, different results were found in two studies of elite female and male distance runners **(Costill et al, 1987; Fink et al, 1988)**. With these elite runners the extremes for percentages of ST fibers were similar (90% to 96% for women and 92% to 98% for men) even though the mean values were different — women had a mean value of 69% ST fibers compared to a mean value of 79% for the men. However, the women had much smaller fiber areas for both ST and FT fibers (mean value of < 4.500 μm^2 in women and > 8100 μm^2 in men.)

Metabolic responses

Beyond puberty the average woman's VO_2 max is only 70% to 75% than the average man's. However, much of this difference might be due to women's less active life-styles. Research with highly trained athletes reveals that much of the difference is due to women's greater fat mass and lower Hb level. Little or no difference in anaerobic threshold is found between the sexes.

PHYSIOLOGICAL ADAPTATION TO EXERCISE TRAINING

Body composition with training — both men and women experience : Losses in total body mass; Losses in fat mass; Losses of relative fat and gains in fat-free mass. The magnitude of the change in body composition appears to be related more to the total energy expenditure associated with training than to do with the participant's sex. As for FFM — Significantly more is gained in response to strength training than with endurance training and magnitude of these responses is much less in women — due primarily to hormonal differences.

Women are more susceptible to injury than men while participating in physical activity and sports has led to concerns about sex-specific differences in joint integrity and the strength of ligament, tendon and bones. The injury could likely be more related to the level of conditioning than to do with the participant's gender.

Neuromuscular adaptation

Women can experience major increases in strength (20% to 40%) as a result of resistance training and the magnitude of these changes is similar to that seen in men. One study compared the training responses of 47 women and 26 men who volunteered to participate in identical progressive resistance weight training programs. The program was conducted twice each week, 40 mins per day for a total of 10 weeks. The strength gains were as follows : Bench press strength : 29% in women, 17% in men, Leg press strength : 30% in women, 26% in men. Muscle girth increase only slightly in the women but the men exhibited classic muscle hypertrophy (**Wilmore, 1974**). The strength gain in female is due to neural factor.

Cardiovascular and respiratory adaptation

Cardiovascular and respiratory changes that accompany cardio-respiratory endurance training do not appear to be sex-specific. The increase in VO_2 max that accompany cardio-respiratory endurance training primarily result from the large increases in maximal Q i.e., small increase in a VO_2 difference. However, Saltin and Rowell state that the major limitation to VO_2 max is VO_2 transport to working muscles (**Saltin and Rowell, 1980**). These researchers believe that the increases is maximal aerobic power that accompany training are primarily due to increased maximal blood flow and muscle capillary density. These changes are irrespective of sex. In fact, one study has demonstrated that endurance trained women have considerably higher capillary to fiber ratio (1.69 capillaries per fiber) than untrained women (1.11 capillaries per fiber) (**Ingjer & Brodal, 1978**). Elite female distance runners in one study had a mean capillary to fiber ratio of 2.5 capillaries per fiber (**Costill et al, 1987**). These values are similar to what has been reported in men of similar trainng status. Although women also experience considerable increases in max VE, reflecting increase in both tidal volume (TV) and breathing frequency (BF) these changes are thought to be unrelated to the increase in VO_2 max.

Metabolic adaptation

Women can experience major increase in endurance capacity (VO_2) max increases of 10% to 40% with aerobic training. These percentages are similar to improvement seen in men. The magnitude of change noted depends on the initial level of fitness; the intensity and duration of training session; the frequency of training and the length of the study. After cardio-respiratory endurance training women's oxygen uptake at the same absolute submaximal work rate does not appear to change, although several studies have reported decrease. Blood lactate levels are reduced at submax effort. Peak lactate levels are generally increased. Lactate threshold increases with training. Free fatty acid utilization increases which is important for glycogen sparing. From the above discussion we can see that women respond to physical training in the same manner as men do. Although the magnitude of their adaptations to training might differ somewhat from those of their male counterparts, the overall trends appear identical.

Athletic ability

Women are outperformed by men in almost all sports, events or activities. In 400 mt free style swim, however, the winning time for women in the 1924 Olympic games was 16% slower than that for men, but these differences decreased to 11.6% in the 1948 Olympics and only 6.9% in the 1984 Olympics. The fastest women in 800 mt free style swimmer in 1979 swam faster than the world record holding man for the same distance in 1972. In competitive sports until 1970s there was an initial reluctance to train women as hard as men. Once girls and women started training as hard as boys and men, their performances improved dramatically. This is illustrated in Fig. 10.3 which shows the records from 1975 to 1991 for women and men in six running events in tract and field. The distance, therefore, in this particular event, gap between the sexes is narrowing — and this is also true in other events and for other sports. On the basis of world record 1991, the female compared to her male counterpart ran 6.4% slower in the 100 mt dash and 11% slower in the 1,500 m run jumped 14.3% lower in the high jump and swam 8.4% slower in the 400 m free style swimming. Do these performance differences result from biological differences? Or do they reflect social and cultural restrictions placed on female during preadolescent and adolescent development? Let us begin by considering basic physiological differences and their impact on performance. Large numbers of girls and women did not participate in 400 m through the Marathon, women's present world records are consistently 10% to 13% slower than men's. Furthermore the improvement in women's records, which was initially quite dramatic, is beginning to level off and parallel the curves for men's record.

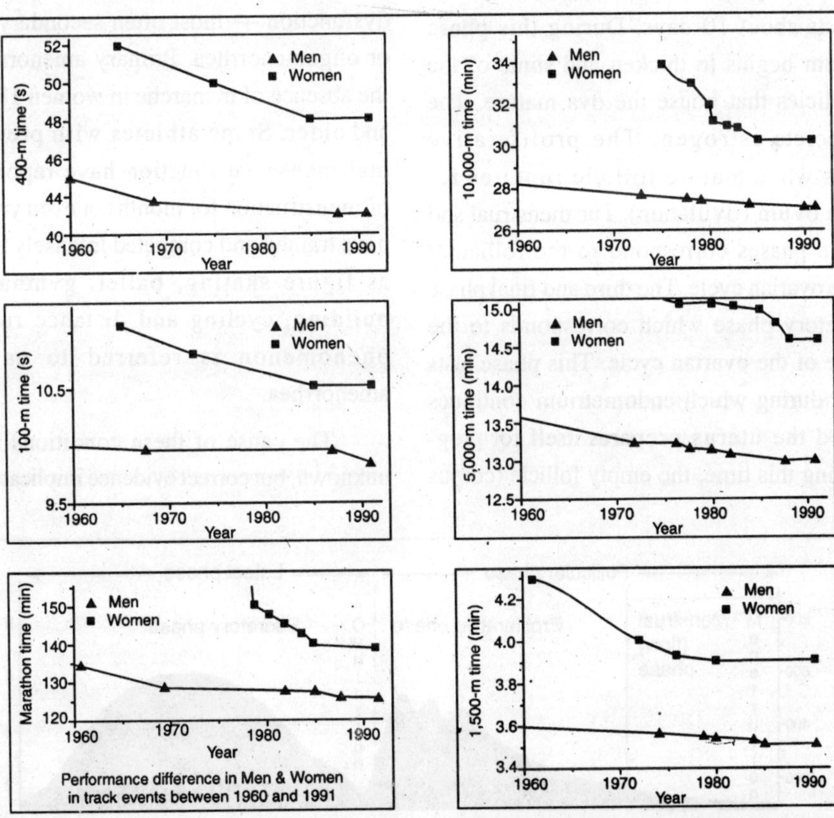

Fig. 10.3 : Performance difference in men and women in track events between 1960 and 1991

SPECIAL CONSIDERATION

Although the sexes respond to acute exercise and adapt to chronic exercise in much the same manner, several additional areas that are unique to females must be considered. Specifically, we will look at menstruation and menstrual dysfunction; pregnancy; osteoporosis; eating disorders and environmental factors.

Pregnancy

The three major phases of the menstrual cycle are illustrated above. The first is the menstrual (flow) phase which last 4-5 days during which time the uterine lining (endometrium) is shed and menstrual flow occurs. The second is the proliferative phase which prepares the uterus for fertilization and lasts about 10 days. During this phase endometrium begins to thicken and some of the ovarian follicles that house the ova mature. The follicles secrete estrogen. The proliferative phase ends when mature follicle ruptures releasing the ovum (ovulation). The menstrual and proliferative phases correspond to the follicular phase of the ovarian cycle. The third and final phase is the secretory phase which corresponds to the luteal phase of the ovarian cycle. This phase lasts 10-14 days during which endometrium continues creases and the uterus prepares itself for pregnancy. During this time, the empty follicle (corpus luteum) secretes progesterone and estrogen secretion also continues. The complete menstruation takes 28 days (**Malina, 1983**). The effect of different phases of the menstruation on performance are subject to considerable individual variation.

In general, the number of women reporting impaired performance in flow phase is about the same as the number reporting no difficulty. Any woman who experiences pre-menstrual syndrome (PMS) or dysmenorrhea is likely to not perform well while experiencing those symptoms. Menarche can be delayed in some young athletes in certain sports viz., gymnastics and ballet. Malina has postulated that the late matures, such as those with delayed menarche, are more likely to be successful in sports such as gymnastics because of their small lean bodies. Female athletes can experience menstrual dysfunction — most often secondary amenorrhea or oligomenorrhea. Primary amenorrhea refers to the absence of menarche in women 18 years of age and older. Some athletes with previously normal menstrual function have reported absence of menstruation for months or even year when they have trained and competed intensely in sports such as figure skating, ballet, gymnastics, body building, cycling and distance running. This phenomenon is referred to as secondary amenorrhea.

The cause of these conditions in athletes is unknown, but correct evidence implicates inadequate

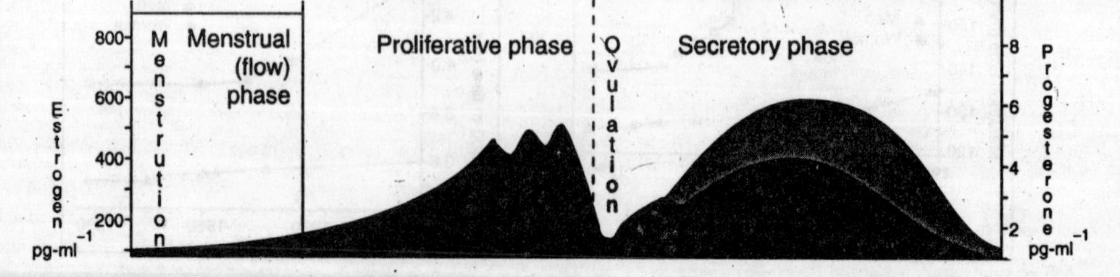

Fig. 10.4 : Phases of the menstrual cycle

nutrition as a primary cause of secondary amenorrhea. This appears to be reversible with reductions in the intensity and volume of training and to increase in calorie intake. In addition, hormonal changes from exercise and training might disrupt gonadotrophin releasing hormone (GnRH) which stops releasing of LH and FSH needed to direct the normal cycle.

During exercise major concerns for the pregnant athlete include the risk of Fetal hypoxia. The acute risk is associated with reduced blood flow to the uterus, as blood diverted to mother's active muscle leading to insufficient oxygen. Fetal hyperthermia (elevated temperature) is associated with the increase in the mother's internal body temperature during prolonged aerobic type exercise under condition of heat stress. Reduced CHO availability to fetus as mother's body use more CHO to fuel her exercise. The benefits of a properly prescribed exercise program during pregnancy out-weigh the potential risk, such as exercise program must be coordinated with woman's obstetrician.

Osteoporosis

Osteoporosis is characterized by decreased bone mineral content, which causes increased bone porosity. Three contributing factors to osteoporosis are estrogen deficiency, inadequate calcium intake and inadequate physical activity. Post-menopausal women, anorexia nervosa have greater risk of osteoporosis.

Eating Disorders

Eating disorders such as anorexia nervosa and bulimia nervosa — are more common in women than in men. Some researchers have estimated the prevalence to be as high as 50% for elite athletes in certain sports (endurance sports, weight classification sports).

Environmental factors

When work rate is adjusted relative to individual $\dot{V}O_2$ max, women and men respond almost identically to heat stress. Any differences noted are likely due to different initial level of conditioning. Women generally have lower sweat rate than men for the same heat stress and this appears to be the result of lower sweat production per sweat gland. However, this reduced sweating capacity does not appear to affect women's ability to tolerate heat, because they have more insulative subcutaneous fat, women have a slight advantage over men during cold exposure, but their smaller muscle mass limits their ability to generate body heat. Studies indicate that responses during exercise at altitude do not differ in women and men.

REFERENCE

Costil, D. L., Fink, W .J., Flynn, M. and Kirwan, J. (1987) : Muscle fiber composition and enzyme activities in elite female distance runners, ***International Journal of Sports Medicine*** 8 (Suppl. 2) 103-106.

Fink, W. J., Costil, D. L. and Pollock, M. L. (1988) : Submaximal and maximal working capacity of elite distance runners part II, muscle fiber composition and enzyme activities. ***Annals of New York Academy of Sciences*** 301, 323-327.

Forbes, G. B., (1972) : Growth of the lean body mass in man, ***Growth*** 36, 325-338.

Hult, J. S., (1986) : The female American runners : A modern quest for visibility. In B. L. Drinkwater (ed) ***Female Endurance Athletes***. Champaign IL. Human Kinetics.

Ingjer, F. and Brodal, P. (1978) : Capillary supply of skeletal muscle fibers in untrained and endurance trained women. ***European Journal of Applied Physiology*** 38-291-299.

Lohman, T. C. (1986) : Application of body composition techniques and constants for children and youth. ***Exercise and Sport Science Review*** 14, 325-357.

Malina, R. M. (1983) : Menarche in athletes : A synthesis and hypothesis : ***Annals of Human Biology*** 10, 1-24.

Saltin, B. and Rowell, L. B. (1980) : Functional adaptations to physical activity and inactivity. ***Federation proceedings*** 39, 1506-1513.

Wilmore, J. H. (1974) : Alterations in strength, body composition and anthropometric measurements consequent to 10 week weight training prog. ***Medicine and Science in Sports*** 6, 133-138.

Weltman, A., Janney, C., Rians, C. B., Strand, K., Berg, B., Tippih, S., Wise, J., Costill, B. R. and Katch, F. (1986) : The effects of hydraulic resistance strength training in pre-pubertal males. ***Medicine and Science in Sports Exercise*** 18, 629-638.

11

THERMOREGULATION AND EXERCISE

Humans are homeothermic which means that they are able to maintain a constant internal body temperature, usually in the range of 36.1° to 37.8°C (97.0 to 100°F). Body heat is transferred by conduction, convection, radiation and evaporation.

Conduction is the process of transfer of heat from one material to another through direct molecular contact. For example, heat generated deep in our body can be conducted through adjacent tissue until it reaches to body surface. It can then be conducted to our clothing or to the air that is in direct contact with our skin. Conversely, if the air around us is hotter than our skin, heat from the air will be conducted to our skin, warming it.

Convection involves transferring heat from one place to another by the motion of a gas or a liquid across the heated surface. As it circulates around us, passing over the skin, it sweeps away the air molecules that have been warmed by their contact with the skin, greater the movement of the air (or liquid such as when we are in water), the greater the rate of heat removal by convection. Although conduction and convection constantly remove body heat when the air temperature is lower than the skin temperature, their contribution to body's total heat loss is only about 10% to 20%. However, if we are submerged in cold water, the amount of heat dissipated by conduction is nearly 26 times greater than when exposed to environmental temperature. At rest, conduction is the primary method for discharging the body's excess heat. At normal temperature the nude body loses about 60% of its excess heat by radiation in the form of infrared rays, a type of electromagnetic wave.

Evaporation is the primary avenue for heat dissipation during exercise, it accounts for about 80% of the total heat loss when you are physically active, but for only about 20% of body heat loss at rest. Insensible heat loss, which happens wherever body fluid is brought into contact with the external environment, such as lungs, mucosa (lining the mouth) and at the skin. Insensible heat loss is relatively constant and removes about 10% of the total metabolic heat produced by our body. As sweat reaches the skin, it is converted from a liquid to a vapour by heat from the skin. Thus sweat evaporation becomes increasingly important as body temperature increases.

Table 1 : Mechanism of heat loss at rest and exercise

	Rest		Exercise	
	% Total	Kcal min^{-1}	% Total	Kcal min^{-1}
Conduction and convection	20	0.3	15	2.2
Radiation	60	0.9	5	0.8
Evaporation	20	0.3	80	12.0

The data presented are taken both at rest, when the body produces about 1.5 Kcal of heat per minute, and during prolonged exercise at 70% of VO_2 max. when the heat production is 10 times higher or about 15 Kcal/min.

The water vapour content, or humidity, of the air plays a major role in heat loss, especially by evaporation. Consider two situations : exposure to dry desert air at 32.2°C (90°F) with 10% relative humidity, compared to the same air temp with 90% relative humidity. We sweat profusely in the dry desert, but evaporation occurs so rapidly that they are not aware that we are sweating. But in latter situation, little sweat can evaporate because the air is already 90% saturated with water, which decreased its capacity to accept more water because the concentration gradient is decreased.

Internal body temperature, when at rest, is kept at approximately 37°C (98.6°F). But during exercise, because the body is often unable to dissipate heat as rapidly as it is produced, a person can develop an internal temperature exceeding 40°C (104°F), with a muscle temperature above 42°C (107.6°F). The muscle's energy systems become more chemically efficient with a small rise in muscle temperature. But internal body temperature above 40°C (104°F) can adversely affect the nervous system and reduce further efforts to unload excess heat.

REGULATION OF INTERNAL BODY TEMPERATURE

Heat production

In extreme cold, heat production is increased and heat loss is retarded to prevent a fall in internal temperature. Thermo-regulation in cold stress is by

(a) Vascular Adjustments

Stimulation of cutaneous cold receptors result in constriction of peripheral blood vessels and reduces the flow of warm blood to cooler surface and redirects it to the warmer core. Hence skin temperature falls — this is known as insulatory benefits of skin (subcutaneous fat).

(b) Muscular activity

Significant metabolic heat is generated though shivering is observed even during exercise if the core temperature is low. O_2 consumption is proportionally higher during this condition.

(c) Hormonal output

Increase heat production → Epinephrine, Norepinephrine

Cold stress (prolonged) → Thyroxine

Sustained elevation in resting metabolism.

ACCLIMATIZATION TO HEAT

Acclimatization changes begin to occur after 4th day and completed on the 14th day.

Changes occur with acclimatization process

Sweating

- Profuse sweat secretion
- Sweat diluted and evaporated rapidly
- Preserve electrolyte in ECF
- Effective distribution of sweat over skin surface, which can cause maximum cooling.
- Sweating contributes about 40% of total adaptation.

Increased plasma volume

Sufficient blood supply to the working muscles without stress on the heart to pump blood. Plasma protein increase with training which hold water by osmosis.

Increased stroke volume

After adaptation stroke volume increases. Blood pressure remains more stable. Appropriate circulation to skin and muscles is maintained to meet the demand of metabolism and thermoregulation.

Improve cutaneous circulation

Metabolic heat transported from deep tissue to the body surface, resulting in lower core temperature.

PHYSIOLOGICAL ADJUSTMENTS DURING HEAT ACCLIMATIZATION

Acclimatization response	Effect
Improved cutaneous blood flow.	Transport metabolic heat from deep tissue to the body's shell.
Effective distribution of cardiac output lower exercise pulse rate.	Stroke volume, blood pressure remain more stable during exercise. Appropriate circulation to skin and muscle to meet demands of metabolism and thermoregulation.
Lowered threshold for start of sweating.	Evaporative cooling begins early in exercise.
More effective distribution of sweat over skin surface.	Optimum use of effective surface for evaporative cooling.
Increased sweat output ↑	Hot environment → skin temperature increased. ↓
Increased plasma volume	
Transmitted to heat loss center in hypothalamus (Anterior)	← Afferent impulse from receptors
Increased heat loss maximizes evaporative cooling	Nerve impulse through nerve fiber to sweat gland. ↓ Increased discharge of vasoconstrictor nerve impulse to skin ↑ Increased blood flow
Lowered salt concentration of sweat	Dilute sweat, preserves electrolytes in extra-cellular fluid.

During exercise metabolic heat production is increased to 15-20 times.
Large part of heat is lost by increased sweat secretion (1.7 L/hour)
Acclimatization changes begin — after 4 days' training and completed in 14 days.

Acclimatization lessens shivering and fine motor task can be done more accurately. The hypothalamus houses our thermoregulatory center. It acts like a thermostat, monitoring our temperature and accelerating heat loss or heat production as needed. Two sets of thermoreceptors provide temperature information to our thermoregulatory center. The peripheral receptors in the skin relay information about the temperature of our skin and the environment around it. Central receptors in hypothalamus transmit information about our internal body temperature.

Effectors can alter body temperature. Increased skeletal muscle activity increases temperature by increasing metabolic heat production. Increased sweat gland activity decreases temperature by increasing evaporative heat loss. Smooth muscle in the arterioles can dilate to direct blood to the skin for heat transfer, or heat production can be increased by the action of hormones like thyroxine and catecholamine. Mean body temperature is a weighted average of our skin temperature and internal body temperature :

$$T\ body = (0.4 \times T\ skin) + (0.6 \times Tr)$$

Body's heat content is the total amount of heat in kilocalories that it contains. Under resting conditions, an average body generally produces 1.25 to 1.5 Kcal per hour. During exercise, heat production can exceed 15 Kcal per minute (900 Kcal/hour). The mechanism for heat dissipation are heavily taxed by evaporating a large amount of sweat. Each liter of evaporated sweat removes 580 Kcal. So body would have to lose 1.55 L of sweat per hour if all the sweat was evaporated and all the metabolic heat was removed by evaporation. (900 Kcal of heat produced/580 Kcal removed per liter of sweat = 1.55 L)

Exercising in hot environments sets up a competition between the active muscles and the skin for the limited blood supply. The muscles need blood and oxygen it delivers to sustain activity, the skin needs blood to facilitate heat loss to keep the body cool. To maintain a constant cardiac output with the shunting of blood to the periphery, the cardiovascular system must make sosme noticeable adjustments. Generally cardiac output increases in the heat when the exercise is moderately severe. During moderate to heavy exercise, cardiac output increases via increases in heart rate. Cardiac output becomes much more difficult to increase during very heavy exercise, when stroke volume and heart rate are at close to maximum (**Nadel, et al, 1980**).

Several authors (**Dill et al, 1973; Fink et al 1975; Irondelle and Freund, 1977; Williams et al 1962**) have observed increases in exercise lactate in hot compared to cool environments. Others (**Klausen et al, 1967, Rowell et al, 1965**) found no significant difference. It has been suggested (**Rowell, 1974**) that increases in lactate were observed in some experiment due to decreased muscle blood flow, reduced removal of lactate by the liver and increased muscle glycogenolysis. Lactate likely to be a factor contributing to fatigue.

Heat elevates heart rate but not oxygen consumption at submaximal exercise intensities. Increase in environmental temperature from 24°C (75.2°F) to 44°C to 54°C (111.2°F-129.2°F) result in proportional increases in heart rate, while oxygen consumption remains stable (**Pandolf et al, 1972**). The elevated heart rate is related to the need to increase cardiac output, whereas the oxygen consumption is responsive to the exercise intensity alone.

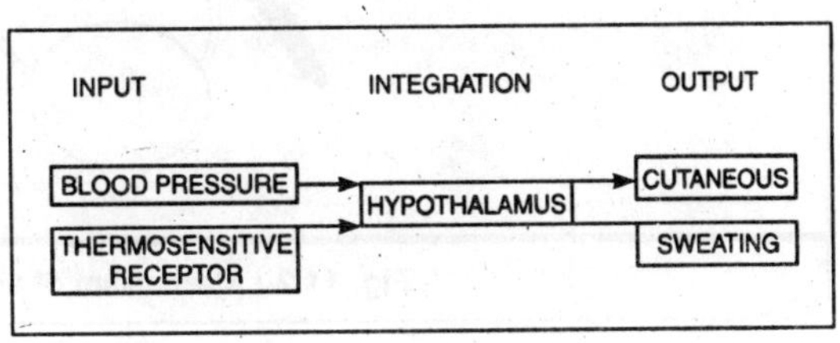

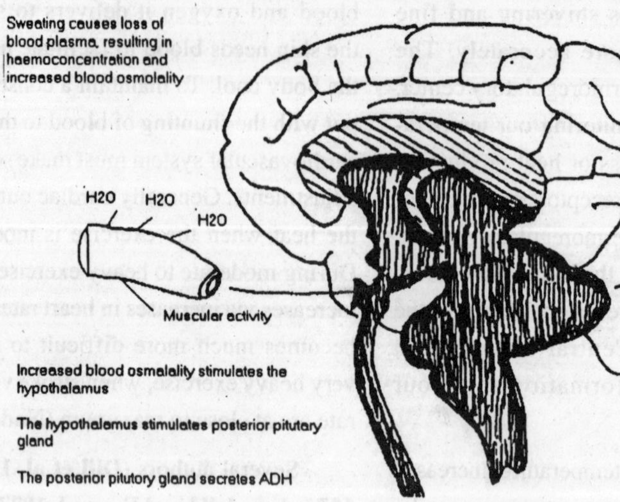

Fig. 11.1 : Balance of osmolality by the hormonal influence of hypothalamus and posterior pituitary

Most investigators agree that maximal oxygen consumption is not affected by heat up to 50°C (122°F) (**Adams et al, 1975, Matsui et al, 1978 Rowell et al, 1965, Saltin et al, 1972**). In addition, it has been shown that group with high VO_2 max (60.1 ml/kg/min) showed better response to submaximal work in the heat (39.4°C) than a group with a low VO_2 max (35.6 ml/kg/min) (**Shvartz et al, 1974**). This observation was based on a lower heart rate and core temperature in the high VO_2 max group. At rest muscle temperature varies between 25°C to 33°C (77°F-91.4°F) depending on environmental conditions (**Faulkner, 1981**). With an average temperature of 37°C (98.6°F), it is clear that the temperature gradient that exists favours the movement of heat from the core to muscles.

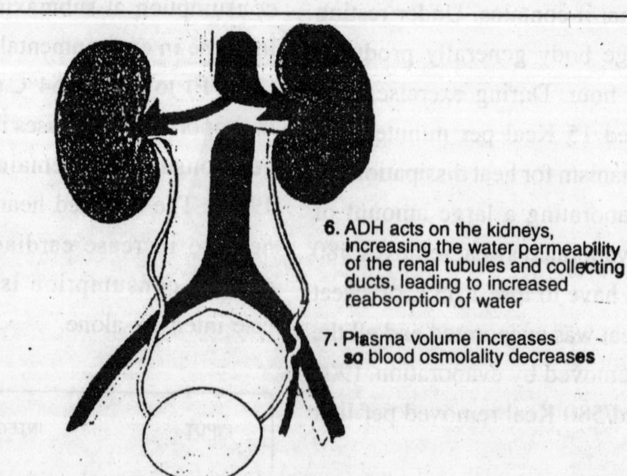

Fig. 11.2 : Mechanism of action of ADH to conserve water

During exercise intensity greater than 25% VO_2 max the temperature 20°C (68°F), a shift in the muscle to core gradient occurs. During high intensity exercise in warm, humid environments, rectal temperature increases continuously (**Saltin et al, 1970**). Therefore the gradient can be interrupted, making it difficult to keep the muscles from overheating. During isometric exercise, endurance decreases when muscle temperature exceeds 32°C (89.6°F) because of the rapid accumulation of metabolites (**Clark et al, 1958**). It seems that optimal muscle temperature for running, cycling and swimming are higher than for isometric exercise (**Faulkner, 1981**). This temperature is approximately 40°C (104°F) (**Brooks et al, 1971**). Aerobic exercise promotes muscle blood flow as well as peripheral blood flow; heat can thus be removed from the core of the body, preventing drastic raise in core temperature. The constructive nature of isometric exercise with reduced or occluded blood flow probably makes it difficult to maintain a muscle/blood temperature gradient that allows efficient heat dissipation.

Under some conditions, the temperature of the environment approaches and can exceed both the skin and deep body temperature. This makes evaporation far more important for heat loss because radiation, convection and conduction are less effective as environmental temperature rises. Increased dependence on evaporation means an increased demand for sweating. The sweat glands are controlled by stimulation of the hypothalamus. Elevated blood temperature causes the hypothalamus to transmit impulses through the sympathetic nerve fibers to the millions of sweat glands distributed over the body's surface. The sweat glands are tubular structure extending through the dermis and epidermis.

Sweat is formed by the filtration of plasma. As the filtrate passes through the duct of the gland, Na^+ and Cl^- are gradually reabsorbed back into the surrounding tissues and then into the blood. During light sweating, the filtrate sweat travels slowly through the tubules, allowing time for almost complete reabsorption of Na^+ and Cl^-. Thus the sweat that forms during light sweating contains very little of these minerals by the time it reaches the skin. However, when the sweating rate increases during exercise, the filtrate moves more quickly through the tubules, allowing less time for reabsorption. As a result Na^+ and Cl^- ion content of the sweat can be considerably higher. Sweat glands apparently do not have a similar mechanism for conserving other electrolytes. K^+, Ca^{++} and Mg^+, for example, are normally found in the same concentration in both sweat and plasma.

While performing heavy exercise in hot conditions, the body can lose more than 1 lt of sweat per hour per square meter of body surface. Sweat rates as high as 2-3 lts per hour have been observed, but these rates cannot be sustained for more than several hours. Maximal daily sweat rates are in the range of 10-15 lts.

During intense effort on a hot and humid day (high level of heat stress), an average sized individual (50-75 kg) might lose 1.5 to 2.5 L of sweat, or about 2% to 4% of body weight each hour. A high rate of sweating reduces blood volume of blood available to supply the needs of the muscles and to prevent heat buildup, which in, turn, reduces performance potential, particularly for endurance activities. In long distance runners, sweat losses can approach 6% to 10% of body weight. Such severe dehydration can limit subsequent sweating and make the individual susceptible to heat related illness.

Loss of both minerals and water by sweating triggers the release of aldosterone and ADH for maintaining appropriate sodium and fluid balance, by retaining Na^+ and water, which can expand the plasma volume.

Heat stress involves more than just the air temperature. Perhaps the most accurate means for measuring it is the wet bulb globe temperature (wbgt) which measures air temperature and accounts for the heat exchange potential through conduction, convection, evaporation, and radiation in a specific environment.

Outdoors WBGT = 0.7(WB) + 0.2(GT) + 0.1(DB)
Indoors WBGT = 0.7(WB) + 0.3(DB)

Where GT is the globe temperature, a measure of radiant heating record from a thermometer enclosed in a black or gray metal sphere. The index as calculated, however, makes no allowance for air movement. A relative air speed of 5 m/s can lower the effective temperature by 5-7°C (41°F-44.6°) (less in warm environment) when organizing distance races such as Marathon competitions it is recommended that the event be cancelled if the WBGT exceeds 28°C (82.4°F). There is a high risk of heat illness in vulnerable individuals if the WBGT lies in the range 23-28°C (73.4°F-82.4°F), moderate risk if the WBGT is 18-23°C (64.4°F-73.4°F) and a low risk at lower temperature (**Noble & Bachman, 1979**). **Wyndham and Strydom** (1972) have suggested that no unacclimatized athlete should run for more than 30 min if the WBGT has reached 25°C (77°F).

Loose fitting and light weight white clothing can protect the body against solar radiation, and it can also conserve sweat that would otherwise roll to the ground. Football fatalities in the USA have often been associated with the wearing of nylon uniforms. While these are easy to wash, they have the serious disadvantage of not allowing the passage of sweat. Natural fibers are much more effective than synthetic materials in this regard.

Sweating may amount to at least 2 lt over the first hour of strenuous activity, dropping to about 1 l/h over more prolonged effort. The first 1.5-2.0 lt can be derived from water associated with the glycogen molecule and water formed by metabolism (**Kavanagh and Shephard, 1978**). However, if the loss amounts to more than 2.5-3.0% of body mass, working capacity is adversely affected, with a greater rise of body temperature and larger increase of exercise heat rate.

Many of the commercially available replacement fluids contain minerals and carbohydrate, but because they are then hyperosmotic the rate of gastric emptying is slowed and the volume of fluid which can be ingested and absorbed is limited. Many factors can affect the rate of gastric emptying, the more important being the volume, temperature and sugar content of the drink. **Costill and Saltin (1974)** showed that a drink volume of about 400-600 ml leaves the stomach more rapidly than smaller volume and that a cold drink (5°C) (41°F) leaves more rapidly than a warm one (35°C) (95°F). Most importantly, they found that heavily sugared drinks in combination with high intensity exercise (over 70% VO_2 max) may combine to block gastric emptying. However, the relative needs for fluids and carbohydrates vary greatly with the athletic events and climatic conditions. In mild exercise in severe heat, fluid replacement is the major concern, and therefore the sugar should be minimized to assure good gastric emptying. But in very heavy exercise over long durations in a cool environment (eg. distance running), maintaining the energy stores may become more important than gastric emptying rate if dehydration is no longer a problem.

Costill suggests the following guidelines for hot weather competition and training (**Costill, D.L. 1977**),

1. Hot weather competition — use cold, palatable drinks in volume of 3 to 10 ounces that are low in sugar concentration (less than 2.5 gm/100 ml of water).
2. Precompetition — drink 13.5 to 20 ounces (two to three glasses) of the above drink thirty minutes before the competition starts.
3. During competition — drink 3 to 6 ounces at 10-15 minute intervals.
4. Post competition — salt foods moderately and use fruit juices such as orange juice and tomato juice to replace electrolytes lost in sweat.

Sweat contains quite large amount of sodium chloride (**Verde et al, 1983**). The normal salt loss is about 12 gm/day, but a competitor who sweats hard can lose up to 8 gm/h from a total pool of some 175 gms. Problems of a cumulative deficit can thus arise through several weeks of competing in a very hot climate. A deficit can be readily detected (**Wyndham and Strydom, 1972**) through a decrease in the salt content of the urine (Fantus test) and a progressive reduction in body mass (due to an associated decrease of body water). A sodium ion loss of 0.5 g/kg causes all athletes to become tired and irritable, with complaints of giddiness, fainting and cramps. Because of the reduced plasma volume, there is a decrease in maximum cardiac output and maximum oxygen intake. If the deficit is allowed to reach 0.75 g/kg, there is apathy, stupor and a marked fall of blood pressure (**Wyndham and Strydom, 1972**). During competition, the blood concentration of sodium and other mineral ions rises, and at this stage water is more important to the body than mineral replacement. During the subsequent recovery period, however, minerals lost in sweat must be replaced (**Kavanagh and Shephard, 1978**). A concentration of 0.1% NaCl can be added to water without an appreciable change in its taste.

In addition to Na^+, sweat contains such minerals as K^+, Ca^{++}, Mg^+ and Fe^{++} (**Verde et al, 1985**). The K^+ concentration is 1.5-2.0 times that is found in the plasma. Fortunately, body K^+ reserves are substantial and most commercial preparations of tablet salt contain K^+. During vigorous exercise, serum K^+ levels rise because of leakage of K^+ from the working muscles. As with Na^+ ions, the appropriate time for replacement of losses is thus in the recovery period, rather than during the exercise bout. (**Kavanagh and Shephard, 1978**)

Heat cramps are probably caused by losses of fluids and minerals that result from excessive sweating. Heat exhaustion is caused by the cardiovascular system's inability to adequately meet the body's needs in active muscles and skin. It is brought on by a reduced blood volume, typically caused by excessive loss of fluids and minerals through prolonged heavy sweating. Thought it is not in itself life-threatening, heat exhaustion can deteriorate to heat stroke if untrained.

Heat stroke is caused by failure of the body's thermoregulatory mechanisms, if untrained it will progress and becomes fatal. Several precautions must be taken when planning to exercise in the heat. These include cancelling the event if the environmental heat stress is too high (WBGT 28°C) (82.4°F), wearing proper clothing, being alert to the signs of hyperthermia, and ensuring adequate fluid. When exercising in the heat, if you suddenly feel chilled and goose bumps form on your skin, stop exercising, get into a cool environment, and drink plenty of cool fluids. The body's thermoregulation system has become confused and thinks that the body temperature needs to increase even more! If left untreated, this condition can lead to heat stroke and death.

Environmental physiologist recommended

- Practise in light weight uniform.
- Provide adequate salt and water replacement.
- Allow for sufficient rest period during practice.
- Workout should be held in early mornings and late evenings.
- Players should be weighed before and after workouts.
- Recommended intensity — (26.6-28.9°C) 80-84°F use — discretion. (29.4-31.6°C) (31.1°C) 85-89°F — Avoid strenuous training. 88°F Avoid training.

Heat acclimatization requires more than mere exposure to a hot environment. It is dependent on : (a) the environmental conditions during each exercise session; the duration of heat exposure, and; the rate of internal heat production (Exercise intensity).

Adaptation to heat increases while undergoing heat acclimatization by exercising in the heat for up to an hour or more each day for 5-10 days. Cardiovascular changes generally occur in the first 3 to 5 days, but changes in the sweating mechanisms generally take much longer, up to 10 days.

A decrease in temperature is sensed by receptors and the message is relayed to the hypothalamus which integrates incoming signals. The effector organs are instructed to respond so that body heat is conserved (Vasoconstriction) or produce shivering and hormonal secretion.

HEAT DISORDERS

Heat stroke : When the body temperature rises beyond a critical temperature into a range of 106-108°F, the person is likely to develop heat stroke.

The symptoms include : Dizziness; abdominal distress, delirium, loss of consciousness, giddiness and headache, blurring of vision. Many of these symptoms probably result from mild degree of circulatory shock due to excessive fluid loss and electrolyte loss. Exceedingly damaging to the body tissues specially to the brain resulting in convulsion. Damage of liver, kidneys and other body organs eventually causes death.

Heat-stroke must be treated immediately.

Aim of the treatment is to bring down temperature to 39°C (102.2°F) quickly.

First Aid — Patient should be moved to a cool, shady area or an air conditioned room and made to lie down.

After removing his clothes, cold wet pads must be applied all over and hospitalized soon.

Heat exhaustion : Unacclimatized athlete, during first hard training session on a hot day exposed to heat wave, there is an in-effective circulatory adjustment, compounded by a reduction in blood volume due to excessive sweating. Blood usually pools in the dilated peripheral vessels, this drastically reduces central blood volume necessary to maintain cardiac output.

Symptoms : Weak rapid pulse, headache, dizziness and general weakness.

First Aid : Person experiencing should stop exercising and move to a cooler environment. Fluid should be administered.

Heat cramp : Cramp occur due to excess fluid and salt loss — through sweating. Body temperature may be normal. It is because salt and water are not replenished adequately.

EFFECTS OF AGE, SEX AND OBESITY

Age : It has been shown that prepubertal girls (**Drink water et al, 1977, Haymes, 198-40**) and prepubertal boys (**Bar-or et al, 1980, Haymes et al, 1975**) have less tolerance for exercise in the heat than adults. This appears to be true even when subjects are matched for aerobic power and working at the same proportion of their maximal capacity (**Drink water, 1977**). There is also evidence that elderly people do not respond as well to heat exposure as do young people (**Drinkwater and Horvath, 1979, Shoenfeld et al, 1978**). (**Drinkwater and Horvath** (**1979**) suggested that for children the greater heat risk is due to the instability of an immature cardio-vascular system, while for the elderly the problem is more likely related to their decreased aerobic capacity.

Sex : Earlier work suggested that at all ages females are less heat tolerant than males (**Haymes et al, 1975; Shoenfeld et al, 1978**). However, recent studies have shown that there are few differences in male and female responses to heat stress when they are matched for VO_2 max. Therefore it seems that the earlier work largely reflected lower fitness levels in women (**Avellini et al, 1980; Shapiro et al, 1980**). However, there are sex differences in that females tolerance hot-wet climates better than males, while males tolerate hot dry conditions better than females (**Shapiro et al, 1980**). This finding is largely explained by the fact that, on the average, females have a higher ratio of body surface area to weight. This is an advantage in hot-wet climates but a disadvantage under hot dry conditions. This is so because heat production is mainly weight dependent, whereas heat dissipation is related to skin surface area. Since evaporation is not a factor in hot wet environment, the more surface area available for radiation and convection losses in relation to heat production, the better the adjustment. In hot dry conditions, a high ratio of surface area to weight is disadvantageous, because it allows more heat gain by convection and radiation.

During distance road races the incidence of heat illness is about the same in men and women (**Haymen et al, 1975**). Repeated prolonged exercise bouts in the heat cause gradual improvement in the ability to eliminate excess body heat, which reduces the risk of heat exhaustion and heat stroke. This process is termed as heat acclimatization.

A series of physiological adjustments designed to minimize disturbances in home stages due to heat stress. The end result of heat acclimatization is a lower heart rate and core temperature — both at rest and during submaximal exercise (**Glsolfi and Cohen, 1979**). The primary adaptations that occur during heat acclimatization are an increased plasma volume, earlier onset of sweating, higher sweat rate, reduced salt loss in sweat and a reduced skin blood flow (**Gosolfi and Cohen, 1979**). It is interesting that heat adaptation occurs rapidly, with almost complete acclimatization being achieved by 7-12 days after the first exposure (**Brengelmann, G 1977; Wyndhan, C 1973**), heat acclimatization results in a 10-12% increase in plasma volume (**Brooks and Fahey 1987**); (**G. Solfi and Cohen, 1979**). The increase in plasma volume is due to an increase in plasma protein. This increased plasma volume **maintains** central blood volume, stroke volume, sweating capacity and allows the body to store more heat with a smaller temperature gain. Heat acclimatization reduces the rate of muscle glycogen use, delaying the onset of fatigue.

As stated previously, heat adaptation results in an earlier onset of sweating. This means that sweating begins rapidly after the commencement of exercise, which translates into less heat storage at the beginning of exercise and a lower core temperature. In addition, heat acclimatization may increase the sweating capacity almost threefold above the rate achievable prior to heat adaptation. Therefore, much more evaporative cooling is possible, which is a major advantage in minimizing heat storage during prolonged work.

Finally, sweat losses of Na^+ and Cl^- are reduced following heat acclimatization due to an increased secretion of aldosterone (**Wyndham 1973**). While this adaptation results in a reduction of electrolyte loss and aids in reducing electrolyte disturbances during exercise in the heat, it does not minimize the need to replace water loss, which is higher than normal.

A summary of heat adaptive responses are as :

1. Increased plasma volume;
2. Earlier onset of sweating;
3. Higher sweat rate;
4. Reduced NaCl loss in sweat;
5. Reduced skin blood flow.

PHYSIOLOGICAL THERMOREGULATION IN THE COLD

The body regulates itself either by heat conservation or heat production. In the first case, the body conserves heat by vasoconstriction of the surface vessels and by shutting down the sweating mechanism. Heat production, increasing metabolite rate, is accomplished by shivering of skeletal muscles or by stimulating increased tissue oxidation by the intervention of various hormones. Cold receptors are located in the skin but they are far fewer than heat receptors. When skin temperature falls below normal, signals from cold receptors increase in frequency (**Thompson, 1977**). Receptors are sensitive to both absolute temperature and the rate of change in temperature (**Webstar, 1974**).

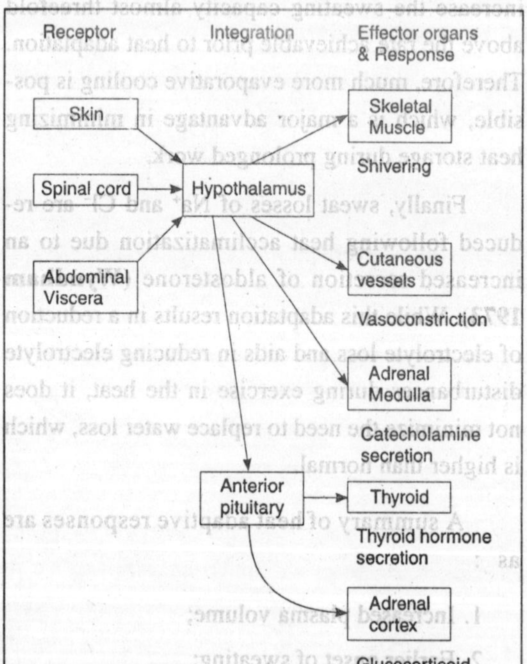

Fig. 11.3 : Regulatory mechanism of cold stress

Cold receptors are located in the spinal cord and abdominal viscera. Signals received by the hypothalamus are integrated and directed by the motor nerves to stimulate muscles to shiver, the sympathetic nervous system to cutaneous blood vessels which vasoconstrict and adrenal cortex to release glucocorticoid (cortisol and corticosterone) (**Webster, 1974**).

Mechanism of heat conservation and production

Vasoconstriction : The major mechanism of heat conservation is vasoconstriction of cutaneous vessels resulting in the flow of heat from the core to the shell to be limited. This results in decreased skin temperature, which decreases the temperature gradient with the environment and thus reduces heat loss. The blood pressure increases and heart rate decreases most likely a parasympathetic (vagus nerve) influence on the heart (**Frisancho, 1979**).

Muscular Shivering : Shivering (involuntary muscle contraction) increases metabolic heat production to help us maintain or increase our temperature, thus reducing muscular heat loss.

Hormonal response : During cold stress the catecholamines are known to increase the release of the free fatty acids that increase oxidative phosphorylation which results in increasing metabolic rate (**Webster, 1974**). Catecholamine also stimulates hyperglycemia, again, producing a condition favouring tissue oxidation. Thyroxine has also been implicated in the increase of metabolic rate in cold acclimatization (**Frisancho, 1974**). Glucocorticoid-Cortisol and cortisone produced by the adrenal cortex stimulate the formation of glucose which increase oxidative metabolism for cold adaptation.

Physiological response to cold stress

Extremities : Since the ear, feet and fingers have very little metabolically active tissue they depend heavily on blood supply for heat. Therefore, when skin vessels constrict, shell temperature decreases to a point close to the environmental temperature. During this condition very little heat is lost by convection and radiation, but the skin become susceptible to frostbite. A hunter's response has been observed in which a cold induced vasodilatation occurs, possibly protecting the skin from injury (**Frisancho, 1979**). Cross-country skiers may have noticed that sensation of periodic warming and cooling of extremities.

Oxygen consumption : VO_2 max is independent of environmental temperature (**Kunk et al, 1980; Matsui et al, 1978**). This condition causes a decrease in muscle temperature (< 38°C) (100.4°F) in which case aerobic power is decreased (**Bergh, 1980**).

Blood lactate and muscle glycogen : Blood lactate levels were elevated in the heat compared to cold and glycogen appears to be spared in the cold, that is exercise is, more aerobic in the cold with more reliance on fat as a fuel.

Strength and endurance during cold stress : Maximal isometric strength does not seem to be affected by the lowering of muscle temperature (**Bergh, 1980**). Peak torque achieved during dynamic muscular contractions, at selected angular velocities, decreases with reduced muscular temperature. Eccentric strength is increased as muscle temperature is lowered (**Asmusen et al, 1976**). Thus the effect of lowered muscle temperature on the development of force seems to be dependent on the type of exercise. When temperature does have an effect it is a result of its influence on the myosin cross-bridges, that is, the rate of breaking and forming actomyosin (**Asmusen et al, 1976**). Muscular endurance has also been studied at various environmental temperatures : 10°C, 13°C, 18°C (50°F, 55.4°F, 64.4°F, 75.2°F) and 24°C (**Clark, Wojciechowic, 1978**). Muscular endurance was improved by 30% in the 10°C (50°F) condition compared to 24°C (75.2°F).

Training during cold conditions

Many people worry about possible damage to lung tissue while exercising in the cold. Environmental air at a temperature of –32°C (89.6°F) is known to be heated to 24°C (75.2°F) before it reaches to bronchi (**Claremont, 1976**). The respiratory discomfort sometimes associated with breathing cold air is most likely related to the fact that cold air is usually very dry. When subjects exercise at submaximal exercise intensities while breathing air cooled to –35°C (95°F), there is not only an absence of harmful tissue effects but VO_2, respiratory rate and rectal temperature are unaffected as well (**Hartung et al, 1980**). Since air is such a good insulator, the athletes require only a tight weight clothing **material** that is porous so that sweat can wick to the surface where it can be removed.

Acclimatization to cold stress

Various physiological adjustments has taken place that would offer an advantage to cold exposed players. It has been suggested that one or more of the following criteria must be met to prove that man has acclimatized (**Webster, 1974**) :

(a) Evidence of an increased metabolic rate in a thermoneutral environment, that is, neither hot nor cold, (b) Evidence of increased tissue insulation, that is, tissue characteristics that reduce heat loss such as fat, (c) A decreased susceptibility to pain, numbness or cold injury in the extremities, (d) A decreased cutaneous threshold for cold thermogenesis.

Subjects placed in a cold chamber begin to show acclimation effect after one week (**Lampietro et al, 1957**). Acclimatization is marked by an increase in metabolic rate (**Lampietro et al, 1957**), a decrease in shivering response, an increase in nonshivering thermogenesis (**Davis, 1975**) and a decrease in skin thickness (**O, Hara et al, 1977**). These changes are related to increased fat mobilization in the cold that reduces skinfolds fat thickness (**O. Hara et al, 1977; O. Hara et al, 1979**).

Cold and performance

Performance of short term events is adversely affected by what is, in essence, the absence of a warm-up. Muscle tone and viscosity are increased and the speed of contraction is slowed, leading to delayed relaxation of the antagonist muscles.

Speed and power events are thus performed poorly and there is an increased risk of injuries due to failure of relaxation, impaired proprioceptive function and hypothermic or hypoglycemic confusion. There may be a small increase in maximum oxygen uptake due to peripheral vascular constriction and an increased physical solution of oxygen in the blood, but any benefit from these changes is offset by the added cost of increased muscle viscosity, shivering, heavy clothing and the need to move over snow or wet terrain. With more prolonged exposure, blood volume is depressed by a cold diuresis and inadequate fluid intake.

During maximal exercise, if core and muscle temperature fall below normal, endurance, VO_2 max and heart rate all decrease linearly with decreasing body temperature. In well-trained male subjects it was shown that VO_2 max declined by 5-6% per degree Centigrade decline in core temperature. Time to exhaustion on a cycle ergometer declined by 20% per degree Centigrade and heart rate decline 8 bpm per degree Centigrade (**Bergh & Ekblom, 1979**). Cold tolerance is modified by age, physical fitness, body surface area and small amount of body fat are the factors that decrease cold tolerance.

REFERENCE

Adams, W. C., Fos, R. H., Fry, A. J. and others. (1975) : Thermoregulation during Marathon running in cool moderate and hot environments. ***Journal of Applied Physiology*** 38 : 1030.

Asmussen, E., Bonde Pattersen, F. and Jorgensen, K. (1976) : Mechano elastic properties of human muscles at different temperature. ***Acta Physiologica Scandanavia*** 96 : 83.

Avellini, B. A., Kamon, E. and Krapewski, J. T. (1980) : Physiological responses of physically fit men and women to acclimation to humid heat. ***Journal of Applied Physiology*** 49 : 254-61.

Bergh, U. and Ekblom, B. (1979) : Physical performance and peak aerobic power at different body temperatures, ***Journal of Applied Physiology*** 46 : 885-891.

Bergh, U. (1979) : Human power at submaximal body temperature, ***Acta Physiologica Scandinavia*** (suppl.) 478 : 1.

Brengelmann, G. (1977) : Control of sweating and skin blood flow during exercise. ***In problems with temperature regulation during exercise***, (E. Nadel eds New York : Academic press).

Brooks, G. A., Hittelman, K. J., Faulkner, J.A. and others, (1971) : Temperature skeletal muscle mitochondrial functions and oxygen debt, ***American Journal of Physiology*** 220 : 1053.

Buskirk, E. R., Kollias, J., Picon Reatigue, E. and others, (1966) : Physiology and performance of track athletes at various altitude in the United States and Peru. In Goddard R.F. editor : The effects of altitude on physical performance. Chicago, ***The Athletic Institute***.

Clancy, L. J., Critchley, J. A. J. H., Leitch, A. G. and others, (1975) : Arterial catecholamines in hypoxic exercise in man, ***Clinical Science Molecular Medicine*** 49 : 503.

Claremont, A. D. (1976) : Taking winter in stride requires proper attire, ***Physical Sports Medicine*** 4 : 65.

Clark, R. S. J., Hellon, R. F. and Lind, A. R. (1958) : The duration of sustained contractions of the human forearm at different muscle temperatures, ***Journal of Physiology*** 143 : 454.

Clark, D. H. and Wojciechowicz, R. A. (1978) : The effect of low environmental temperature on local muscular fatigue parameters. ***Am. Correct. Ther. J.*** 32 : 35.

Costill, D. L. (1977) : Fluids for athletic performance. Why and what should you drink during prolonged exercise. In Toward understanding Human performance. ed. E. J. Burke Ithaca, ***New York Movement Publication***.

Daniels, J. and Oldridge, N. (1970) : Effect of alternate exposure to altitude and sea level on world class middle distance runners : ***Medicine and Science in Sports*** 2 : 107-112.v.

Davis, T. R. A. (1982) : Chamber cold acclimatization in man. ***Journal of Applied Physiology*** 16 ; 1011.

Dill, D. B., Yousef, M. K. and Nelson, J. D. (1973) : Response of men and women to two hour walk in desert heat, ***Journal Applied Physiology*** 35 : 231.

Dill, D. B. and Adams, W. C. F. (1972) : Maximal oxygen uptake at sea level and at 3,090 in altitude in high school champion runners. ***Journal of Applied Physiology*** 30 : 854.

Drinkwater, B. L., Kupprat, I. C., Denton, J. E., Crist, J. L. and Horvath, S. M. (1977) : Response of prepubertal girls and college women to work in the heat. ***Journal of Applied Physiology*** 43 : 1046-53.

Drinkwater, B. L. and Horvath, S. M. (1979) : Heat tolerance and aging, ***Medicine and Science in Sports*** 11 : 49-55.

Drinkwater B.L., Folinsbee L.J., Bedi T.F. and others, (1979) : Response of women mountaineers to maximal exercise during hypoxia. ***Aviation Space Environment Medicine*** 50 : 657.

Faulkner, J. A. (1981) : ***Heat and contractile properties of skeletal muscles.*** In Horvath S.M. and Yousef M.K. editors, Environmental physiology : aging, Heat and altitude, Amsterdam, Elsevierl North Holland.

Fink, W. J., Costill, D. L. and Van Handel, P. J. (1975) : Leg metabolism during exercise in the heat and cold. ***European Journal of Applied Physiology*** 34 : 183.

Frisancho, A. R. (1979) : **Human adaptation : a functional interpretation,** St. Louis, The C. V. Mosby.Co.

Gisoifi, C. and Cohen, (1979) : Relationship among training, heat acclimatization, and heat tolerance in men and women : The controversy revisited, ***Medicine and Science in Sports 11.*** 56-59.

Grover, R. F., Reeves, J. T., Grover, E. B. and others, (1967) : Muscular exercise in young men native to 3100 m altitude. ***Journal of Applied Physiology*** 22 : 555.

Hartung, G. H., Myhre, L. G. and Nunneley, S. A. (1980) : Physiological effects of cold air inhalation during exercise. ***Aviation Space Environmental Medicine*** 51 : 591.

Haymes, E. M. (1984) : Physiological response of female athletes to heat stress : A review, ***Physician and Sports Medicine*** 12(March) 43-59.

Haymes, E. M., Mc Cornic, R. J. and Buskirk, E. R. (1975) : Heat tolerance of exercising lean and obese prepubertal boys. ***Journal of Applied Physiology*** 39 : 457-61.

Horstman, D. H., Weiskopf, R. and Robinson, S. (1979) : The nature of perception of effort at sea level and high altitude. ***Medicine Science Sports*** 11 : 150.

Irondelle, M. and Freund, H. (1977) : Carbohydrate and Fat metabolism of unacclimated men during and after submaximal exercise in cool and hot environments, ***European Journal of Applied Physiology*** 37 : 27.

Kavanagh, T. and Shephard, R. J. (1978) : ***Fluid and mineral needs of post coronary distance runners.*** In F. Landry & WAR orban (Eds) Sports Medicine Symposia Specialists, Miami.

Klausen, K., Dill, D. B., Phillips, E. E. and others, (1967) : Metabolic reactions to work in the heat, ***Journal of Applied Physiology*** 22 : 292.

Lahiri, S. (1977) : ***Physiological responses and adaptations to high altitude.*** In Robertshow D., Ed. **Environmental Physiology II,** Baltimore, University Park Press.

Lampietro, P. F., Bass, D. E. and Buskirk, E. R. (1957) : Diurnal oxygen consumption and rectal temperature of man during cold exposure. ***Journal of Applied Physiology*** 10 : 198.

Maresh, C. M. (1981) : ***Influence of moderate altitude residents (2200 mts) on the acute mountain sickness and exercise response during early hypobaric hypoxia (4270 mt),*** Laramie, Wyoming, University of Wyoming Doctoral, Dissertation.

Matsui, H., Shimaska, K., Miyamura, M. and othoro, (1978) : ***Seasonal variation of aerobic work capacity in ambient and constant temperature.*** In Folinsbee, J. J. and others, editors. **Environmental Stress,** New York, Academic Press. Inc.

Nadel, E. R., Fortrey, S. M. and Wenger, C. B. (1980) : *Effect of hydration state on circulatory and thermal regulations.* ***Journal of Applied Physiology*** 49 (4) : 715.

Noble, H. B. & Bachman, D. (1979) : Medical aspects of distance race planning. ***Physician Sports Medicine*** 7 (6).78.

O Hara, W. J., Allen, C., Shephard, R. J. (1977) : Loss of body weight and fat during exercise in a cold chamber. ***European Journal Applied Physiology*** 37 : 205.

O Hara, W. J., Allen, C., Shephard, R. J. and others, (1979) : Fat loss in the cold — a controlled study, ***Journal of Applied Physiology*** 46 : 872.

Pandolf, K. B., Cafarelli, E., Noble, B. J. and others, (1972) : Perceptual responses during prolonged work, ***Perception Motor Skills*** 35 (975).

Pugh, L. G. C. E. (1964) : Cardiac output in muscular exercise at 5,800 mt (19000ft). ***Journal of Applied Physiology*** 19 : 441.

Pugh, L. C. G. E. (1964) : Muscular exercise at great altitude. ***Journal of Applied Physiology*** 19 : 431.

Rowell, L. B., Blackman, J. R., Martin, R. H. and others, (1965) : Hepatic clearance of indocyane green in man under thermal and exercise stress. ***Journal of Applied Physiology*** 20 : 384.

Rowell, L. B. (1970) : Human cardio-vascular adjustments to exercise and thermal stress, ***Physiology Review*** 54 (1) : 75.

Saltin, B. Grover, R. F. Blomquist, C. G. and others, (1968) Maximal oxygen uptake and cardiac output after 2 weeks at 4300 mt. ***Journal of Applied Physiology*** 25 : 400.

Saltin, B., Gagge, A. P. and Stdwijk, J. A. S. (1970) : Body temperature and sweating during thermal transients caused by exercise. ***Journal of Applied Physiology*** 28 : 318.

Shapiro, Y., Pandolf, K. B., Avellini, B. A., Pimental, N. A. and Goldman, R. F. (1980) : Physiological responses of men and women to humid and dry heat. ***Journal of Applied Physiology*** 49 : 1-8.

Shephard, R. J. (1980) : Altitude, ***Olympic Book of Sports Medicine*** (Ed. A Dirix, H. G. Knuttgen and K. Tittel. 168.

Shoenfeld, Y., Udassin, R., Shapira, Y., Ohri, A. and Sohar, E. (1978) : Age and sex differences in response to short exposure to extreme dry heat. ***Journal of Applied Physiology*** 44 : 1-4.

Shvartz, E., Magazanic, A. and Glick, Z. (1974) : Thermal responses during training in a temperate climate. ***Journal of Applied Physiology*** 36 : 572.

Stock, M. J., Chopman, C., Stirling, J. L. and others, (1978) : Effect of exercise, altitude and food on blood hormone and metabolites levels. ***Journal of Applied Physiology*** 45 : 350.

Thompson, G. E. (1977) : Physiological effects of cold exposure. In Robertshaw, D. (ed) ***Environmental Physiology II***, Baltimore, University Park Press.

Verde, T., Shephard, R .J., Corey, R. and Moore, R. (1983) : Sweat composition in exercise and heat. In N Bachl, L. Prokop and R. Suckert (eds) ***Current topics in Sports Medicine***, Urban and Schwarzenburg, Vienna.

Vogel, J. A. and Hansen, J. E. (1966) : Cardio-vascular function during exercise at high altitude. In Goddard R.F. (ed). ***The Effect of Altitude on Physical Performance***. Chicago, The Athletic Institute.

Vogel, J. A., Hartley, L. H., Cruz, J. C. and others, (1974) : Cardiac output during exercise in sea level residents at sea level and altitude. ***Journal of Applied Physiology*** 36 : 169.

Webster, A. I. F. (1974) : Adaptation to cold in Robertshaw, D. ***Environmental Physiology I***, Baltimore, University Park Press.

West, J. B., Boyer, S. J., Graber, D. J., Hackett, P. H., Maret, K. H., Milledge, J. S., Peters Jr, R. M., Pizzo, C. J., Samaja, M., Sarnquist, F. H., Schoene, R. B. and Winslow, R. M., (1983) : Maximal exercise at extreme altitudes on Mount Everest. ***Journal of Applied Physiology*** 55 : 688-698.

Williams, C. G., Bredell, G. A. G., Wyndham, C. H. & Others, (1962) : Circulatory metabolic reactions to work in heat, ***Journal of Applied Physiology*** 17 : 625.

Wyndham, C. (1973) : The physiology of exercise under heat stress. ***Annual Review of Physiology*** 35 : 193-220.

Wyndham, C. H. and Strydon, N. B. (1972) : Korpertiche Arbeit bei hoher Temperature. In W Hollmann (ed). ***Zentrale Themen der Sportmedzin Springer***, Berlin.

12

ALTITUDE AND PERFORMANCE

Gravity

The physical strain imposed on the body with increasing altitude is caused by decreasing barometric pressure. The acceleration due to gravity diminishes by some 0.3 cm/s^2 for every 1,000 mt of altitude. A high competition site thus confers an advantage on many classes of athlete including jumpers, pole vultures, hurdlers and throwers. However even at 4,000 mt the benefit (0.13%) is smaller than that obtained from a higher altitude, gravitational forces increasing by 0-53% from the equator to the poles.

Wind Resistance

The wind resistance encountered by the athletes is largely due to turbulent air movement over the body surface and it is thus proportional to 1/2 pv^2, where p is the density of the atmosphere and v is the relative velocity of air movement. Density decreases by 19.9% of 1830 mt, 25.7% at 2,440 mt and 31.2% at 3,050 mt. At sea level wind resistance accounts for some 11% of the energy expanded in running 5,000 mt, thus the decrease of atmospheric density boosts the potential 5,000 mt performance by about 3.4% at an altitude of 3,000 mt. Since work against turbulent resistance is proportional to the third power of relative air speed, the advantage of high-altitude competition is much larger in the faster events, about 14.3% in a 100 mt run, and even greater in cycling, skiing and speed skating contests.

Temperature

The ambient temperature decreases by about 2°C for every additional 300 mt of altitude. Cold air can hold little water, so the air at altitude is dry. These two factors increase the susceptibility to cold related disorders and dehydration when at altitude. Because the atmosphere is thinner and drier at altitude, solar radiation is more intense at higher elevations.

Oxygen Partial Pressure

The percentage of gases in the air we breathe at altitude is identical to that at sea level — O_2 is 20.93%, CO_2 0.03% and N_2 is 79.04% of the total air. The partial pressure of each gas, however, is reduced in direct proportion to the increase in altitude. Partial pressure of oxygen at sea level is 159 mm.Hg. But it drops to 125 mm.Hg at an elevation of 2,439 mt (8,000 ft). As a result, partial pressure of oxygen within alveoli and the pulmonary capillaries also decrease. Arterial pO_2 at sea level is about 94 mm.Hg, and the partial pressure of oxygen in body tissues is consequently about 20 mm.Hg, so the pressure gradient between arterial and tissue pO_2 at sea level is about 74 mm.Hg. At 2,439 mt (8,000 ft), the arterial pO_2 drops to about 60 mm.Hg, while tissue pO_2 remains at 20 mm.Hg. Thus the pressure gradient decreases from 74 mm.Hg to 40 mm.Hg. This is nearly 50% reduction in diffusion gradient. Thus, there is some 31% less oxygen per unit volume of air available to the athlete at 3,000 mt than at sea level.

Such hypoxia has little direct impact on the performance of the sprinter provided that a somewhat longer recovery interval is allowed between heats. However, the endurance competition is appreciably handicapped. Advantages due to a lesser wind resistance and reduced gravitational forces are outweighed by hypoxia if an event lasts more than 7 min, and a substantial loss of performance is seen 5 km and 10 km races. In Mexico City, times for the last two events are commonly about 8% poorer than at sea level. The corresponding diminution in the partial pressure of atmospheric oxygen is about 24%, indicating that various physiological mechanisms provide even a temporary altitude resident with some compensation against hypoxia.

PHYSIOLOGICAL RESPONSE TO ALTITUDE

Hemoglobin, Hematocrit, Plasma Volume and Blood Glucose

During the first week at altitude there is a increase in the number of circulating erythrocytes (RBC). Hypoxia stimulates the release of erythropoietin, which is responsible for stimulating erythrocyte production. Hemoglobin and Hematocrit levels are both increased by acute exposure to altitude, primarily due to dehydration (**Frisancho, 1979**). This would be expected given the need to maximize the oxygen carrying capacity of the blood.

Plasma volume decreases within a few hours of arrival at altitude as a result of fluid shifts and respiratory water loss. This causes dehydration, which decreases the plasma volume. This reduction in plasma volume concentrates the erythrocytes, even further increasing the blood's oxygen carrying capacity. This adaptation is beneficial at rest and during low levels of exercise but it reduces endurance capacity at near maximal or maximal level of exercise. Blood glucose levels are depressed at high altitude (3,650 mt, 11,976 ft) and the normal rise in free fatty acid lévels during exercise is potentiated (**Stock et al, 1978**).

Pulmonary Ventilation

On exposure to hypoxia, an increase in resting pulmonary ventilation (VE) is observed when alveolar oxygen tension (PAO_2) reaches 60 mm of Hg or less, usually at altitude greater than 3,040 mt (10,000 ft) due to an increment of tidal volume, not the respiratory rate. Hypoxia stimulates the carotid bodies, causing the elevated VE (**Frisancho, 1979**). Increased pulmonary ventialtion by 65% have been reported. This causes the body fluids to become more alkaline due to reduction in CO_2 with hyperventilation (immediate effect). This is compensated by excretion of base via the kidney and concomitant reduction in alkaline reserve (delayed effect). Maximal VE is increased at moderate altitude in both men and women. Increased exercise ventilation may be related to increased noradrenaline levels (**Clancy, et al, 1975**). Some investigators have observed increases in maximal pulmonary ventilation at high altitude (>4,000 mt) compared to sea level (**Buskirk et al, 1966, Horstman et al, 1979**) and other investigators have observed no increase

(**Drinkwater et al, 1979, Maresh, 1981**). The pulmonary diffusion is not hindered by altitude, but oxygen transports slightly impaired because hemoglobin saturation at altitude is reduced, although by only a small amount. The diffusion gradient that allows oxygen exchange between the blood and active tissue is substantially reduced at elevation, thus oxygen uptake is impaired. This is partially compensated for by a decrease in plasma volume, concentrating the RBCs and allowing more oxygen to be transported per unit of blood.

Cardiovascular system

Immediate	Longer term
Increase in submaximal heart rate (HR)	Submaximal heart rate remain elevated
Increase in submaximal cardiac output	Submaximal Cardiac output (Q) falls to or below sea level
Maximum cardiac output (Q) remains the same or slightly lowered	Maximum cardiac output is lowered
Stroke volume remains same or slightly lowered	Stroke volume is lowered
Maximum heart rate remains the same or slightly lowered	Maximum heart rate is lowered

Cardiac Output

It is unclear whether submaximal exercise cardiac output changes with altitude. However, maximal cardiac output definitely is decreased due to decrement of maximum stroke volume and variable decrease in maximal heart rate (**Pugh, 1964; Saltin et al, 1968; Vogel et al, 1974**).

Aerobic Response

Submaximal oxygen consumption in men is unaffected by high altitude (4100 mt., 13448 ft) when the exercise intensity at altitude is adjusted to the same relative intensity used at sea level. However significantly different oxygen consumption are observed between normoxia and hypoxia (4,100 mt = 13,448 ft) in women. Aerobic power is significantly depressed by hypoxia in both sexes. It is estimated that aerobic power is reduced by 3.2% for each 300 mt (1,000 ft) above 1,600 mt (5,000 ft.) (**Buskirk et al, 1966**). VO_2 max decreases little until the atmospheric pO_2 drops below 125 mmHg. This generally occurs at an altitude of 1,600 mt (5,248 ft). However, above 1600 mt VO_2 max decreases approximately 11% for every 1,000 mt (3,281 ft) increase (**West et al, 1983**). Men climbing Mount Everest in a 1981 expedition experienced a change in VO_2 max from about 62 ml/kg/min at sea level to only about 15 ml/kg/min near the mountain's peak. Normal resting O_2 consumption are about 5 ml/kg/min. So without supplemental O_2 these men had little capacity for physical effort at this elevation. A study by **Pugh (1964)** showed that men with VO_2 max value of 50 ml/kg/min at sea level would be unable to exercise or even to move near the peak of Mount Everest because their VO_2 max values at that altitude would drop to 5 ml/kg/min.

Anaerobic Response

Anaerobic pathway (glycolytic system) appears to be affected when a person performs submaximal activity. This may be due to lower O_2 tension which requires a higher contribution from glycolysis than at sea level, which results in a significant increase in blood lactic acid concentration (**Klausen et al, 1970**).

ACCLIMATIZATION TO ALTITUDE

Physiological changes associated with acclimatization can be classified into fast response, occurring within a few weeks; and slow response, occurring over many years (**Lahiri, 1977**). A typical fast acclimatization response is the reflex hyperventilation observed almost immediately on high altitude exposure (**Lahiri, 1977**). Because the number of oxygen molecule in a given volume of air is less at higher altitude, more air must be inspired there to supply as much oxygen as during normal breathing at sea level. In hyperventilation too much CO_2 can be cleared, leading to respiratory alkalosis. In response, the kidneys excrete more bicarbonate ion, so less acid can be buffered. Additionally, hemoglobin (**Frisancho, 1979**) and Hematocrit levels have been observed to make an adaptive response increase within 3 weeks of exposure to altitude (**Vogel, 1966**). Hypoxic condition stimulates the release of erythropoietin, which increase erythrocyte (RBC) production. More RBC means more hemoglobin. Although, plasma volume decreases initially (few hour of arrival) as a result of fluid shift and respiratory water loss. More water is lost by evaporation during respiration at altitude because the air entering the lungs is very dry. This causes dehydration which decreases the plasma volume, which also concentrates the hemoglobin — it eventually returns to normal. Normal plasma volume plus additional red blood cells increase total blood volume. All of these changes increase blood's oxygen carrying capacity. Slow acclimatization response involve hypertrophy of tissues and cells and changes in subcellular material (**Lahiri et al, 1977**). Tissue adaptation to altitude include an increase in the myoglobin content of the muscles, and an augmentation in the activity of various enzyme systems. These responses occur over 1 or 2 weeks, helping to compensate sprinter for loss of tissue-buffering capacity and speedy recovery from exhaustive exercise. Other school of thought indicate that muscle fiber areas decreased, thus decreasing total muscle area. Part of this is from dehydration and appetite suppression which leads to protein breakdown in the muscle. Capillary density in the muscle, increase which allow more blood and oxygen to be delivered to them. (The cause for these changes is currently being debated). The mitochondria and glycolytic enzyme activities of the leg muscles (Vastus lateralis and Gastrocnemius) are significantly reduced after 3 to 4 weeks. This suggests that, in addition to receiving less oxygen, muscles lose some of their capacity to perform oxidative phosphorylation and perform both aerobic and anaerobic exercise.

Table 1 : Changes in Muscle Structure and Metabolic Potential during 4-6 weeks of chronic Hypoxia

Parameters	Change	% Change
Muscle area	Decreased	11 - 13
ST fiber area	-do-	21 - 25
FT fiber area	-do-	19
Capillary density (Capillary per mm²)	Increased	13
Succinate dehydrogenase	Decreased	25
Citrate synthetase	-do-	21
Phosphorylase	-do-	32
Phosphofructokinase	-do-	48

Examples of slow response adaptations are increased capillary density and pulmonary diffusion capacity (**Buskirk E.R., 1978**) and increased concentration of mitochondria and respiratory chain enzyme (**Lahiri, 1977**).

Short Term Physiological and Performance Responses

Runners exposed to 17 days at 3,090 mt (10,135 ft) showed a small return of VO_2 max toward sea level values, but these values still remained significantly depressed (**Dill and Adams, 1971**). Although pCO_2 and % SO_2 returned toward sea level values after 3 weeks at 4,300 mt (14,108 ft), the change is minimal (**Vogel and Hansen, 1966**).

Table 2 : Changes in arterial partial pressure of oxygen (PaO_2) and O_2 saturation (SO_2) at rest and maximal exercise during acute acclimatization to high altitude

	Resting Response		Maximal exercise response	
	PaO_2 (mm.Hg)	SO_2 (%)	PaO_2 (mm.Hg)	SO_2 (%)
Sea level	93	95	106	96
1st week	44	82	45	79
3rd week	53	86	55	82

Cardiac output values do return to sea level values after 3 weeks at 4,300 mt. The continued depression of VO_2 max must, therefore, be related to tissue level changes. Depressed maximal lactate values do not normalize after 22 days at 2,300 mt (7455 ft), in fact, they are depressed by 51%. Submaximal (75% of VO_2 max) endurance time appears to be improved by 12 days' exposure to altitude. It is revealed that the oxygen transport system is not impaired during light and moderate exercise at high altitude. Only when the aerobic system is maximally stimulated does an impairment appear.

Time of acclimatization

Depends on the height of altitude. 3-4 weeks are required for adaptation at 3,000 mt. Acclimatization for competitive events should be longer as the altitude becomes higher. Time required to acclimatize to altitude is related to the individual as well as the preceding training state of the individual.

Intensity required for training

While executing training programs similar to those used at training at high altitude, one should be aware that because muscular fatigue sets in earlier at altitude, one is forced to accept a slower tempo as well as a reduced intensity and duration.

Altitude training may improve performance at sea level for the unconditioned, non-athletic person, but the training intensity and duration that is required for the highly trained athlete (in order to reach peak performance) cannot be achieved the same at altitude as it can at sea level. Thus improved performance is not found for highly conditioned athletes.

ALTITUDE TRAINING AND EXERCISE PERFORMANCE

Can altitude training improve sea level performance? Most studies have shown no improvement in sea level performance following altitude training. In the few studies where altitude training was found to influence post-altitude sea level performance, this may be due to the fact that subjects were not well trained before going to altitude. This makes it difficult to determine post-altitude improvement rate, and the improvement was due solely to training, independent of altitude. Studying athletes at altitude poses a difficult problem as the athletes are often unable to train at the same volume and intensity of effort as compared to sea level and in moderate to high altitude training often causes dehydration and loss of fat free mass. These conditions tend to diminish the athlete's fitness and their tolerance to intense training. As a result, the studies which are focused as "Altitude training improve sea level performance" are difficult to interpret, and the debate continues.

A strong theoretical argument can be made for altitude training. The oxygen transport system of conditioned altitude newcomers is similar to natives. Athletes from Lexington Kentucky (sea level) won all the tract events against native athletes from Leadville. Of course, they won the same events in Lexington **(Grover et al, 1967)**. The best athlete wins at altitude even though aerobic performance times are decreased. Some people believe athletes who must perform at altitude must compete within 24 hr of arrival at higher altitudes. This does not provide much acclimatization because the altitude exposure is brief enough and the classic symptoms of altitude sickness not become totally manifested. The other opinion is to train at higher altitudes for at least two weeks before competing. But not even two weeks are sufficient for total acclimatization. It would require minimum of 4-6 weeks. For team sports requiring considerable endurance (viz., Volleyball, Football, Basketball), several weeks of intense aerobic training at sea level is necessery to increase the athletes VO_2 max levels. This will let them compete at altitude at a lower relative intensity than those who haven't prepared in a similar manner.

Alternatively, athletes who must perform at altitude should train at an altitude of 1,500 m (4,921 ft) to 3,000 m (9,843 ft) for at least 2 weeks prior to performing. This allows their bodies time to adapt to hypoxia and other environmental conditions at altitude. Work capacity will be reduced during the initial days at altitude. For this reason, when reaching higher altitude, workout intensities should be reduced to 60% and 70% of sea level intensity, and then gradually working up to full intensity. **Daniel and Oldridgeh (1970)** observed that alternate periods of training at 2,287 m (7,503 ft) and at sea level adequately stimulated altitude acclimatization. Staying at sea level for up to 11 days did not interfere with the usual adjustments to altitude as long as training was maintained.

The physiological objectives has been to time the return to sea level, so that the altitude polycythemia is preserved, but body buffers are restored to their initial values while there is a theoretical possibility of gaining some advantage of oxygen transport 4-20 days following altitude exposure. The hematological changes are transient, lasting only for several days. This may provide a slight advantage for the athlete. To resolve the debate we must await more definitive results. Many coaches and athletes are convinced that altitude training enhances performance, but with little fact and figure. This form of training is expensive due to transportation, housing, food and other cost and its effectiveness is not fully supported by the existing research on endurance runners.

ACUTE MOUNTAIN SICKNESS

Acute mountain sickness (AMS) is observed in people at an altitude as high as 1,500 mt (4,920 ft) and in virtually everyone above 5,000 mt (16,400 ft). Symptoms are at their maximum after 24 or 48 hrs and disappear in 6-8 days. The symptoms include anorexia, headache, nausea, lassitude, insomnia and fatigue. The exact cause of acute altitude sickness is not known but many researchers suspect that the symptoms may result from CO_2 accumulation in the tissues. Acute altitude sickness can usually be avoided by a gradual ascent to altitude, climbing no more than 300 mt (984 ft) per day at elevations above 3,000 m (9,843 ft). Medication such as acetazolamide can also be used to reduce the symptoms. Pulmonary edema and cerebral edema, which involve accumulation of fluid in the lungs and the cranial cavity, respectively, are life threatening conditions. Both are treated by O_2 administration and descent.

REFERENCE

Frisancho, A. R. (1979) : ***Human adaptation : a functional interpretations***, St. Louis, The C.V. Mosby.Co.

Clancy, L. J., Critchley, J. A. J. H., Leitch, A. G. and others (1975) : Arterial catecholamine in hypoxic exercise in man, ***Clinical Science Molecular Medicine*** 49 : 503.

Buskirk, E. R., Kollias, J., Picon, Reatigue, E and others (1966) : Physiology and performance of track athletes at various altitude in the United States and Peru. In Goddard, R. F. editor : ***The effects of altitude on Physical performance***, Chicago, The Athletic Institute.

Horstman, D. H., Weiskopf, R. and Robinson, S. (1979) : The nature of perception of effort at sea level and high altitude. ***Medicine Science in Sports*** 11 : 150.

Drinkwater, B. L., Folinsbee, L. J., Bedi, T. F. and others (1979) : Response of women mountaineers to maximal exercise during hypoxia. ***Aviation Space Environment Medicine*** 50 : 657.

Maresh, C. M. (1981) : Influence of moderate altitude residents (2200 mts) on the acute mountain sickness and exercise response during early hypobaric hypoxia (4,270 mt), Laramie, Wyoming University of Wyoming *Doctoral Dissertation*.

West, J. B., Boyer, S. J., Graber, D. J., Hackett, P. H., Maret, K. H., Milledge, J. S., Peters, Jr, R. M., Pizzo, C. J., Samaja, M., Sarnquist, F. H., Schoene, R. B. and Winslow, R. M. (1983) : Maximal exercise at extreme altitudes on Mount Everest. ***Journal of Applied Physiology*** 55 : 688-698.

Pugh, L. C. G. E. (1964) : Muscular exercise at great altitude. ***Journal of Applied Physiology*** 19 : 431.

Pugh, L. G. C. E. (1964) : Cardiac output in muscular exercise at 5,800 mt (19000 ft). ***Journal of Applied Physiology*** 19 : 441.

Saltin, B., Grover, R. F., Blomquist, C. G. and others (1968) : Maximal oxygen uptake and cardiac output after 2 weeks at 4,300 mt. ***Journal of Applied Physiology*** 25 : 400.

Vogel, J. A., Hartley, L. H., Cruz, J. C. and others (1974) : Cardiac output during exercise in sea level residents at sea level and altitude. ***Journal of Applied Physiology*** 36 : 169.

Stock, M. J., Chopman, C., Stirling, J. L. and others (1978) : Effect of exercise, altitude and food on blood hormone and metabolites levels. ***Journal of Applied Physiology*** 45 : 350.

Klausen, K., Dill, D. B., Phillips, E. E. and others (1967) : Metabolic reactions to work in the heat, ***Journal of Applied Physiology*** 22 : 292.

Lahiri, S. (1977) : Physiological responses and adaptations to high altitude. In Robertshow D. Ed. ***Environmental Physiology* II**, Baltimore, University Park Press.

Vogel, J. A. and Hansen, J. E. (1966) : Cardio-vascular function during exercise at high altitude. In Goddard, R. F. Ed. ***The Effect of Altitude on Physical Performance***. Chicago, The Athletic Institute.

Buskirk, E. R., Kollias, J., Picon Reatigue, E. and others (1966) : Physiology and performance of track athletes at various altitudes in the United States and Peru. In Goddard R.F. editor : ***The Effects of Altitude on Physical Performance***, Chicago, The Athletic Institute.

Dill, D. B. and Adams, W. C. (1971) : Maximal oxygen uptake at sea level and at 3,090 mt. altitude in high school champion runners. ***Journal of Applied Physiology*** 30 : 854.

Grover, R. F., Reeves, J. T., Grover, E. B. and others (1979) : Muscular exercise in young men native to 3100 m altitude. ***Journal of Applied Physiology*** 22 : 555, 1967. Frisancho.

13

HORMONAL REGULATION OF EXERCISE

Endocrine glands release hormones directly into the blood to alter the activity of tissues possessing receptors to which hormones can bind. These substances were released in minor amounts resulting in very low concentrations in the blood (<1 mmol) and they exerted their function on tissues in other region of the body (**Laycockwise, 1983**). The plasma hormone concentration determines the magnitude of the effect at the tissue level. The hormone concentration can be changed by altering the rate of secretion or inactivation of the hormone, the quality of transport protein and the plasma volume. The rate of excretion of a hormone in the urine has been used as an indicator of its rate of secretion during exercise (**Bonen, 1976, Euler, 1969, Howley, 1976**). An increase in the quantity capacity or affinity of transport protein would reduce the amount of free hormone and its effect on tissue (**Ganong, 1979, Keizer & Rogal, 1990**). After binding to a receptor on a membrane, the major effect of some hormones is to activate carrier molecules in or near the membrane to increase the movement of substrates or ions from outside to inside of the cell, for example, insulin binds to receptors on the surface membrane of the cell and can mobilize glucose transporters located in the membrane. The transporters link up with glucose on the outside of the cell membrane where the concentration of glucose is high and the glucose transporter diffuses to the inside of the membrane to release glucose for use in the cell (**James, 1995**).

CLASSIFICATION OF HORMONES

Hormones can be classified as either steroid or non-steroid. Steroid hormones are lipid soluble, and most of them are formed from cholesterol. This group includes the adrenal cortex (cortisol and aldosterone), the ovaries (estrogen and progesterone), the placenta (estrogen and progesterone). Non-steroid hormones are proteins peptide or amino acid. Two hormones from thyroid gland (thyroxine and triiodothyronine) and two from adrenal medulla (epinephrine and non epinephrine) are amino acid hormone. All other non-steroid hormones are protein and peptide hormones.

Steroid Hormones

Steroid hormones pass through cell membranes. Once inside the cell, a steroid hormone binds to its specific receptors. The hormone receptor complex then enters the nucleus, binds to part of the cell's DNA and activates certain genes (direct gene activation). In response to this activation, mRNA then enters the cytoplasm within the nucleus. The mRNA enters the cytoplasm and promotes protein synthesis. This protein may be enzymes that can have numerous effects on cellular processes — Structural proteins to be used for tissue growth and repair, Regulatory proteins that can alter enzyme function.

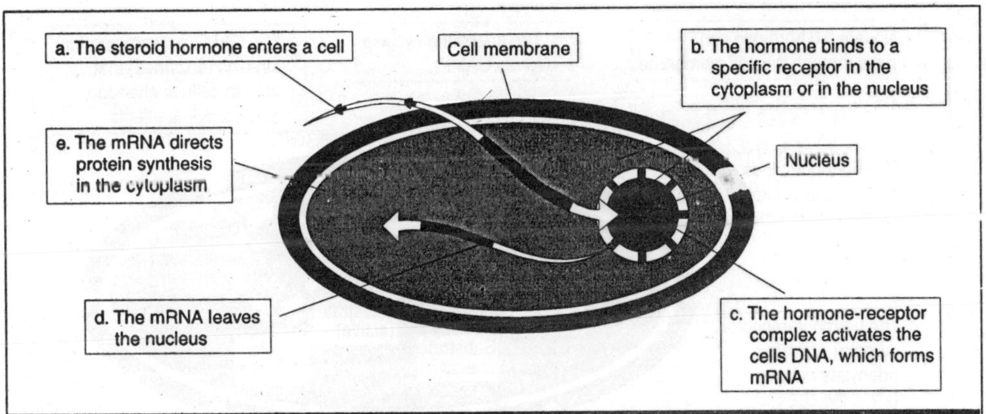

Fig. 13.1 : The mechanism of action of a steroid hormone, leading to direct gene activation

These processes, the activation of DNA and the synthesis of specific protein — take time to turn on (making the hormones involved 'slow acting hormones' but their effects are longer lasting than those generated by second messenger **(Guyton AC 1986)**. Many hormones, because or their size of highly charged structure, cannot easily pass cell membranes. These hormones exert their effects by binding to a receptor on the membrane surface and activating a G-protein located in the membrane of a cell. The G-protein is the link between the hormone receptor interaction on the surface of the membrane and the subsequent events inside the cell. The G-protein may open an ion channel to allow Ca^{++} to enter the cell or it may activate an enzyme in the membrane. If the G-protein activates adenylate cyclase then cyclic AMP (Cyclic 3' 5' adenosine monophosphate) is formed from ATP, in turn, the cyclic AMP concentration increases in the cell and activates protein which directly alters cellular activity.

If the G-protein activates a Ca^{++} ion channel, then Ca^{++} enters the cell and binds to and activates a protein called calmodulin. The activated calmodulin influences cellular activity in much the same way as cyclic AMP does. Lastly, a G-protein may activate a membrane-bound enzyme phospholipase C. When this occurs, a phospholipid in the membrane, phosphatidylinositol, is hydrolysed into two intracellular molecules, inositol triphosphate, which causes Ca^{++} release from intracellular molecules, and inositol triphosphate, which causes Ca^{++} release from intracellular stores and diacylglycerol. The diacylglycerol activates protein kinase C that, in turn, activate protein in the cell. Cyclic AMP Ca^{++} inositol triphosphate and diacylglycerol are viewed second messengers in the events following the hormone's binding to the receptors on the cell membrane. These second messengers should not be viewed as being independent of one another, because the changes in one can affect the action of the others **(Voet and Voet, 1990)**.

Non-steroid hormones

Non-steroid hormones cannot enter the cell easily, so they bind to receptors on the cell membrane, which triggers a series of enzymatic reactions that lead to the formation of an intracellular second messenger (Gama). Attachment of the hormone to the appropriate membrane receptor activates an enzyme adenyl cyclase, situated within the cell membrane. This enzyme catalyzes the formation of CAMP from cellular ATP.

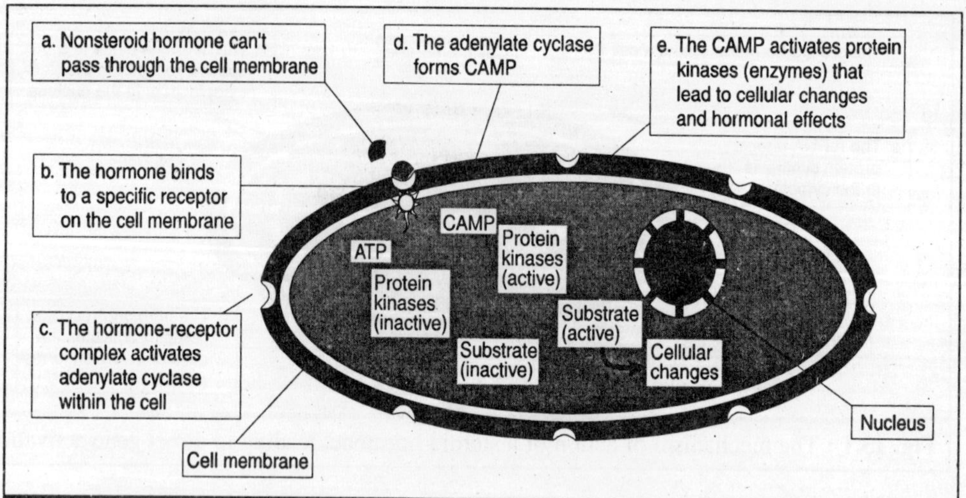

Fig. 13.2 : The mechanism of action of a non-steroid hormone, utilizing a second messenger (CAMP)

CAMP can then produce specific physiological responses that include — activation of cellular enzymes; change in membrane permeability; promotion of protein synthesis; change in cellular metabolism; stimulation of cellular secretions.

PITUITARY

The pituitary gland was once thought to be the master endocrine gland controlling many other glands and organs. It is now recognized that pituitary gland is largely controlled by hypothalamus. Muscular activity promotes sweating, and sweating causes loss of blood plasma, resulting in hemoconcentration and increased blood osmolality. Increased blood osmolality stimulates the hypothalamus. The hypothalamus, in turn, stimulates the posterior pituitary gland, which secretes ADH. ADH acts on kidneys increasing the water permeability of the renal tubules and collecting duct, leading to increased reabsorption of water. Plasma volume increases, resulting in blood osmolality decrease.

Exercise appears to be strong stimulant to the hypothalamus, because exercise increases the release of all anterior pituitary hormones. Of the six anterior pituitary hormones four are tropic hormones, meaning they affect the functioning of other endocrine glands. The exception to this is GH and PRL. GH is a potent anabolic agent. It promotes muscle growth and hypertrophy by facilitating amino acid transport into the cell. In addition, GH directly stimulates fat metabolism (Lipolysis) by increasing synthesis of enzyme involved in this process. Growth hormone levels are elevated during aerobic exercise, apparently in proportion to the exercise intensity and typically remain elevated for some time after exercise.

THYROID

Release of TSH from the anterior pituitary increases during exercise. TSH controls the release of triiodothyronine and thyroxine. So exercise-induced increase in TSH would be expected to stimulate the thyroid gland. Exercise indeed produces an increase in plasma thyroxine levels, but a delay occurs between the rise in TSH levels during exercise and the increase in plasma thyroxine levels. Furthermore, during prolonged submaximal exercise, thyroxine level remains relatively constant after a sharp initial increase as exercise begins and triiodothyronine levels tend to decrease. The two hormones increase the basal metabolic rate by as much as 60% to 100%. These hormones also increase protein synthesis (Synthesis of enzyme), increase the size and number of mitochondria in most cells, promote rapid cellular uptake of glucose, enhance glycolysis and gluconeogenesis and enhance lipid metabolism, increasing FFA availability for oxidation.

Calcitonin decreases plasma calcium concentration. It acts primarily on two targets — the bone and the kidney. In bone, calcitonin inhibits the activity of the osteoclast (the bone resorbing cells), thus inhibiting bone resorption. In the kidney, calcitonin increases urinary excretion of Ca^{++} by decreasing Ca^{++} reabsorption from the renal tubules. Calcitonin is primarily important in children, while their bones are rapidly growing and developing strength. This hormone is not a major regulator of Ca^{++} homeostasis in adult. But it does appear to offer some protection against excessive bone reabsorption.

As the plasma concentration of T3 and T4 increases, they inhibit the release of TSH releasing hormone from the hypothalamus as well TSH. This self-regulating system ensures the necessary level of T3 and T4 for the maintenance of normal metabolic rate. Recent evidence suggests that resistance training has little effect on pituitary (TSH) — thyroid (T3, T4) functions (**Alen et al, 1993**).

PARATHYROID

Parathormone is a principal regulator of plasma Ca^{++} concentration and it also regulates plasma phosphate. Its release is stimulate by a decrease in plasma Ca^{++} level. PTH has 3 targets — bone, intestine and kidney. In the bone, PTH stimulates osteoclast activity. This increases bone resorption, which releases both Ca^{++} and phosphate into the blood. In the intestine PTH increases Ca^{++} absorption indirectly by stimulating an enzyme that is required for the process of increased intestinal Ca^{++} absorption. Because PTH raises plasma level of phosphate, the additional phosphate must be removed. In kidney, it (PTH) increases Ca^{++} reabsorption but decreases phosphate reabsorption, which promotes urinary excretion to phosphate. Over an extended period, exercise increases bone formation. This results primarily from increased intestinal absorption of Ca^{++}, decreased urinary excretion of Ca^{++} and increased PTH levels. Conversely, immobilization or complete bed rest promotes bone resorption. During such a period, PTH level decreases.

The hormone stimulates bone to release Ca^{++} into the plasma, and simultaneously increases the renal absorption of Ca^{++}, both raise the plasma Ca^{++} level. Parathyroid hormone also stimulates the kidney to convert a form of vitamin D (Vitamin D3) into a hormone that increases the absorption of Ca^{++} from the gastrointestinal tract. Exercise increases the concentration of parathyroid hormone in the plasma (**Ljunghall et al, 1986, Ljunghall et al, 1988**).

ADRENAL GLAND (ADRENAL MEDULLA)

When the adrenal medulla is stimulated by sympathetic nervous system, approximately 80% of the secretion is epinephrine and 20% is norepinephrine, although these percentages vary with different physiological conditions. Epinephrine and norepinephrine help to face a real or perceived crisis. Although some of the specific actions of these two hormones differ, the two work together. Their combined effect includes — increased rate and force of heart contraction; increased metabolic rate; increased glycogenolysis in the liver and muscles; increased release of glucose and FFA into blood; redistribution of blood to the skeletal muscle; increased blood pressure; increased respiration.

Epinephrine and norepinephrine binds to α and β adrenergic receptors and bring about changes in cellular activity (eg increased heart rate, mobilization of fatty acids from adipose tissue) via second messengers. The different receptors cause changes in the cell's Ca^{++} concentrations. With increasing exercise intensity, plasma norepinephrine level increase markedly at work rate above 50% of VO_2 max. During steady state activity, lasting more than 3 hrs at 60% of VO_2 max, plasma level of both hormones rise. When the exercise bout ends, epinephrine levels return to resting levels within few minute of recovery, but nor-epinephrine can remain elevated for several hours.

ADRENAL CORTEX

Adrenal cortex secretes over 30 different steroid hormones referred to as corticosteroids. These are generally classified into 3 major types :

1. Mineralocorticoid
2. Glucocorticoid
3. Gonadocorticoid.

Mineralocorticoid maintains electrolyte balance in the ECF, especially Na^+ and K^+. Aldosterone (95% of all mineralocorticoid) works primarily by promoting renal reabsorption of Na^+, thus causing the body to retain Na^+. When Na^+ is retained so as water, thus aldosterone fights dehydration. Na^+ retention also leads to enhanced K^+ excretion. So aldosterone plays a role in potassium balance as well. For these reason, aldosterone secretion which is stimulated by many factors, including decreased plasma Na^+, decreased blood pressure and increased plasma K^+ concentration.

Glucocorticoids are essential for life, and maintain fairly constant plasma glucose level. Cortisol (95% of all glucocorticoid activity subserved) is known to stimulate gluconeogenesis to ensure adequate fuel supply; increase mobilization of FFA, making them a more available energy source; decrease glucose utilization, sparing it for the brain; stimulate protein catabolism to release amino acids for use in repair, enzyme synthesis and energy production. It acts as an inflammatory agent. It depresses immune reaction and increases the vasoconstriction caused by epinephrine.

Gonadocorticoids : These hormones are the same as those produced by reproductive organs. Apparently these cortical secretion have little effect in adults. The amount secreted is insignificant.

PANCREAS

Pancreas secretes two major hormones — insulin and glucagon. When plasma glucose level are elevated (hyperglycemia), such as after meal, pancreas receives signals to release insulin into the blood. Among its action, insulin facilitates glucose transport into the cell, specially those in muscle and connective tissue; promotes glycogenesis; inhibits gluconeogenesis. Pancreas secretes glucagon when the plasma glucose concentration falls below normal level (Hypoglycemia). Glucagon promotes increased breakdown of liver glycogen to glucose and increased gluconeogenesis. Both processes increase plasma glucose level. During exercise lasting 30 mins or longer, insulin level tends to decline, although plasma glucose conc. may remain relatively constant. Research has shown that the no. of availability of insulin receptors increases during exercise, increasing the body's sensitivity to insulin. This reduces the need to maintain high plasma insulin level for transporting glucose into the muscle cells. Plasma glucagon shows a gradual rise throughout the period of exercise. Glucagon primarily maintains plasma glucose concentrations by stimulating liver glycogenolysis and maintaining adequate plasma glucose level.

GONADS

The testes secrete androgen testosterone which is responsible for the development of male secondary sex characteristics and spermatogenesis. The critical role of the androgen is the promotion of skeletal muscle growth, which is particularly important to our understanding of strength training and gender difference in muscle growth. The androgenic effects of testosterone are responsible for muscle protein retention and muscle hypertrophy observed during strength training.

The ovaries secrete estrogen and progesterone. Estrogen promote development of the female secondary sex characteristics, the proliferative phase of the menstrual cycle, oogenesis, ovulation and many changes during pregnancy. Progesterone promote the secretory phase of the menstrual cycle, prepare the uterus for pregnancy and prepare the breast for lactation.

KIDNEY

Kidney releases erythropoietin which stimulates bone marrow and regulates RBC production. Research has shown that part of the adaptation when training at high altitude is an increased release of erythropoietin which, in turn, stimulates more RBC production and increases blood oxygen carrying capacity.

ENDOCRINE RESPONSE TO EXERCISE

CHO and fat metabolism are responsible for maintaining muscle ATP level. During prolonged exercise plasma glucose is increased by the combined action of glucagon, epinephrine, norepinephrine and cortisol. These hormones promote glycogenolysis and gluconeogenesis thus increasing the amount of glucose available for use as a fuel source. GH and thyroid hormone share these functions. Insulin helps the released glucose to enter the cells where it can be used for energy production. But insulin level declines during prolonged exercise, indicating that exercise facilitates the action of insulin so that less hormone is required during exercise than when at rest. Exercise may enhance insulin binding to receptors on muscle fibers (**Sutton and Farrell, 1988**).

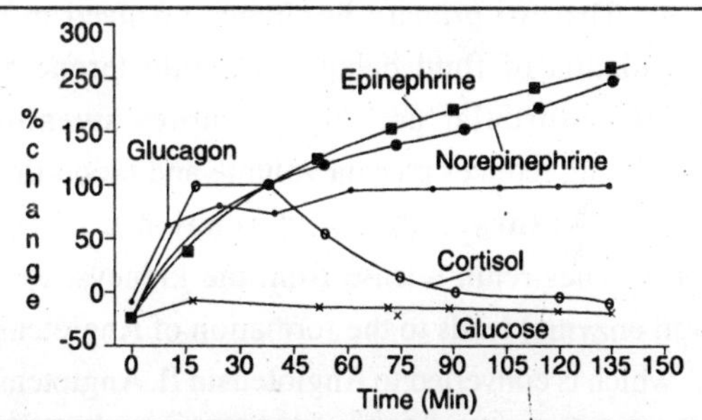

Fig. 13.3 : Changes in plasma level of epinephrine, glucagon, cortisol and glucose during three hours of cycling at 65% of VO_2 max

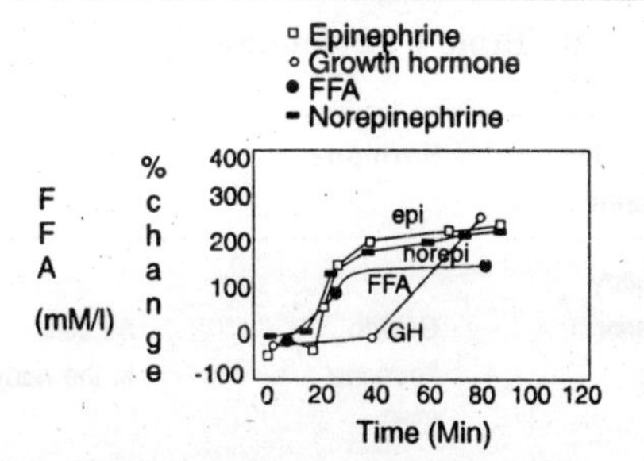

Fig. 13.4 : % changes of 4 major hormones during exercise

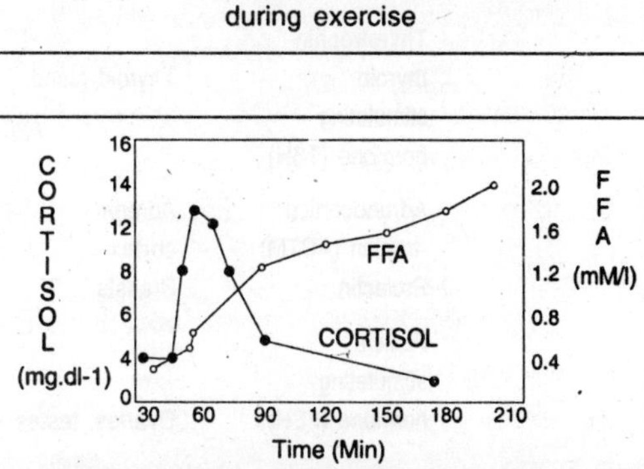

Fig. 13.5 : Response of cortisol during exercise

When CHO reserves are low, the body turns more to fat oxidation for energy, and this process is facilitated by cortisol, norepinephrine and GH. Cortisol accelerates lipolysis, resulting free fatty acids into the blood, so they can be taken up by the cells and used for energy production. But cortisol levels peak and then return to near normal levels during prolonged exercise. When this happens the catecholamine and GH take over cortisol's role.

The two primary hormones involved in the regulation of fluid balance are aldosterone and ADH. Muscular activity promotes sweating. Sweating reduces plasma volume and blood flows to the kidneys. Reduced renal blood flow stimulates renin release from the kidneys. Renin (an enzyme) leads to the formation of Angiotensin 1 which is converted to Angiotensin II. Angiotensin II stimulates the release of aldosterone from the adrenal cortex. Aldosterone increases Na^+ and H_2O reabsorption from the renal tubular plasma volume increases. ADH is released in response to increased plasma osmolality. When osmoreceptor in the hypothalamus senses this increase, the hypothalamus triggers ADH release from posterior pituitary. ADH acts on the kidney, promoting water conservation. Through this mechanism plasma volume is increased, which results in dilution of the plasma solutes. Blood osmolality decreases.

Loss of fluid (plasma) from the blood results in a concentration of the constituents of the blood, a phenomenon referred to as hemoconcentration. Conversely, a gain of fluid into the blood results in a dilution of the constituents of the blood, which is referred to as hemodilution. Hemoglobin is one of the substances diluted by plasma expansion. For this reason some athletes who actually have normal Hb level may appear to be anemic as a consequence of this Na^+ induced hemodilution. This condition must not be confused with true anemia, and can be remedied with few days of rest, allowing time for aldosterone levels to return to normal and the kidneys to unload the extra Na^+ and water.

Table 1 : Brief description of hormonal gland target organ and major functions

Endocrine Gland	Hormone	Target organ	Major Functions
Pituitary Anterior lobe	Growth hormone (GH)	All cells in the body	— Promotes development and enlargement of all body tissues up through maturations. — Increases rate of protein synthesis — Increases mobilization of fats and uses fat as an energy source. — Decreases rate of CHO utilization.
	Thyrotrophin thyroid stimulating hormone (TSH)	Thyroid gland	— Controls the amount of thyroxin and tri-iodothyronine produced and released by the thyroid gland.
	Adrenocortico -trophin (ACTM)	Adrenal cortex	— Controls the secretion of hormone from adrenal cortex.
	Prolactin	Breasts	— Stimulates breast development and milk secretion.
	Follicle stimulating hormone (FSH)	Ovaries, testes	— Initiate growth of follicles in the ovaries and promotes secretion of estrogen from the ovaries. — Promotes development of sperm in testes.

Endocrine Gland	Hormone	Target organ	Major Functions
	Luteinizing hormone (LH)	Ovaries, testes	— Promotes secretion of estrogen, progesterone and causes follicle to rupture, releasing the ovum — Causes testes to secrete testosterone, Posterior lobe
From hypo-thalamus	Antidiuretic Hormone (ADH) (or vasopressin)	Kidney	— Assists in controlling water excretion by the kidney — Elevates blood pressure by contracting blood vessels
	Oxytocin	Uterus, Breasts	— Stimulate contraction of uterine muscles; — Milk secretion
Thyroid	Thyroxine & Triiodothyronine	All cells in the body	(a) Increases the rate of cellular metabolism, increases the rate of contractility of the heart
	Calcitonin	Bones	(b) Controls calcium ion concentration in the blood
Parathyroid	Parathormone	Bones, Intestine & Kidneys	(c) Controls calcium ion concentration in ECF through its influence on bone, intestine and kidney
Adrenal Medulla	Epinephrine non-epinephrine	Most cells in the body Most cells in the body	— Mobilizes glycogen, increases skeletal muscle blood flow — Increases HR and contractility, O_2 consumption — Contracts arterioles and venules thereby BP
Cortex	Mineralocorticoid (aldosterone)	Kidney	— Increase Na^+ retention and K^+ excretion through kidney
	Glucocorticoid (cortisol)	Most cells in the body	— Control metabolism of CHO, Fat, Protein, anti-inflammatory action
	Androgen and Estrogen	Ovaries, breasts, testes	— Assists in the development of the female and male sex characteristics
Pancreas	Insulin	All cells in the body	— Control blood glucose level by lowering glucose level — Increases utilization of glucose and the synthesis of fat
	Glucagon	All cells in the body	— Increases blood glucose, stimulates the breakdown of protein & fat
	Somatostatin	Islets of Langerhans and G.I. tract	— Depresses the secretion of both insulin and glucagon
Gonads (testes)	Testosterone	Sex organ muscle	(a) Promote the development of male sex characteristics change in voice, promote muscle growth
Ovaries	Estrogen	Sex organ adipose tissue	(b) Promote development of female sex characteristics provide increased storage of fat Assist in regulating the menstrual cycle
Kidney	Renin Erythropoietin	Adrenal cortex Bone marrow	(c) Assists in BP control (d) Erythrocyte production

REFERENCE

Alen, M., Pakarinen, A. and Hakkinen, K. (1993) : Effects of prolonged training on serum thyrotropin and thyroid hormone in elite strength athletes, ***Journal of sports science*** 11 : 493-97.

Bonen, A. (1976) : Effect of exercise on excretion rates of urinary free cortisol, ***Journal of Applied Physiology*** 40 : 155-158.

Euler, US. Von (1969) : Sympatho-adrenal activity and physical exercise. ***In Biochemistry of Exercise, Medicine and Sports***, 3rd ed, J.R. Poortman, 170-81, New York, Karger, Basal.

Ganong, W. F. (1979) : ***Review of Medical Physiology***, Los Affas CA Lange Medical Publications

Guyton, A. C. (1986) : ***Test Book of Medical Physiology***, 7th eds, Philadelphia : W.B. Saunders.

Howley, E. T. (1976) : The effect of different intensities of exercise on the excretion of epinephrine, ***Medicine and Science in Sports*** 8 : 219-22.

James, D. E. (1995) : The mammalian facilitative glucose transporter family. International union physiology sciences, ***American Physiology Society*** 10 : 67-71.

Keizer, H. A. and A. D. Rogal (1990) : Physical exercise and menstrual cycle alterations : what are the mechanism? ***Sports Medicine*** 10 (4) : 218-35.

Laycock, J. F. and Wise, P. H. (1983) ***Essential Endocrinology***, New York, Oxford University Press.

Ljunghall, S. et al (1988) : Increase in serum parathyroid hormone levels after prolonged exercise. ***Medicine and Science in Sports and Exercise*** 20 : 122-25.

Ljunghall, S. et al, (1986) : Prolonged low intensity exercise raises the serum parathyroid hormone levels, ***Clinical Endocrinology*** 25 : 535-42.

Sutton, JR. and Farrell, P. (1988) : Endocrine responses to prolonged exercise; Exercise science and sports medicine, vol.I, Edited by D.R. Lamb and Murray : Indianapolis, Benchmark Press 1.

Voet, D. and Voet, J. G. (1990) : ***Biochemistry***, New York, John Wiley and Sons).

14

FOOD, NUTRITION AND SPORTS PERFORMANCE

Introduction

Diet significantly influences athletic performance. An adequate diet, in terms of quantity and quality, before during and after training and competition will maximise performance. In the optimum diet for most sports, carbohydrate (CHO) is likely to contribute about 60-70% of roal energy intake and protein about 12%, with the remainder coming from fat. Total energy intake must be raised to meet the increased energy expended during training and maintenance of energy balance can be assessed by monitoring body weight, body composition and food intake. Where there is a need to reduce body weight this should be done gradually, and not immediately before competition. In athletic events of high intensity and long duration (such as multiple sprint sports and endurance sports) performance is generally limited by carbohydrate availability. High carbohydrate diet (even in excess of two-thirds of total energy) maximum carbohydrate (glycogen) stores improve performance in such activity. A high carbohydrate diet is also necessary to sustain high intensity training on daily basis. After each bout of exercise, the diet should contain sufficient carbohydrate to replenish the glycogen stores and to maximise subsequent performance. The requirement for sugars and starch, in both solid and liquid forms, will vary, depending on the timing and nature of the physical activity. Increased fluid intake is necessary to avoid dehydration, and may improve performance during prolonged exercise, especially when sweat loss is high. These fluid may contain some carbohydrate, the concentration of which will be formulated considering the duration of exercise and climatic conditions. If exercise is of short duration and sweat loss is small, the replacement of salts can be achieved from a normal food intake after exercise. Protein requirements are higher in individuals involved in physical training programs than in inactive people. However, most athletes already consume sufficient protein as a consequence of their increased energy intake. Fat consumption should not be greater than 30% of total energy intake. Supplementary fat intake beyond this limit is not recommended for training or competition because the body is able to mobilise its large reserve of this energy store. Except where there is a need to reduce body fat content, it is important to maintain these stores by ingesting sufficient energy between periods of exercise. Vitamin supplementation are not necessary for athletes eating a diet adequate in respect of quantity and quality of the diet. Minerals and trace elements are essential for health, particular attention should be paid to iron and calcium status in those individuals who may be at risk. There is no good evidence to support the use of other nutritional supplements, including those commonly assumed by athletes to have ergogenic effects.

Limit of energy turnover in relation to physical performance, achievement of energy balance on a daily basis (1KJ = 0.2388KC)

Table 1 : Energy intake data of different endurance, strength and team sports athletes from Erp Barrt et al, 1989

Type of Sports	Sex	Energy intake (Kj Kg^{-1} day^{-1}) Mean	Range
Endurance			
Cycling	M	253	207 - 314
Swimming	M	221	119 - 300
Rowing	M	189	167 - 225
Running	M	193	127 - 311
Triathlon	M	272	246 - 295
Cycling	F	164	115 - 215
Running	F	168	123 - 218
Swimming	M	200	92 - 338
Strength			
Body building	M	157	106 - 183
Judo	M	157	76 - 210
Weight Lifting	M	167	99 - 203
Gymnastics	F	158	91 - 216
Body building	F	110	91 - 133
Team Sports			
Water polo	M	194	92 - 299
Soccer	M	192	118 - 287
Hockey	M	181	167 - 217
Volleyball	F	140	101 - 229
Hockey	F	145	91 - 199
Handball	F	142	78 - 271

(Subjects were elite athletes including European, world and Olympic medal winner. Data were obtained by 4 or 7 days' food diary. The main component of daily energy turnover(ADMR—average daily metabolic rate).

In the average subject, the energy expenditure for maintenance processes is usually called basal metabolic rate (BMR). This is the energy expenditure for the ongoing processes in the body at resting state, when no food is digested and no energy is needed for temperature regulation, i.e., in the post-absorptive state in a thermo-neutral environment. The remaining components of ADMR are the diet induced thermogenesis (DIT) and the energy expenditure for physical activity (EEA). DIT is a fraction of energy intake of about 10% depending on the micronutrient composition of the food consumed. EEA is the most valuable component of the daily energy turnover, ranging between an average value 25-30% up to 75% in extreme situation during heavy sustained exercise. Table 1 shows some examples of energy intake in endurance strength and team sports athletes.

Energy turnover in relation to physical performance during sports activity is limited to body composition. Body composition is a limiting factor in sports like gymnastics, body building and judo, where a low body mass or fat mass is preferable for performance when competing in specific weight class. In these types of sports, subjects often try to maintain a negative energy balance to lose weight. The other extreme includes endurance sports like cycling and triathlon, where the only way to success is the maintenance of energy balance at the upper limit of human performance in terms of energy turnover. Both topics — the consequence of a limiting energy intake on energy turnover and the upper limit of energy turnover during endurance exercises — will be discussed. Finally we will focus on two topics encountered by the average athlete, namely, changes in energy metabolism during the preparatory period when physical activity is gradually increased and how energy intake is regulated at a changing energy expenditure from day to day.

The lower limit of energy expenditure

Energy intake, especially for females, gymnasts and ballet dancers is often extremely low (**Erp-Baar et al, 1989, Dahlstrom et al, 1990**). Energy expenditure in the average sedentary subject ranges between 1.4 BMR and 1.6 BMR (**WHO, 1985**), while reported energy intake in top gymnast is usually below this level despite the fact that they trained for 3-4 hours a day. Whether the intake data are realistic or not, in some sports the athletes often limit energy intake to reduce body mass and fat mass with consequences for energy turnover and probably performance. The lower limit of ADMR is set by the sum of BMR, DIT and a minimum EEA. Reducing intake to lose mass reduces directly DIT and indirectly BMR while it is probably different to mobilise energy for physical activity, resulting in a lowered EEA as well. Subjects on a weight reducing diet show a reduction in their resting metabolic rate, not only through a loss of metabolic active tissue but also per unit active tissue. The efficiency of energy turnover goes up. There are indications that this phenomenon is more pronounced when energy restriction periods are repeated as practiced in some sports where weight control takes place before matches and required afterwards. The result is weight cycling and it may get increasingly difficult to lose weight while regaining it is facilitated (**Steen et al, 1988**).

Intensely training female athletes often encounter other problems when energy intake is restricted, namely menstrual dysfunction related decrease in bone density and iron deficiency anemia. There is a close relation between total energy intake and iron intake. Most male athletes meet their requirement, whereas some women, mainly due to menstruation losses may have a negative balance between intake and losses. This may lead to iron deficiency anemia. A high percentage of elite female athletes experience secondary amenorrhea. Though energy restriction is probably not the only reason, nutritional intake in amenorrheic athletes tends to be lower than in eumenorrheic athletes (**Deuster et al, 1986**). One of the important consequences of the amenorrhea is a decrease in bone density which predisposes a subject to stress fracture. Resumption of the menstrual function does not result in a complete regain of lost bone mass (**Drinkwater et al, 1990**).

Some studies indicate that performance capacity decreases either as a consequence of reduced carbohydrate intake and availability or as a result of the effects on fluid balance. There is also evidence for a reduction in spontaneous activity and so the body defends itself against a negative energy balance through a reduction of resting energy expenditure. People in a negative energy balance get slower and this cannot be the goal of an athlete. The long term effect of a negative energy balance is not only the loss of body fat but also the loss of fat free mass, i.e., of muscle mass. Wrestlers wanting to reduce their weight by a decrease in energy intake show a diminished protein nutritional status (**Craig et al, 1990**). The practice of starvation in order to achieve a rapid weight loss in the days before competition in weight category sports is well-known. Several methods are used including an increase in exercise instead of tapering off the training intensity and food restriction sometimes combined with deprivation or total absence of fluid intake. Besides the excessive losses of lean body mass, depletion of glycogen stores, the most important energy substrate for high intensity performance will occur. Therefore the net result is diminished body reserve for athletic events which more than offsets any advantage of competing in a lower weight classification (**Houston et al, 1981**).

The upper limit of energy expenditure

It is not known what sets the upper limit of energy turnover, energy intake or energy expenditure, i.e., the capacity to eat and produce food or the capacity to supply energy through oxidation. It is evident that the power output of the human muscle is higher on carbohydrate than on fat and protein and that the body store of carbohydrate energy in the form of glycogen can cover energy expenditure over 1-2 hours only. Thus the upper limit of power output during endurance exercise with an intensity higher than 60% of the aerobic power is increased when one can eat energy dense carbohydrate rich foods while one works, a common practice in cycle races.

It is clear that the energy turnover is directly related to the power output of the body. **Brouns et al, (1989)** did a simulation study, measuring the influence of diet manipulation on performance in subjects cycling for 2 days reaching a level of energy expenditure of 26 MJ per day. Subjects received a conventional solid diet with a high carbohydrate content (62.5% En) supplemented with water or the same diet supplemented with a 20% enriched carbohydrate liquid (total carbohydrate 80% En) subjects were able to maintain energy balance during the exercise days on the carbohydrate supplemented diet while on the water supplemented solid diet the energy intake was 5-10 MJ per day too low. Under such conditions the athlete must drink and eat to maintain body carbohydrate stores during the exercise as well as to replete the stores within 18H for the exercise performance on the next day. From respiratory exchange measurements, an oxidation rate of nearly 139 carbohydrate kg^{-1} day^{-1} was calculated.

The actual intake in the carbohydrate supplemented experiment was 16 g carbohydrate kg^{-1} day^{-1} suggesting that, also with respect to carbohydrate intake, there is a ceiling in the energy intake above which other factors play a role in relation to fatigue. The alternative, a higher intake of fat, which has a higher energy density is not appropriate in top sports performance because for maximal power output the muscle needs carbohydrate instead of fat. From these experiments it become clear that energy intake cannot meet energy expenditure at high working levels even when high carbohydrate conventional foods are consumed unless energy-dense, carbohydrate-rich liquid formulae are supplemented, which can be ingested in large enough quantities. Subjects working long hours at high intensity do not have enough time to consume the process food outside the exercise period to balance the energy expenditure. Therefore the practice of consuming large quantities of liquid carbohydrate rich formulations is one of the appropriate nutritional strategies to optimise performance during extreme sustained exercise.

Changes in energy expenditure during a training program

Novice athletes starting a training program change their physical activity with consequences for the energy turnover depending on the intensity and the duration of training bouts. Two studies provide data on this both in novice athletes preparing for running a marathon **(Janssen et al, 1989)** and half marathon **(Westerterp et al, 1991)**. Energy expenditure, as measured before 8, 20 and 40 weeks after the start of the training period with doubly labelled water, showed an initial increase of an average 30% and remained stable afterward. The training volume of the subjects doubled after the energy turnover had stabilised at 1.3 times the pre-training level. It is revealed that the subjects already in the beginning of the training period, after 8 weeks-reached a natural limit of their daily energy turnover. Afterwards, they could increase their training volume without the increase of the energy expenditure by an increasing efficiency as a mere result of the training.

Initially the increase in ADMR was two to three times higher than one would expect from training distance and the running cost measured on a treadmill (**Meijer, 1990**). There were no indications that the training had an influence on the level of spontaneous physical activity (**Meijer et al, 1991**).

Subjects in the two studies were real novice athletes. At the start of the training period they were sedentary as can be seen from their physical activity index (PAI = ADMR/BMR) the initial PAI value was 1.66 ± 0.07 (Mean ± SD) close to the value of 1.54 for sedentary subjects (**WHO, 1985**). The PAI value after 8 weeks of training was 2.03 ± 0.18 close to the value of 2.14 for the subjects engaged in hard work.

One indication for the increase in the efficiency of energy turnover after the start of the training, apart from changes during the training itself, is a change in resting metabolic rate. Though there are indications for an increase in resting metabolic rate directly after an exercise bout, in the long term, subjects showed a decrease in their resting energy expenditure. In male resting metabolic rate as measured in a respiratory chamber, was 4% lower ($p < 0.05$) after 40 weeks of training. In female the same tendency was observed (**Westerlerp and Saris, 1992**). The decrease in resting metabolic rate combined with the increase in lean body mass, especially in the males who even gained significantly more LBM than the females ($p < 0.05$), is more evidence for an increase in energy efficiency during the training period.

Despite the lack of change in the quantity of energy consumed as measured by self report there are systematic changes in the quality of food consumption in dietary records in the course of a training program. **Jenssen et al (1989)** reported an increase in the precentage En CHO from 47 to 55% and 48-52% in females and males, respectively, over 18 months while preparing for marathon. The increase in CHO consumption was at the expense of dietary fat. Thus the increase in physical activity caused a favourable change in food habits with regard to the nutritional guideline for good health. There were no indications of a gender difference in substrate utilization as suggested by **Tarnapolsky et al, 1990**. They got indications of a higher capacity for fat utilization during endurance exercise in females compared with males, suggesting a lower need for dietary CHO in the former group.

CARBOHYDRATE AND EXERCISE

Over the past decade, sports nutrition dogma was that high carbohydrate (CHO) diet (consisting of 60-70% of total energy intake) were necessary for optimal performance (**William, 1995, Costill, 1992**). This high CHO diet was recommended in order to maintain muscle glycogen stores during intense training and enable athletes to work at higher training loads (**William, 1993**). However, studies have found that athletes are not following this advice. The range of CHO intake generally falls between 40-60% (**Fabes et al, 1990; Hawler et al, 1995**). Recently, it has been discussed whether CHO diet of over 60% total energy intake are necessary or not (**Hawley et al, 1995**). **Hawley et al (1995)** pointed out that if an athlete ingests 20.92 MJ/day (5000 Kcal/day) with only 45% CHO, the average athlete will then consume more than 550 g CHO per day. This amount appears sufficient to restore muscle glycogen within a 24 hour period. Furthermore, chronically elevating CHO to 60-70%s of total energy for athletes who are restricting calorie intake (female long distance runners, dancers, gymnasts), may reduce fat or protein intake that would jeopardies health and performance. For example, very low fat intake may impair the status of fat soluble vitamins.

Recent attention has also focussed on possible benefits of a high fat diet (**Sherman and Leenders, 1995**). The basis for suggesting that high fat diet will improve performance probably developed from studies that raised fatty acid levels in the blood and documented an increased rate of fat oxidation. Both infusion and ingestion of fat were found to elevate plasma-free fatty acids and spare muscle glycogen during exercise (**Dyck et al, 1993; Vukovich et al, 1993, Griffith et al, 1994**).

Several studies have examined effects of short term high fat diets on exercise performance and results have been equivocal (**Sherman and Leenders, 1995**). **Guezennec (1992)** reviewed the role of lipids in endurance exercise and questioned the theoretical basis for ingesting a high fat diet for ergogenic effects. **Sherman and Leenders (1995)** in a more recent review concluded that high fat diets may not be effective in enhancing performance. Endurance performance was examined after 7 moderately trained participants ingested either a high fat (76%) or a high CHO (76%) diet for 4 days (**Johannessen et al, 1981**). The participants on the high fat diet showed a shorter time to exhaustion when running on a treadmill. Another study also found that a high fat diet ingested by 5 trained cyclists did not improve endurance time (**Dhinney et al, 1983**). In contrast, a diet of 38% fat ingested by 6 trained runners for 7 days resulted in greater endurance time compared with a 24% fat diet (**Muoio et al, 1994**). These authors suggested that restriction of dietary fat (by ingesting a high CHO diet) may be detrimental to endurance performance. Ingesting a high fat diet (70% fat) for two weeks improved endurance time during moderately intense cycling in 5 trained cyclists compared with a high CHO diet (12% fat) (**Lambart et al, 1994**). Interestingly, an improvement in endurance after the high fat diet occurred although the initial muscle glycogen levels were twice as low as with the high CHO diet.

At present there are insufficient data to state with certainty that high fat diet can improve performance, and there are some data to suggest that these diets could be detrimental to performance. However, the relationship of high blood fat levels and cardiovascular disease questions the practice of using a high fat diet to alter performance when it may negatively affect health.

Carbohydrate utilization during exercise

Muscle glycogen initially degraded to glucose-1-phosphate by the action of phosphorylase and then converted to glucose-6-phosphate. Glucose is taken from the blood by a carrier mediated process and phosphorelated to glucose-6-phosphate in a reaction catalysed by hexokinase. Thus glucose-6-phosphate represents a common entry point for glucose and glycogen into the series of cytosotic reactions, known as glycolysis or the Embden-Meyerhof pathway, which produces pyruvate. The major fate of pyruvate is oxidation in the Kreb's cycle and electron transport chain. However, if the rate of pyruvate formation exceeds the rate of pyruvate oxidation lactate will be produced. The degradation of 1 mole of glucose and glycogen to lactate results in the generation of 2 and 3 moles of ATP, respectively. In contrast the complete oxidation of glucose and glycogen to CO_2 and H_2O produces 38 and 39 moles of ATP, respectively. The oxidation of CHO yields 21.1 KJ (5.05 Kcal) per liter of oxygen consumed.

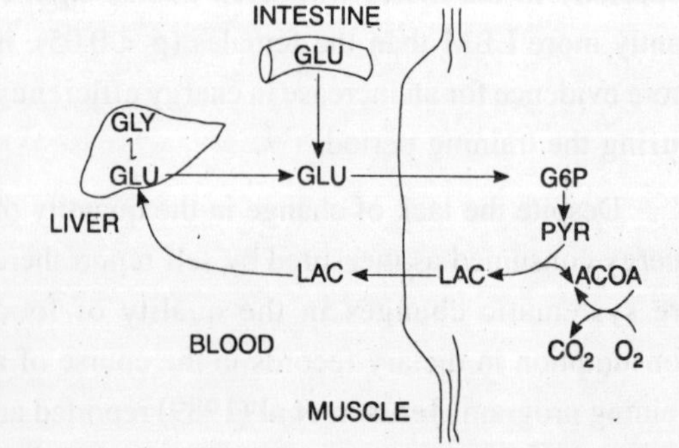

Fig. 14.1 : Overview of carbohydrate interactions during exercise

During high intensity dynamic exercise (eg sprinting, track cycling, interval training multiple sprint sports such as football, hockey), the breakdown of high energy phosphates (ATP-CP) and degradation of glycogen are the predominant energy yielding pathways. It is possible that subpopulation of the fast twitch muscle fibers are depleted of glycogen during intense exercise. Furthermore, it has been demonstrated that increased dietary CHO intake can improve high intensity exercise performance while inadequate CHO intake impair performance (**Maughan, 1990**). There is also greater reliance on phosphogens and muscle glycogen during static contraction above 20-30% MVC, where increased intramuscular pressure results in occlusion of the arterial blood supply, thereby limiting oxygen and blood bound substrate delivery. During prolonged exercise requiring 60-85% of maximal oxygen uptake, muscle glycogen is an important substrate for oxidative metabolism. Its rate of utilization is most rapid during the early stages of exercise (**Yollestad et al, 1984**) and is exponentially related to exercise intensity (**Saltin and Karlsson, 1971; Vollestad and Bln, 1985**).

Fatigue during such exercise is often associated with depletion of glycogen in the contracting muscle, specially in those fibers recruited during exercise (**Harmansen et al, 1967**); (**Vollestad et al, 1989**). In addition, the pattern of muscle glycogen depletion is influenced by the mode of exercise. Cycling exercise results in glycogen loss predominantly in vastus lateralis, during running it is greater in gastrocnemius and soleus. The close relationship between muscle glycogen depletion and fatigue appears to be due to the inability of glycogen depleted muscle cells to maintain a sufficient rate of ATP re-synthesis. Recent studies have observed increase in the ATP breakdown products IMP and ammonia in muscle depleted of glycogen (**Broberg and Saltin 1989; Norman et al, 1987**). Furthermore another possible effects of lowered muscle glycogen availability is the loss of substrate in particular pyruvate, for anaplerotic reactions that provide Krebs cycle intermediates necessary for the continued oxidation of acetyl units derived from other substrate (**Sahlin et al, 1990**).

The increase in skeletal muscle glycogenolysis that occurs during exercise is the result of a number of local and systemic regulatory factors. These include calcium and cyclic AMP mediated activation of phosphorylase, allosteric activation of phosphorylase and phosphofructokinase by a number of muscle metabolites and alterations in substrate availability (**Hargreaves and Richter, 1988; Hargreaves, 1990**). Although muscle glycogen is the predominant carbohydrate energy source during the early stages of exercise, blood glucose becomes more important as exercise continued (**Wahren et al, 1971**). Muscle glucose uptake can increase up to 30-40 times the resting levels depending upon the exercise intensity during (**Katz et al, 1986; Wahren et al, 1971**). This increase in glucose uptake is achieved by activation of the membrane mechanisms involved in glucose transport and the enzyme responsible for glucose disposal. The important regulatory factors include membrane glucose transporter numbers and activity, sarcoplasmic calcium, circulation insulin levels and glucose availability (**Hargreaves, 1990; Holloszy et al, 1986**). Accompanying the increased peripheral utilisation of glucose during exercise is an increase in hepatic glucose output. Initially this is due to accelerated glycogenolysis, but, as exercise continues, gluconeogenesis becomes more important with lactate, pyruvate glycerol and alanine being major gluconeogenic precursors (**Fetig and Wahren, 1975**). During prolonged exercise lasting several hours, hepatic glucose output may fall behind peripheral glucose utilisation resulting in hypoglycemia (**Fetig et al, 1982**). Although the breakdown of muscle glycogen and blood glucose provides pyruvate for oxidation, another important function during exercise is the generation of lactate which can be used as a gluconeogenic precursor and a substrate for contracting muscle (**Brooks, 1986**).

In view of the importance of CHO during exercise, the resynthesis of the CHO reserves, in particular muscle glycogen, following exercise is a critical metabolic process in the recovery period. Although exercise will activate glycogen synthase in muscle (**Bak and Padersen, 1990**). Full restoration of muscle glycogen during recovery is dependent upon an adequate CHO intake. There are a number of factors influencing the rate of muscle glycogen resynthesis, most notably the type and amount of CHO ingested and the timing of CHO ingestion (**Costill, 1988**). It has been reported that exercise induced muscle damage can impair muscle glycogen resynthesis, an effect that in partially overcome by increasing CHO intake (**Costill et al, 1990**). There appears to be preferential resynthesis of muscle glycogen reserves following exhaustive exercise; however, once this process is complete, liver glycogen levels will return to normal as long as CHO intake is adequate.

Factors influencing CHO utilisation during exercise

Muscle glycogen and glucose utilisation is influenced by a number of factors. These include exercise intensity and duration, training status diet, environment, age and gender.

Exercise intensity and duration

As exercise intensity reaches and exceeds maximal oxygen uptake, muscle glycogen utilisation increases markedly and blood glucose utilisation declines. This provides an energetic advantage, since slightly more ATP is generated from the breakdown of glycogen than glucose. The critical role of CHO, in particular muscle glycogen, during exercise above 65-70% of maximal oxygen uptake is demonstrated by the observation that patients suffering from a glycogen phosphorylase deficiency (McArdle's disease) have a maximal exercise capacity that is 40-50% of the expected normal value (**Lewis and Haller, 1986**). Furthermore, there is evidence that the dominant use of fat as a substrate cannot normally support exercise above 60-65% of maximal oxygen uptake (**Davies and Thompson, 1979**). Thus the intense training loads undertaken by competitive athletes place a large demand on their CHO reserves and necessitate increased dietary CHO intake if they are to avoid CHO deficiency that will impair their ability to train effectively.

As exercise duration increases, there is a declining contribution from CHO and increased availability of plasma-free fatty acids. Nevertheless, even during prolonged exercise lasting several hours, there is a reliance on CHO to provide pyruvate for ongoing free fatty acid oxidation. In game situation, intermittent high intensity efforts are performed over 30-90 min and under such conditions there is also likely to be heavy dependence upon CHO reserves.

Training Status

There is a marked decrease in muscle glycogen utilisation and lactate production during exercise at the same absolute and relative intensity following endurance training (**Hurley et al, 1986; Janson and Kaijser, 1987**). The reduction in glucose turnover is likely to result in smaller liver glycogen utilisation during exercise. The reduction in carbohydrate utilisation is generally believed to be due to the increase in muscle oxidative capacity that occurs in response to training. Such adaptation promotes an increase in the aerobic breakdown of CHO, an increase reliance on fat oxidation and less stimulation of glycolysis during exercise (**Holloszy and Coyle, 1984**). Although the reliance on CHO is lower following training, athletes still need to be aware of the need for adequate dietary CHO, since, as a consequence of training, they will be able to train and compete at higher exercise intensities.

Diet

Carbohydrate oxidation and muscle glycogen utilisation during exercise are greater following consumption of a high CHO diet, presumably due to the relative hyperinsulinemia and increased CHO availability. The increase in muscle glycogen utilisation (**Sherman et al, 1981**) appears to be counteracted by the greater glycogen availability, since endurance performance is enhanced by glycogen loading (**Bergstrom et al, 1967. Karlsson and Saltin, 1971**). In contrast, following consumption of a high fat diet or after 3-4 days fast, carbohydrate oxidation, muscle glycogen utilisation and glucose turnover during exercise are lower than after a mixed diet or in the post-absorptive state, respectively (**Bergstrom et al, 1967; Janson and Kijser 1982; Knapic et al, 1988**). These effects appears to be due to a reduction in CHO availability and the inhibitory effects of lipid metabolites on CHO utilisation, the so-called "glucose-fatty acid cycle". Recent work has demonstrated reduced muscle glucose uptake during exercise in the presence of elevated plasma levels of lipid metabolites (**Hargreaves et al, 1991**), although their effect on muscle glycogen utilisation during exercise is less clear (**Costill et al, 1977; Hargreaves et al, 1991**).

Environment

During exercise in the heat there is an increase in muscle glycogen utilisation (**Fink et al, 1975**), although this has not been observed in all studies (**Nielsen et al, 1990, Young et al, 1985**). A reduction in muscle blood flow, although controversial (**Nielsen et al, 1990**), increased muscle temperature and elevated catecholamines may all contribute to a stimulation of muscle

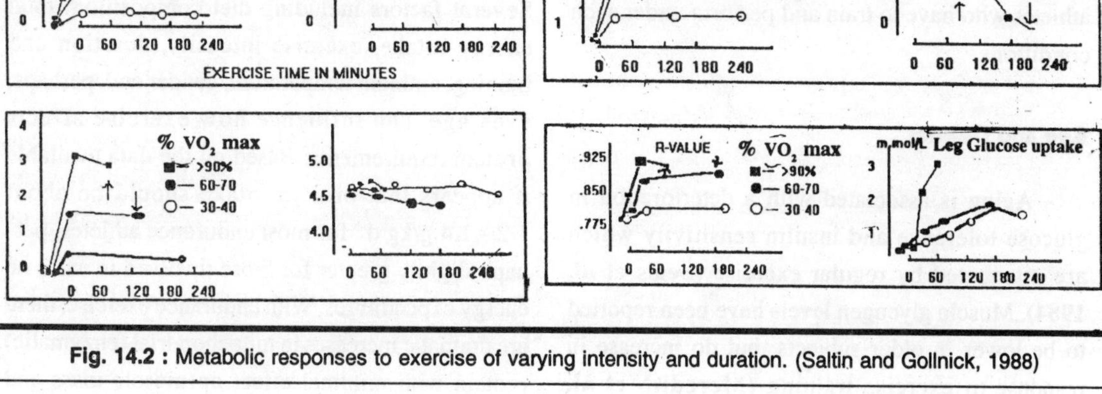

Fig. 14.2 : Metabolic responses to exercise of varying intensity and duration. (Saltin and Gollnick, 1988)

glycogenolysis during exercise in the heat. It has recently been demonstrated that muscle glycogen is an important substrate for shivering thermogenesis in humans during cold exposure (**Martinean and Jacob, 1988**) and that muscle glycogen utilisation is greater during high exercise at 9°C compared with 21°C, although this difference is not seen at higher exercise intensities (**Jacobs et al, 1985**). The increased circulating catecholamines observed in cold environment may account in part for these observations. Expose to hypoxic environments is associated with an increase in blood lactate, which may reflect an accelerated glycogenolysis or a reduction in lactate clearance. Glucose disposal, as measured using tracer technique, is greater during exercise under hypoxic conditions (**Cooper et al, 1986**). However, this may not necessarily result in increased blood glucose utilisation, since there is intracellular accumulation of glucose in contracting muscle under such condition (**Kats and Sahlin, 1989**). Following adaptation to altitude there appears to be 'Sparing' of muscle glycogen (**Young et al, 1982**), which may reflect either increased mobilisation and utilisation of free fatty acid (**Young et al, 1982**) or an inability to fully activate skeletal muscle during exercise (**Green et al, 1989**). These observed effects of environment on CHO metabolism during exercise may well have implications for the dietary CHO-requirements of athletes who have to train and perform under such conditions.

Age and Gender

Aging is associated with a deterioration in glucose tolerance and insulin sensitivity which are attenuated by regular exercise (**Seals et al, 1984**). Muscle glycogen levels have been reported to be lower in older subjects, but do increase in response to exercise training (**Meredith et al, 1989**). Glycogen utilisation, expressed per unit of unit of energy expenditure during submaximal exercise, is higher in the elderly (**Meredith et al, 1989**).

It has often been suggested that there is a greater reliance on fat oxidation during exercise in female compared with male subject, although studies have produced conflicting results (**Costill et al, 1979; Froberg and Pedersen, 1984**). In a recent study the metabolic responses of male and female subject, matched for training status and diet, were studied during exercise at 60-65% of maximal oxygen uptake (**Tarnopol sky et al, 1990**). Muscle glycogen utilisation was 25% lower and estimated total CHO oxidation was 43% lower in the female subjects. In contrast, (**Brewar et al, 1988**) have observed no differences in the metabolic responses to treadmill running and increased dietary carbohydrate intake between male and female runners. Further work is required to examine the extent of gender differences in the metabolic response to exercise and whether such differences, if they exist, result in differences in dietary CHO requirements.

EFFECT OF EXERCISE ON PROTEIN REQUIREMENT

Existing evidence strongly indicate that daily protein needs are increased as a result of either regular strength speed or endurance exercise. Several factors including diet composition, total energy intake, exercise intensity, duration and training, ambient temperature, gender and, perhaps, even age, can influence how exercise affects protein requirements. Based on the data available it appears that protein intake should be about 1.2 - 1.4 g/kg d^{-1} for most endurance athletes, perhaps slightly greater for those involved in extreme energy expenditures. With endurance exercise, there are dramatic increases in mitochondrial (enzymatic) protein with minimal effect on muscle mass and strength (myofibrillar protein) while, in strength or speed exercise, there is little change in mitochondrial protein but the gain in muscle mass and strength are truly phenomenal. In situations, where energy demands are high for prolonged time, protein may provide a significant quantity of amino acids for use an auxiliary exercise fuel (Fig. 14.2). If so, inadequate dietary protein and/or overtraining could lead to losses of endogenous protein (probably both liver and muscle) and, eventually, to impaired exercise performance. In contrast, when an attempt is made to increase cell mass (hypertrophy), additional dietary protein may be necessary to provide sufficient amino acids to maximize protein synthesis (Fig. 14.2-4). As with endurance training, strength or speed training can also be done too frequently. In this case, the exercise catabolic response exceeds the subsequent anabolic response and the overall result is either reduced gains or even decreases muscle mass and strength. Perhaps additional dietary protein can minimize this effect and, therefore, produced greater exercise induced hypertrophy. In addition, some degree of muscle soreness is frequently present following exercise, specially with eccentric exercise, and both structural changes in muscle (mitochondrial swelling, degenerating fibers, contractile protein disorientation, etc.) and efflux of muscle specific enzymes into the vascular system have been reported (**Berg and Haralambai, 1978; Janssen et al, 1989 Kuipers et al, 1989**). Additional dietary protein might help to promote the recovery/repair process and, as a result, improve exercise performance.

For strength, speed athletes protein intakes of 1.2-1.7g/kg d^{-1} should be sufficient to maintain positive nitrogen balance. Although it is frequently stated that high protein intakes are harmful there is no reason to suspect intake at these levels will cause any problem (**Lemon, 1991, b**). Finally, despite the fact that these protein intakes exceeds most current recommendations for sedentary individuals, it is not necessary for all athletes to increase their protein intake because, as a result of very high energy intakes, many athletes routinely consume 1.2-2.0 g/kg d^{-1}. Therefore, before deciding to increase protein intake a complete dietary evaluation should be performed to determine if addition is necessary.

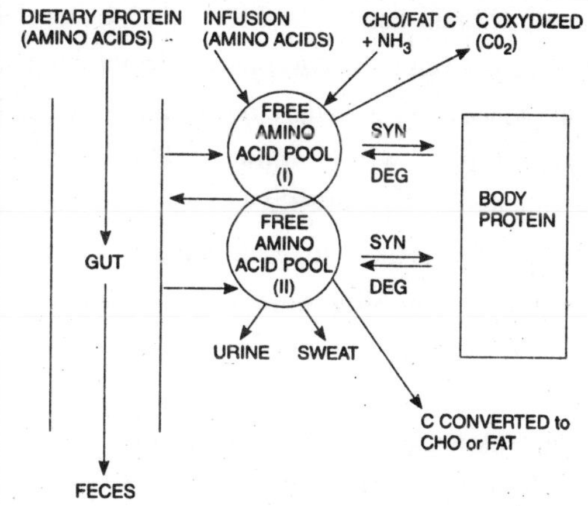

Fig. 14.3 : Schematic representation of protein metabolism

Exercising muscle can take up branch chain amino acids (BCAAs) from the blood and oxidise them (**Ahlborg et al, 1974, Hag et al, 1982; Wolfe et al 1982**). Ingestion of BCAAs resulted in greater muscle production of ammonia and it was suggested that BCAA should provide significant source of ammonia to the exercising muscle, but any ergogenic effect this might have has not been proven (**Maclean et al, 1994**). **Davis, 1995 (a, b)** proposed that BCAAs may be involved in reducing central fatigue due to increased brain level of serotonin (5-hydroxytryptamine 5-HT). Serotonin levels are increased by circulating levels of the amino acid tryptophan. BCAAs in the blood compete with tryptophan for transport across the blood-brain barrier. In theory, the greater the circulating levels of BCAAs, the smaller the amount of tryptophan will cross the blood-brain barrier, and central fatigue will be reduced. However, ingesting the amounts of BCAAs necessary to exert such an effect is likely to result in gastrointestinal disturbances and slow water transport across the gut, both being disadvantageous during exercise.

IMPORTANCE OF FAT AS A SUPPORT NUTRIENT FOR ENERGY METABOLISM OF ATHLETES

In contrast to limited CHO stores, the lipid stores in the human body are, from a practical standpoint, unlimited to take some examples to illustrate this point, jogging at about 2/3rd of maximal aerobic power requires in the order of 1.2 to 2 MJ (3-500 Kcal/h). Similarly, a Marathon run of 4-5 h duration would require less than 1 kg of body fat, provided only fat was utilized for combustion. The problem with lipid utilisation during exercise is not the physical availability of fat as an energy source, but to bring the lipid to the site of oxidation in the muscles, and actually have it used in the oxidative process to furnish energy. Lipid for utilisation during exercise is present in three forms : triglycerides in adipose tissue (the main store); triglycerides within the muscle and circulating triglycerides, primarily in very low density lipoprotein, produced by the liver as well as chylomicron transporting exogenous, absorbed lipid.

The intermediate triglyceride stores in muscle, which are limited in sine to about 10-40 mol/kg/W.W (**Essen et al, 1977; Hurley et al, 1986; Broun et al, 1989**) are utilized during work, because they decrease in mass under appropriate exercise condition. There is evidence that fatty acid reesterification is also going on in muscle during exercise. The latter probably occurs during conditions of excess mobilisation of adipose tissue triglycerides. It seems most likely that the local muscular stores are tagged of their energy during exercise and that the net mass of these depots is dependent on the balance between influx from circulating free fatty acids (FFA) from adipose tissue, and efflux to the machinery from transforming fat to utilize energy in the muscle. The main sources of lipid energy comes from adipose tissue, which contains almost 400 MJ (100,000 Kcal) in a sedentary person.

This lipid is stored as triglyceride which first has to be hydrolyzed to FA and glycerol before being mobilized. The fat depots drained by portal vein as the FA produced will reach the liver directly and in high concentrations. The liver will transform the excess of these FA, which are not needed for oxidation purpose in the liver to very low density lipoprotein (VLDL). These VLDL are then utilized in the periphery for energy purposes in muscle during exercise. These circulating triglycerides also have to be hydrolyzed before they enter the muscle tissue. This is catalysed by lipoprotein lipase localized at the level of the capillary endothelium, where circulating VLDL are captured for hydrolysis of their triglyceride. This enzyme has an increased activity in muscle and heart during fasting conditions, while the adipose tissue enzyme is activated in the postprandial state to facilitate uptake of circulating exogenous lipid by adipose tissue.

The main mobilizer of fat for exercise purpose is the sympathetic nervous system, with varying capacity to stimulate the lipase system. The beta adrenergic receptors have been found in three different forms (BAR 1, BAR 2 and BAR 3). The nerve endings release the lipolytic hormone norepinephrine, which stimulates triglyceride hydrolysis by activation of a specific hormone-sensitive lipase. In addition, there are adrenergic receptors, also of different kinds (AAR, and AAR2) where clearly the AAR2 inhibit lipolysis. The end result in terms of net lipolysis is dependent on which of these receptors are stimulated. The regula tion of the net balance of the density of the lipolytic BAR's and antilipolytic AAR's is poorly known but it seems likely that steroid hormone might be involved in these processes.

After stimulation of the adrenergic receptors, signals are sent through a system of stimulatory (GS) or inhibitory (G1) proteins which activate or inhibit a cyclase enzyme in the adipocyte membrane. Through a protein kinase system the hormone sensitive lipase protein is phosphorylated and becomes active to facilitate triglyceride cleavage in the 1, 3 (outer) positions of the triglyceride. The 2 (middle) position is then hydrolyzed by a monoglyceride lipase which is apparently not rate limiting for triglyceride hydrolysis.

Once liberated by these hydrolytic process the glycerol molecule diffuses out of adipose tissue and is used mainly for gluconeogenetic purposes in the liver. The fatty acids also diffuse out and are then bind to albumin and transported to various end organs. Some of them are reesterified within the adipocyte to from new triglycerides. This process is dependent on the availability of glucose transported into the adipocyte by the action of insulin. During exercises the majority of fatty acids hydrolyzed are mobilized from the adipocyte and transported as FFA bound to albumin, to be used by the contracting muscle.

The lipolytic process is stimulated by exercise, but this occurs gradually and does not cease when exercise has ended. The main stimulator of FFA mobilisation by lipolysis is the SNS. There are also inhibitory factors which keep the system in balance. Insulin is the most important counter regulatory hormone for this process and act mainly by stimulating phosphodiesterase, which breaks down CAMP to AMP, thereby preventing the stimulation by CAMP of the hormone sensitive lipase. Insulin concentrations are suppressed during exercise, with the SNS inhibiting release of insulin, facilitating lipid mobilisation by diminishing the inhibitory effect of insulin. Lactate may also directly inhibit the lipolytic process. Beta adrenergic blocking drugs and nicotinic acid derivatives inhibit lipolytic process, and thereby the availability of FFA for working muscle, might be hazardous when the glycogen stores and circulating glucose are limited with training the lipolytic process becomes more sensitive to stimulate by adaptation at the level of the adrenergic receptors. The BAR's increase in density and the cyclase system is also more active. Insulin and lactate production depicted low, both shifting towards a more efficient delivery of lipid substrate to the oxidative process in the muscle. Finally the signals from the SANS for lipid metabolisations are less pronounced at the same submaximal work load. In other words, the whole system has adapted towards more economy and efficiency than before physical training.

NUTRITION FOR IMPROVED SPORTS PERFORMANCE

Many athletes look to various nutritional manipulations to improve their performance. While some manipulations have been scientifically documented to enhance performance, others, like high fat diets, are controversial. Many supplements marketed as ergogenic aids are based on data from animal studies or in vitro experiments with little or no scientific evidence that they are effective performance enhancer in humans. An overview of nutritional manipulations designed to improve performance that have received recent attention in the literature as well as notoriety in the athletic community are discussed. The discussion also focused at the possible mechanism of action of these nutritional manipulations and their effectiveness.

Branched-Chain Amino Acids (BCAAs)

Exercising muscle can take up BCAAs from the blood and oxidise them (**Ahlborg et al, 1974; Haggs et al, 1982; Wolfe et al, 1982**). Although it was speculated that ingestion of BCAAs should result in improved performance by supplying muscle with another usable substrate, studies have not confirmed this even when BCAAs were infused (**Blomstrand et al, 1995; Vanier et al, 1994**). Ingestion of BCAAs resulted in greater muscle production of ammonia, and it was suggested that BCAAs could provide a significant source of ammonia to the exercising muscle, but any ergogenic effect this might have has not been proven (**MacLean et al, 1994**).

Davis (1995 & 1995a) proposed that BCAAs may be involved in reducing central fatigue due to increased brain levels of serotonin (5-hydroxytryptamine; 5-HT). Serotonin level are increased by circulating levels of the amino acid tryptophan. BCAAs in the blood compete with tryptophan for transport across the blood-brain barrier. In theory, the greater the circulating levels of BCAAs, the smaller the amount of tryptophan will cross the blood-brain barrier, and central fatigue will be reduced. However, ingesting the amount of BCAAs necessary to exert such an effect is likely to result in gastrointestinal disturbances and slow water transport across the gut, both being disadvantageous during exercise. Studies of the mechanism BCAAs function are intriguing and may provide us with a better understanding of events occurring during exercise. However, at present, there are little data to support an ergogenic effect of BCAAs using dosages that are physically tolerable.

Creatine

Recent attention has focussed on the use of creatine as an ergogenic aid for short term strenuous exercise. Several British track athletes, including 1 gold medalist, may have used creatine supplements before the 1992 Olympic games in Barcelona (**Anderson, 1993**). Creatine does not appear to have adverse effects, and it is not prohibited by the International Olympic Committee (IOC). Creatine exists in muscle as creatine phosphate providing the high energy phosphate for adenosine diphosphate to restore adenosine triphosphate levels quickly. The theoretical basis for creatine as an ergogenic aid is that more creatine phosphate (CP) will be stored in muscle, and hence there will be a greater capacity for immediate energy production. The CP reaction also serves as a buffer during high intensity exercise where lactic acid is produced. However, mechanisms to explain the ergogenic effects have not been proven (**Greenhaff, 1995; Maughan, 1995**).

Creatine ingestion appears to increase muscle creatine levels. Ingestion of 20 g creatine (5 g, qid) resulted in marked increases of muscle creatine levels in 4-5 days (**Harris et al, 1992**). Furthermore 1 hour of hard exercise per day using 1 leg produced an increase in muscle creatine in the exercised leg but not the contralateral leg. Ingestion of creatine 20 g/day for 5 days resulted in faster phosphocreatine resynthesis in the two minutes of recovery from intense electrically evoked isometric contractions (**Greenhaff et al, 1993**).

Five days of creatine 20 g/day produced greater torque production during a bout of maximal isokinetic contractions compared with placebo (**Greenhaff and Casey, 1993**). Performance of a resistance exercise task was improved after 14 to 28 days of supplementation of creatine 20 g/day compared with placebo (**Earnest et al, 1995**). Other studies have confirmed that about 20-30 g of creatine per day for about a week or more enhanced performance of short term strenuous exercise

(**Balsom et al, 1993; Soderlund et al, 1994**). Whether there would be any benefit for endurance exercise is questionable (**Balsom et al, 1993**). Several studies reported that creatine supplementation resulted in increased body weight (**Greenhaff et al, 1993; Earnest et al, 1995; Balsom et al, 1993**), which could be related to an increase in fat free mass or an increase in water retention. Further research on change in body composition after creatine supplementation appears warranted.

Carnitine

Carnitine is thought to serve as an ergogenic aid in its role as a component of several enzymes responsible for the transport of long chain fatty acids into the mitochondria (**Cerretelli and Marconi, 1990; Clarkson, 1992**). In theory, an increase in carnitine availability to the muscle could increase fatty acid oxidation and spare glycogen. It helps in optimal functioning of the Krebs Cycle by increasing CoA availability.

Carnitine 2 g/day for four weeks produced an increase in carnitine levels in the muscle and increased the activity of respiratory chain enzymes (**Huertas et al, 1992**). Supplementation of 14 days or less had no effect on muscle carnitine levels (**Barnett et al, 1994; Soop et al, 1988; Vukovich et al, 1994**). Ingestion of 2.5 g/day of carnitine for 10 days produced insignificant increase of carnitine in the blood, but carnitine was found in the urine (**Baker et al, 1992**). The low absorption of carnitine suggests that oral doses of carnitine have little effect on body stores so that it may take large doses (2 g/day) for a long period of time (more than four weeks) to significantly increase muscle carnitine stores (**Arenas et al, 1991**). Some studies found a slight improvement in lipid oxidation after carnitine supplementation, most studies did not, even when muscle carnitine were elevated (**Vukovich et al, 1994; Decombaz et al, 1993; Oyono-Enguelle et al, 1988**). Carnitine has been reported to result in increase maximal oxygen consumption (**Marconi et al, 1985; Vecehiet et al, 1990**) and lowered respiratory quotient. Studies have found no effect of carnitine supplements on VO_2 max, work output during an endurance cycling task and time to exhaustion on a treadmill. These studies examined doses of 2-4 g/day for 2-4 weeks (**Greig et al, 1987; Kasper, 1994**). In another study it was showed that 2 g carnitine taken 1 hour before exercise VO_2 max (**Vecchiet et al, 1990**). It is unlikely that carnitine would be incorporated into the muscle in the short time period. Another study infused 1-3 g of carnitine intravenously 40 minutes before exercise and reported increase, lipid oxidation (**Natali et al, 1993**). Such short time period between ingestion and exercise suggests that carnitine must act on site other than the muscle, such as the liver (**Brass and Hiatt, 1994**). Overall there are some evidences supporting improvement in performance in carnitine supplementation but studies are still inconclusive.

Bicarbonate Loading

Numerous studies investigated the effect of bicarbonate to improve performance (**Horswil, 1995**). The bicarbonate is thought to act as a buffer and reduce the effects of lactic acidosis during high intensity exercise. The pH of the blood at rest is 7.35, and after high intensity exercise can fall to 6.8. Ingestion of bicarbonate results in increased bicarbonate level in the blood and enhanced blood-buffering capacity. The results of studies examining bicarbonate ingestion have been equivocal. In recent review article (**Horswill 1995**) compared the percentage change in performance in 21 studies to the doses of sodium bicarbonate ($NaHCO_3$) that was used. He reported a positive relationship (**Matson and Tran, 1993**). Generally, studies that found an ergogenic effect used doses of 300 mg $NaHCO_3$ per kg body weight, while studies using 200 mg/kg or less showed no effect (**Coombes and McNaughton, 1993**). The meta analysis showed that $NaHCO_3$ resulted the mean improvement of 27% in time to exhaustion.

$NaHCO_3$ ingestion of 300 mg/kg body weight resulted in participant performing more work during 2 sets 60 repetition isokinetic knee flexon and extension (**Coombes and McNaughton, 1993**). Studies that have examined multiple sprints with short recovery periods appeared to show beneficial effects of $NaHCO_3$ while studies using only a single sprint do not (**Horswill, 1995**). The exercises that benefit are those that produce high lactic acid level. The increased $NaHCO_3$ level in the extracellular may promote H^+ efflux from muscle and produce enhanced recovery between repeated bouts (**Horswill, 1995**). Recently it has been suggested that the mechanism to explain the ergogenic effect may not lie in the bicarbonate ion but instead may be due to the accompanying sodium load (**Kozak-Collins et al, 1994**). Sodium could produce a change in intravascular volume which could alter performance. To test this, effects of ingestion either $NaHCO_3$ (300 mg/kg) or NaCl (207 mg/kg), both containing equimolar amounts of sodium, on repeated one minute cycling sprints were examined.

No difference between the conditions was found in the number of intervals completed. However, blood pH was significantly higher for the $NaHCO_3$ condition compared to the NaCl condition. Thus, although blood was less acidic, performance was not enhanced. The hematocrit increased to the same extent in both conditions suggesting that the intravascular fluid status was altered similarly. If this is the case, then the improvement in performance attributed to $NaHCO_3$ may well be due to intravascular volume enhancement from the sodium.

Williams (1995) noted that doses of 300 mg/kg $NaHCO_3$ could be disadvantageous because of development of gastrointestinal distress leading to nausea and diarrhoea. One study found that 300 mg/kg $NaHCO_3$ resulted in a faster time to complete a 15 hundred mtr run, yet two of the twelve participants reported gastrointestinal disturbances and did not show improvement in the bicarbonate loading condition compared with placebo (**Williams, 1995**). Other than gastrointestinal problems in some athletes, the dosages appeared to be medically safe for acute ingestion.

Phosphate loading

Early studies suggested that phosphate supplements would delay fatigue due to their buffering capacity (**Bucci, 1989**). The results of more recent studies are equivocal and the mechanism of action unclear (**Clarkson, 1991; Tremblay et al, 1994**). A well-designed study found that one gram of natural buffered phosphate supplement four times per day for three days delayed the onset of anerobic metabolism in a run to exhaustion and increased VO_2 max (6-12%) (**Cade et al, 1984**). Erythrocyte 2, 3 diphosphoglycerate content increased, and it was speculated that this increase may have been responsible for the improvement in aerobic capacity. Another study found that phosphate loading (1 gm tribasic sodium phosphate, taken four times per day for six days) resulted in a 7.9% increase in VO_2 max, a 10.5% increase in ventilatory anerobic threshold and a trend toward improvement on 8 km. run performance (**kreider et al, 1990**). However, no change in 2, 3 diphosphoglycerate was found. A subsequent study reported that 4 gm of tribasic sodium phosphate for 3-4 days resulted in a 9% increase in VO_2 max, 10% increase in anerobic threshold and 8% improvement in cyclic performance time. In contrast, some studies found no beneficial effect of phosphate loading (**Ahlberg et al, 1986; Weatherwax et al, 1986; Bredle et al, 1988; Mannix et al, 1990**). Recent comprehensive review addressed the problems and inconsistencies in the studies on phosphate loading. Also, another study examined the effect of an acute (1.24 gm given 1 hour before exercise) or chronic (3.73 gm per day for six days before the exercise) ingestion of a commercially available product containing mono and dibasic sodium phosphate, tribasic potassium phosphate, and ascorbic acid (Vitamin C) (**Duffy and Conlee, 1986**). No significant effect of the phosphate product was found on treadmill run time to exhaustion or leg power measured by a isokinetic dynamometer.

A recent comprehensive review (**Tremblay et al, 1994**) addressed the problems and inconsistencies in the studies on phosphate loading. Phosphate loading produces only small changes in plasma phosphate levels. **Tremblay et al, 1994**, Point out that it is difficult to interpret the results of the studies overall because of several confounding variables. These include: differences in mode and intensity of exercise, dietary intakes, type/amount/length of dosage, wash-out period, participants' fitness level, and sample collection and analysis techniques that could affect results. Although it was concluded that the literature does not sufficiently support phosphate loading as an ergogenic aid, several studies have documented ergogenic effects and the degree to which performance is enchanced is similar among the studies. Further studies with rigorous methodological controls are warranted to fully document the effectiveness of phosphate loading and, if it does have performance benefits, to ascertain the mechanism.

Caffeine

Caffeine has no nutritional value and is classified as a drug with pharmacological effects, specifically as a stimulant (**Clarkson, 1993; Conlee, 1991**). Because of this action and studies which showed that caffeine benefitted endurance performance, caffeine is included on the IOC's list of restricted substances. Anecdotal evidence, however, suggests that caffeine is widely consumed by athletes (**Rogers, 1985**). The Center for Drug-Free Sport found that 26% of 16,000 Canadian youths (aged from 11 to 18 years) used caffeine to enhance performance (**Graham et al, 1994**).

Caffeine is rapidly absorbed by the gut, and peak values in the blood appear 1 hour after ingestion. Although most of the ingested caffeine is degraded in the liver and excreted byproducts, a small percentage of caffeine (0.5 to 4%) is excreted unchanged. Detection of this small amount in the urine is relatively easy, allowing the IOC to set a limit of 12 mg/L of caffeine in the urine. Several detailed reviews of caffeine and performance are available (**Clarkson, 1993; Conlee, 1991; Graham et al, 1994; Spriet, 1995; Van Handel, 1983; Wilcox, 1990**).

The mechanism of caffeine action as a stimulant is not entirely known but it may involve stimulation of the sympathetic nervous system and increase in adrenaline (epinephrine) release and action (**Bucci, 1989**). Caffeine could also enhance performance via an alteration in fuel supply and usage. Caffeine increases energy expenditure, (**Astrup et al, 1990**) and there appears to be enhanced fat oxidation which increases citrate and the acetyl CoA : CoA-SH ratio, thereby sparing muscle glycogen (**Tarnopolshy, 1994**). Whether caffeine increases blood levels of catecholamines is controversial. Other mechanisms may also contribute to the effect of caffeine on performance, such as a direct effect on muscle (**Graham and Spriet, 1991**). Costill and colleagues were the first to demonstrate that caffeine ingestion resulted in increased endurance. Since then, several studies have assessed the effects of caffeine on performance, and the results have been equivocal. Three well-designed and controlled studies have been done by the same laboratory. In the first study, it was found that a high caffeine dosage (8mg/kg), given to well-trained competitive distance runners

1 hour before exercise, at about 85% VO_2 max, resulted in increased endurance times by about 50% (**Graham and Spriet, 1995**). In other study (**Spriet et al, 1992**), the same dosage was given to recreational athletes, and their endurance time improved by about 27%. More recently (**Graham and Spriet, 1995**) dosages of 3,6 or 9 mgs/kg were compared, and it was found that endurance was enhanced in the first 2 conditions (3 and 6 mg/kg) but not the 9 mg/kg condition, which differs from their pervious study. The authors explained this discrepancy by the fact that more athletes in the later study were light caffeine users (< 250 mg/day), and it appeared that the lightest users had smaller responses and complained of mental 'confusion.'

Dosage of 5 to 13 mg/kg all resulted in increased endurance during cycling at 80% VO_2 max (**Pasman et al, 1995**). Another study showed that 6 mg/kg produced faster swim times for the 1,500 m swim (**Macintosh and Wright, 1995**). Caffeine may have an even greater effect on sports performance at high altitudes (**Fulco et al, 1994**). Recent studies have documented that caffeine ingestion at levels of about 6 mg/kg will enhance endurance performance at intensities of about 80% VO_2 max. Most studies have been performed using male athletes, so the effects for female athletes are largely unknown. Short term intense exercise has not been consistently found to be improved by caffeine ingestion (**Tarnopolshy, 1994**).

It must be stressed that ingestion of levels above about 7 mg/kg can produce urinary level glucose to or at the IOC limit. Because caffeine is a drug and has no nutritional value, the ethics of using caffeine must be addressed. It has been suggested that the IOC limits be lowered to 8 mg/L to discourage athletes from taking ergogenic doses yet allow for moderate habitual consumption (**Tarnopolshy, 1994**).

CONCLUSIONS

Over the past decade (in eighties), high CHO diets have been advised for athletes, with some recommendations as high as 70% of total energy intake. Recently (in nineties) long term use of high CHO diets during training has been questioned. Athletes with high caloric intakes would appear to ingest sufficient CHO if the diet is only 45% CHO. Perhaps this chink in the armour of the high CHO diet made it possible for other diets to attract attention, particularly the high fat diet. Despite a theoretical basis for high fat diets to be effective as performance enhancers, data regarding high fat diets and performance are equivocal regardless, it should be recognized that long term use of a high fat diet may have adverse effects on health.

Various substances purported to have ergogenic effects have been discussed in this review. While caffeine is easily available in products already marketed, most of the other substances have found their way into products marketed specifically for athletes. There is a theoretical basis to believe that each of the products could have an ergogenic effect, but there is no overwhelming scientific evidence suggesting that carnitine, phosphate, and BCAAs are effective. Companies take advantage of theoretical effects based on animal studies — or even in vitro experiments — to market products with little or no scientific evidence that they improve performance. Nutritional supplements, unlike drugs, are not required to have strong scientific clinical evidence that they are effective before they are allowed to be marketed.

Data are fairly convincing that caffeine will enhance endurance performance ant that bicarbonate and creatine will benefit short duration strenuous exercise. Although it may appear that many of the ergogenic aids cited herein are safe, there have been few stuides of the effects of long term supplementation. In addition to requiring strong scientific support that diet modifications or supplements will benefit performance, the sports medicine community must determine health consequences of their long term use before they are recommended.

15

TRAINING FOR PERFORMANCE

Performance in any sports or event depends on the various factors. Proper planning for training is the primary factor. Objective for sports training is to improve performance by increasing the maximum energy output during a particular movement. A conditioning program should allocate the appropriate amount of training time to match the aerobic and anerobic energy demands of the sport.

BASIC PHYSIOLOGICAL PRINCIPLES FOR TRAINING

According to the principle of individuality, each person must be recognized as unique and such individual variation must be allowed for designing training programs. Different people will response to a given training program in different ways. According to the principle of specificity, to maximize the benefits, training must be specifically matched to the type of activity the person normally engages in. An athlete involved in a sports that requires tremendous strength, such as weight lifting, would not expect great strength gains from endurance running. According to the principle of disuse, training benefit is lost if training is either discontinued or reduced too abruptly. To avoid this, all training programs must include a maintenance program. According to the principle of progressive overload, training must involve working the body (muscle and cardiovascular system) harder than normal; as the body adapts, training progresses to a higher work lèvel. As an example, consider a boy who can perform only 10 reps of a bench press before reaching fatigue using 40 kgs of weight. With a week or two resistance training he can probably increase to 12-15 reps with the same weight. He then adds 2.3 kg to the bar, and his repetitions drop to 8-10 as he continues to train, the repetitions continue to increase and within another week or two he is ready to add an additional 2-3 kgs. Thus, there is a progressive increase for the weight lifted. Similarly with aerobic and anerobic training, training volume can be increased progressively; manipulating intensity and duration. Resistance training increases strength, power and muscular endurance. The workout is designed around sets, repetition and resistance.

Table 1 : Two arm curl resistance training program

Set 1	Resistance	80 lb
	Repetition	8
Set 2	Resistance	90 lb
	Repetition	10
Set 3	Resistance	100 lb
	Repetition	12

In this example, the 12 RM is 80 lb. A resistance of 90 lbs of the 10 RM (90 lbs) is used for second set and 100% of 10 RM (80 lb) is used for the third. Interval training involves alternating period of work with rest or reduced activity. It allows more work with rest or reduced activity. It allows more work to be performed overall, because some recovery occurs during the activity.

Table 2 : Sample Interval Training Program for Middle Distance Runner

Set	Repetitions	Distance time	Interval time	Recovery activity	Recovery
1	6	400 M	75 s	75 s	Jog
2	6	800 M	180 s	180 s	Jog/walk

Interval training can be used in almost any sport activity but most often used in track, cross-country and swimming. **Fox and Mathews (1974)** have identified the major variables that must be individually adjusted for each athlete :

Rate and distance of the work interval (Load and duration of resistance training).

Number of repetition and sets during each training session.

Duration of the rest interval (Recovery).

Type of activity during the rest interval.

Frequency of training per week.

Continuous training is a non-stop workout with no rest intervals. High intensity continuous training is performed at high intensities (85-95% of HR max) and is very effective for endurance training without requiring highly stressful and uncomfortable work levels. Long Slow Distance (LSD) training used relatively low intensity work (60% to 80% of HR max) performed for a very long distance or duration, which places less stress on the cardiovascular and respiratory system but can cause joint and muscle discomfort or injury. Training at a constant near competition pace enhances a runner's ability to maintain an even pace during a race and typically results in the best race times. Furthermore, serious runners need to regularly train or race at or near their race paces to develop leg speed, leg strength and muscular endurance. The demand of such training programs are extraordinary, particularly when extended over weeks and months. Slower pace variation should be introduced periodically, such as once or twice per week to give the athlete some relief from exhaustive high intensity continuous training.

LSD training is probably the most common endurance conditioning used by people who want to stay in condition for health-related purpose. The athlete who participates in team and sports endurance trains only for general conditioning, and the athlete who wants to maintain endurance conditioning during the off-season.

Fartlek training (speed play), used primarily by distance runners, is continuous training done in an interval fashion. Runners can vary their pace at will from high speed to slow jogging. Runs are normally performed 45 min or longer. Many coaches have used Fartlek training because it provides variety.

Circuit training involves a series of stations forming a circuit through which a person progresses as rapidly as possible. A different activity is performed at each station. Most circuit training allows modest increases in aerobic endurance and major increase in strength, muscular endurance and flexibility. Cardiovascular conditions can be enhanced by increasing the speed through the circuit and by placing stations far the apart.

TRAINING PHYSIOLOGICAL ENERGY SYSTEM

Training to improve 'Anerobic Power'

Training to improve 'Anerobic Power' centers around the need to enhance **'ATP-CP System'**. Short high intensity intervals work outs of 5-10 sec duration stresses the ATP-CP metabolic pathway. Short durations of this type of interval produce little lactic acid and recovery is fast. Rest interval ranges between 30-60 sec. The number of repetitions would be determined by athlete's fitness level.

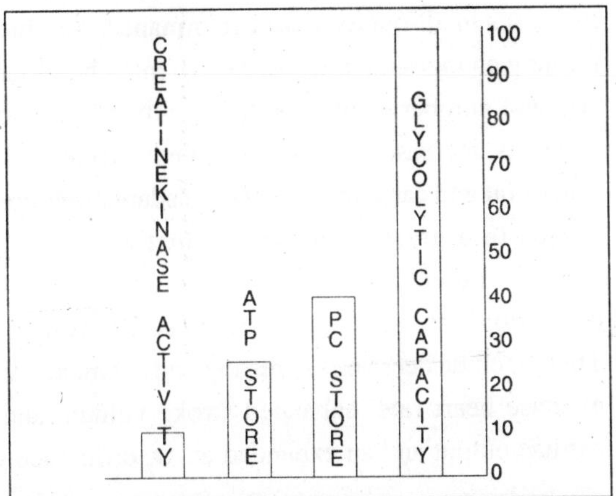

Fig. 15.1 : Changes of energy store after methodical training

Studies have shown that muscular ATP stores increase 25% (3.8 mM to 4.8 mM/kg of wet muscle) following a training program of 7 months, 2-3 days per week. Concentration of PC in the muscle (Boy 11-13 years) has been reported to increase nearly by 40% after 4 months of training. Studies have shown that 36% increase of creatine kinase following an 8-week training program was also reported.

Training to improve glycolytic system

In a maximal effort of more than 10 secs., there is a growing dependence on energy production from Anerobic Glycolysis. In order to improve the 'energy system' high intensity intervals of 20-60 sec duration are useful in overloading this metabolic pathway. This type of training drastically reduces muscle glycogen stores. For this reason that athlete often alternates hard interval training days and light training sessions. Increased Glycolytic capacity, greater quantity of blood lactate during maximum work. The increased glycolytic enzyme activities speed up the rate and quantity of glycogen broken down to lactic acid. ATP derived from lactic acid system is increased.

Evidence : Maximum lactate tolerance is increased following maximal exercise of short duration in 6-8 weeks.

Training To Improve Aerobic Capacity

Interval training is the performance of repeated exercise bouts. 'Longer work interval' has a greater involvement of aerobic energy production. Intense interval provides greater participation of 'Anerobic Metabolism'. Generally it is believed that high intensity intervals are more effective in improving Aerobic power and Lactate Threshold than low intensity interval — Long, Slow Distance (70% of HR max) high Intensity, Continuous exercise (85% and above). The objective during high intensity continuous program is to exercise at a heart rate near 'Lactate Threshold' for approx. 25-50 min. As the athlete improves, it may become necessary to repeat the 'Speed Lactate' test to alter the training intensity.

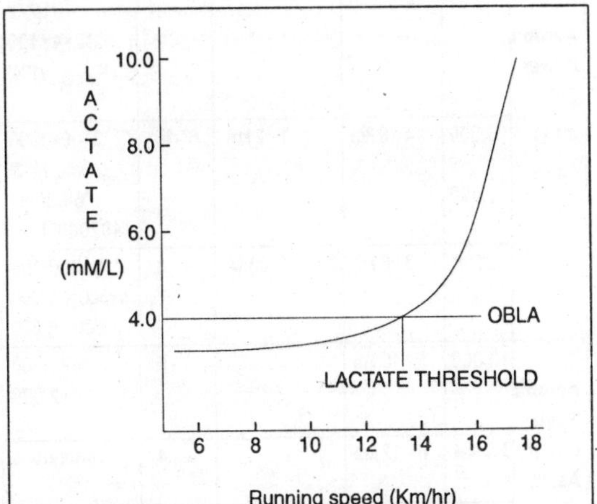

Fig. 15.2 : Speed-Lactate relationship

Training causes a greater release of fatty acid from adipose tissue i.e., availability of fat as a fuel is increased and the activity of enzyme involved in the activation, transport and breakdown of fatty acid is increased. At a given work load, trained person oxidizes more fat and less carbohydrate that untrained person (**Saltin and Karlsson, 1971; Saltin et al, 1969**). Greater fat oxidation would mean less lactic acid accumulation and thus less fatigue.

Table 4 : Training Examples to Improve Speed, Speed Endurance, Aerobic Power and Anerobic Threshold

	Event	Total Quant. in one session	Main distance	Lactate	Training Examples
Speed	100	1,000 M	30 - 80	6	*2 - 4×4×60 /2'/4' *3*4×80/3'/6'
Speed End. (-la)	200	1,500 M	150 - 200	6 -12	*10×Flying 100 M/3' *8×150/3' *4×200/8'
	400	1,800 M	200 - 300	>18	*3×2×200 /2/'8' *38(3008150 /2')/8'
	800	2,500 M	200 - 600	15 - 18	*10*200/2' *6×300/4' *3×400/5' ×500/8' 2-3×600
Aerobic Power (VO_2 max)	1,500	4,000 M	200 - 600	8 -12	*4×4×200 /15"/3' *2×4×400 /1'/4'
	3,000 5,000	4 - 8 km	1 - 2 km	6 -10	*3 - 6×1000 /1'-3' *6-600/3', *402000/1'-3"
	Uphill	3 - 6 km	300 - 1000 M	4 - 8	*10×300/300 *5×500 - 1,000 /500 - 1,000
Aerobic Basis (An. th) Ae. th	10,000	5 - 10 km		4 - 6	*6×1,000 *4×2,000
	Fartlek	8 - 12 km		2 - 4	Continuous
	Mara-thon	15 - 30 km		2	Continuous

PHYSIOLOGICAL EFFECT OF TRAINING

Exercise training brings about specific metabolic and physiological adaptations that involve subcellular as well as gross physiologic changes. Anerobic training increases glycolytic enzymes. This is usually accompanied by concomitant increases in all-out exercise performance. Aerobic training changes include increase in mitochondrial size and number as well as the activity of aerobic enzymes, increase myoglobin and enhance oxidation of fat and carbohydrate. These adaptations are geared to a greater aerobic production of ATP. Aerobic training brings about both functional and dimensional changes in the cardiovascular system. These include decreases in resting and submaximal exercise heart rate, enhanced stroke volume and cardiac output and an expanded av-O_2 difference.

METABOLIC ADAPTATION TO TRAINING

Endurance training stresses ST muscle fibers. In response to the training stimulus these fibers become 7% to 22% larger (**Costill et al, 1976**) than the corresponding FT fibers. Although the percentage of ST and FT fibers do not appear to change, endurance training may cause FTb fibers to take on more FTa fibers characteristics.

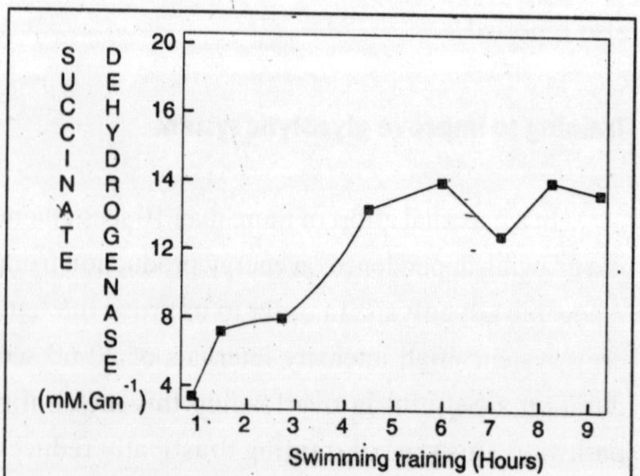

Fig. 15.3 : Enzyme activity and swim training

Endurance trained athlete can have 5% to 10% more capillaries in their leg muscle than sedentary individual (**Harmansen and Wachtlova 1971; Ingjer, 1979**). With longer periods of endurance training, the number of capillaries have shown to increase by as much as 15% (**Harmansen and Wachtlova 1971**). Having more capillaries allows greater exchange of gases, heat, wastes and nutrients between the blood and the working muscle fibers.

This maintains an environment well-suited to energy production and repeated muscle contractions. Substantial increase in muscle capillary number occur within the first few weeks or months of training. Endurance training increases muscle myoglobin content by about 75% to 80%. Myoglobin stores O_2. Endurance training increases both the number and the size of the mitochondria.

The number of mitochondria increases proportionally with the increasing volume of aerobic training. Activities of many oxidative enzymes are increased with training. SDH, one of the muscles key oxidative enzymes, increased with swim training. Interestingly, although these enzyme activities continued to rise throughout the period of training, little change in the body's maximal O_2 uptake (VO_2) occurred during the final six weeks of training. This suggests that VO_2 max might be more influenced by the circulatory system's limitations for transporting O_2 than by the muscle's oxidative potentials. Citrate synthetase also dramatically influenced by endurance training. Jogging or cycling for as little as 20 min per day has been shown to increase leg muscle's SDH activity by more than 25% above that in sedentary individuals. Training more vigorously such as 60-90 min per day produces a 2.6 fold increase in this activity. All these changes occurring in the muscles combined with adaptation in the O_2 transport system lead to enhanced functioning of the oxidative system and improve endurance. Aerobic training places repeated demands on muscles stores of both glycogen and fat. Endurance trained muscle stores considerably more glycogen storage allows the athlete to better tolerate the subsequent demand of training because more fuel is available for use. Endurance trained muscle also stores more fat (Triglyceride) than does untrained muscle. The activities of may enzymes involved in β-oxidation of fat increase with training, thus FFA levels increase. This leads to increased use of fat as an energy source, sparing glycogen.

TRAINING THE AEROBIC SYSTEM

The ideal training regimen should have a caloric expenditure of about 5,000 to 6,000 Kcal. week^{-1}. There seems to be little benefit beyond this level. This translates in between 80 km to 95 km of running per week (**Costill, 1986**). To achieve the same aerobic benefits, swimmers would need to swim roughly 4,000 to 6,000 mt. day^{-1} (**Costill et al, 1991**) of course these are only estimates of the stimulus required for muscular conditioning. As we increase our total body's aerobic capacity, there is also an increase in the maximal oxidative or respiratory capacity (QO_2) of our muscle. The highest average QO_2 values reported in human muscle (5.2 hr^{-1} g^{-1}) are those in the deltoid muscles of swimmers who had expanded more than 10,000 Kcal week^{-1} during training (**Costill, 1985**).

Intensity is a critical factor in improving performance adaptations are specific to the speed and duration of training bouts. So those who perform at higher intensities must train at higher intensity. High intensity speed training can include either intermittent exercise at near competition pace. Aerobic interval training involves repeated bouts of high intensity performance separated by brief rest periods. This training although traditionally considered only anerobic, generates aerobic benefits because the rest period in so brief that full recovery cannot occur, thus the aerobic system is stressed. In competitive swimming, repeated short efforts lasting from 30 S to 5 Min (50-400 M of swimming) performed slightly slower than race pace, but with very brief rest interval (5-15s). Such short rest intervals force the participant to exercise at an aerobic level, placing little reliance as glycolytic lactate producing system.

Table 4 : Example of Aerobic interval training

Best 10 km (min)	Reps	Interval Distance	Rest(s) (min)	Pace	Rest between set
46:00	20	400	10 - 15	2:00	3-5 min
43:00	20	400	10 - 15	1:52	"
40:00	20	400	10 - 15	1:45	"
37:00	20	400	10 - 15	1.37	"
34:00	20	400	10 - 15	1:37	"

Volume is the key to successful aerobic training, the runner must perform a large number of these repeated runs. In this example 20 reps of 400 m are performed, resulting in a total sun of 8,000 mt (approx. 5 min). The pace mentioned is slightly slower than that used during the 10 km race. In this case, slower by 8-10 s per 400 M. Yet this pace is generally faster and could be sustained easily during a continuous 8,000 mt run. The difficulty of this interval set is that the rest period is relatively brief — only about 10-15 s. Such short rest intervals allow little time for muscle to recover, yet they provide a brief respite from the muscular stress. Continuous training is done as one prolonged bout of exercise, but many athletes find it boring. Direct evidence shows that aerobic interval training produces greater muscular adaptations than continuous training bout.

ANEROBIC TRAINING (ADAPTATIONS IN THE ATP-PCR SYSTEM)

Few studies have examined the training adaptations to short, maximal exercise bouts that are aimed specifically at developing the ATP-PCr system.

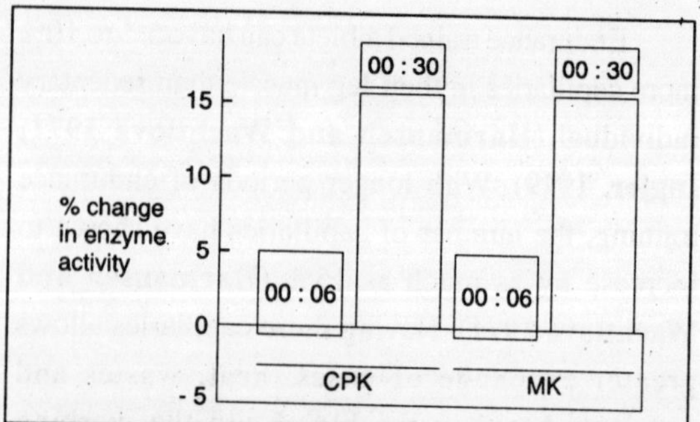

Fig. 15.4 : The activities of the muscle enzymes Creatine phosphokinase (CPK) and Myokinase (MK)

Costill et al (1979) reported their finding from one of such study. The participants performed maximal knee extension for training. One leg was trained using 6 s maximal work bouts that were repeated 10 times. This type of training preferentially stresses the ATP-PCr energy system. The other leg was trained with repeated 30s maximal bouts which, instead, preferentially stresses the glycolytic system. Both form of training produced the same muscular strength gain and the same resistance to fatigue. As shown in Fig. 15.4, the activities of the muscle enzymes Creatine phosphokinase (CPK) and Myokinase (MK) increased as a result of the 30 sec. training bouts, but were unchanged in the leg trained with repeated 6 s maximal effort. These findings lead us to conclude that maximal sprint bout (6s) might improve muscular strength, but little to the mechanism responsible for ATP break down. Such training will enhance performance by improving strength, but will result in little or no improvement in the enegy release from ATP and PCr. Such strength gain enable an individual to perform a given task with less effort which reduces the risk of fatigue. Whether or not those changes allow the muscle to perform more anerobic work remain unanswered, although a 60s sprint fatigue list suggests that short sprint type anerobic training does not enhance anerobic endurance.

ADAPTATION TO GLYCOLYTIC SYSTEM

Anerobic training (30s) increases the activities of several key glycolytic and oxidative enzymes. The frequently studied glycolytic enzymes are phosphofructokinase (PFK), phosphorylase and lactate dehydrogenase (LDH). The activity of these three enzymes increase 10% to 25% with repeated 30 s training bout (**Costill et al, 1979**).

OTHER ADAPTATIONS TO ANEROBIC TRAINING

Anerobic training enhances performance through efficiency of movement, aerobic energetics, buffering capacity. Training at high speeds improves skill and coordination for performing at higher intensities, anerobic training optimises fiber recruitment to allow more efficient movement and movement economization. Consequently, repeated bouts of sprint training (30s maximal effort bout) increase the muscle's aerobic capacity (**Costill et al, 1979**). This enhancement of muscle's oxidative potential will assist the anerobic energy system, efforts to meet muscle energy needs during highly anerobic effort. Anerobic training improves the muscles' capacity to tolerate the acid that accumulate within them during anerobic glycolysis. Buffers (viz., HCO_3 and phosphate) combine with H^+ to reduce the fibers' activity, thus they delay the onset of fatigue during anerobic exercise. Eight weeks of anerobic training has been shown to increase muscle buffering capacity by 12% to 50% (**Sharp et al, 1986**).

Interestingly, under similar circumstances endurance, trained subject neither accumulate as much muscle lactate as nor experience the usually low pH value seen in sprint trained men — muscle pH does not appear to limit sprint performance for endurance trained athlete.

Table 5 : Selected muscle enzyme activity ($mmol.\ g^{-1}\ min$) for untrained, anerobic trained and aerobically trained men

	Untrained	Aerobically trained	Anerobically trained
Aerobic Enzymes			
Oxidative system			
SDH	8.1	20.8*	8.0
Malate dehydrogenase	45.5	65.5*	46.0
Carnitine pamityl transferase	1.5	2.3*	1.5
Anerobic Enzymes			
ATP-PCr system			
Creatine phosphokinase	609.0	589.0	702.0*
Myokinase	309.0	297.0	350.0*
Glycolytic System			
Phosphorylase	5.3	3.7*	5.8
Phosphofructokinase	19.9	18.9	29.2*
Lactate dehydrogenase	766.0	621.0	811.0

MONITORING TRAINING CHANGES

Many have considered VO_2 max to be the best means for evaluating training adaptation. But the test is too impractical for widespread use and it cannot measure muscle adaptation to training. Multiple measurements of blood lactate levels during an exercise bout of increasing intensity has been proposed as a good means for monitoring progress of training.

Various methods for monitoring training adaptations have been tried, but the easiest seems to be comparing single blood lactate values taken at various times during a training period, after a fixed pace activity is performed blood lactate accumulation following such a standard test (200 mt. swing) decline steadily in these swimmers over a seven month training period. This suggests that they were developing either a greater aerobic capacity or a reduced reliance on the glycolytic system for energy, and, perhaps, both. Even with this method, many questions remain unanswered about what actually happens within the body in response to the training stimulus.

CARDIORESPIRATORY ADAPTATION

Respiratory system

(i) Maximum minute ventilation is increased following training. The increase in ventilation should be considered secondary to the increase in Max VO_2. Increment is brought about by increase in both Tidal Volume and Breathing Frequency.

(ii) Training causes an increased ventilatory efficiency. The amount of air ventilated at the same O_2 consumption level is lower in trained athletes as compare to their untrained counterparts. Since the O_2 cost of ventilation increases greatly with increasing ventilation causing a greater ventilatory efficiency, particularly over a prolonged effort (e.g., the Marathon), it would result in less oxygen to the respiratory muscles and more to the working skeletal muscles.

(iii) The various lung volumes measured under resting conditions (except tidal volume) are larger in trained than in untrained individuals. The majority of these changes can be attributed to the fact that training results in improved pulmonary function and, therefore, in larger lung volume.

(iv) Athletes tend to have larger diffusion capacities at rest and during exercise than do non-athletes (e.g. endurance runners). Diffusion capacity is not directly affected by training, but, rather the larger lung volume of athletes provide a greater alveolar-capillary surface area.

Cardiovascular system

The effects of training are influenced by many factors. Generally, the optimum intensity, frequency and duration of the training program lead to a greater improvement in most functions. The training effects are specific to the type of training program. Genetic limitations are also influential in determining the final magnitude of the training effect. The training effect addressed to improve cardiovascular function at rest, at submaximal and maximal workout is discussed below.

Cardiovascular changes at rest

Change in heart size (cardiac hypertrophy)

Endurance athletes	Non-endurance athletes
A large ventricular cavity	A normal sized ventricular cavity
Normal thickness of ventricular wall	A thicker ventricular wall
Filling of blood in the ventricle during diastole is more and greater than non-endurance athletes	Ventricular force of contraction is more compared to their endurance counterpart

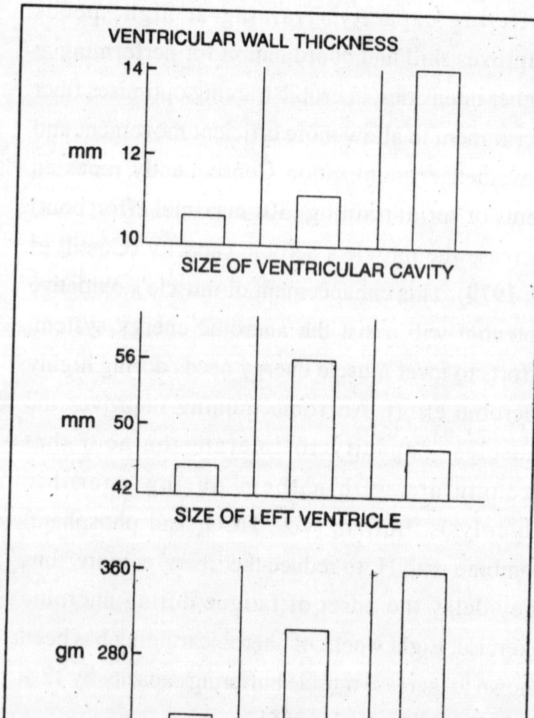

Fig. 15.5 : Diagrammatic representation of ventricular wall thickness, size of ventricular cavity, size of left ventricle of endurance power athletes and normal population

Heart volume is not genetically dependent. An intensive training can improve the heart volume. In endurance activity due to prolong effort, cardiac output is sustained at high level which causes volume stress resulting in cardiac hypertrophy through an increase in the size of ventricular cavity. In power activity, intermittent elevation of arterial pressure causes pressure stimulus which, in turn, results in hypertrophy through thickening of ventricular wall.

Decreased heart rate

Resting bradycardia resulting from training. It is evident when athletes and non-athletes are compared and less evident but still clear when sedentary subjects undergo training program and less evident when athletes are studied in the untrained versus trained state. Resting bradycardia dependent upon (a) long time period of intensive training and (b) inversely proportional to the level of fitness. What causes the training bradycardia? It may due to parasympathetic inhibition (increased vagal tone), decreased sympathetic influence or combination of both. This is probably mediated by an increase in parasympathetic activity and a concomitant decrease in sympathetic discharge. In addition training may also decrease the intrinsic rate of firing of the SA node (**Bolter et al, 1973; Scheuer et al, 1974**).

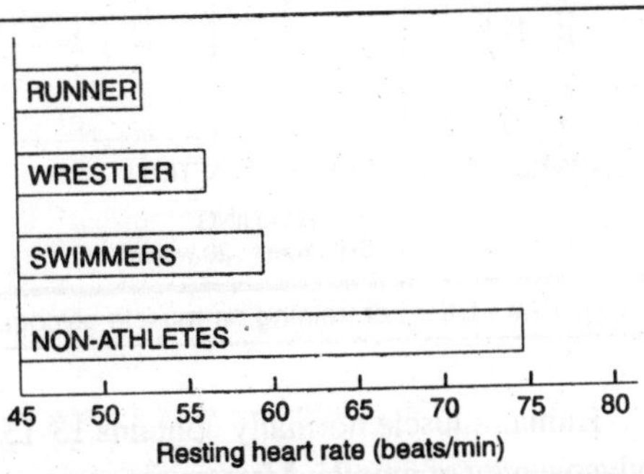

Fig. 15.6 : Diagrammatic representation of resting bradycardia in various sports and events

Increased stroke volume

Increased stroke volume (SV) is more pronounced in endurance athletes due to increased ventricular cavity. More blood refilling during diastole increases SV. Long term intensive training program increased myocardial contractility. Pronounced increment of SV is observed when Athletes are compared with Non-Athletes.

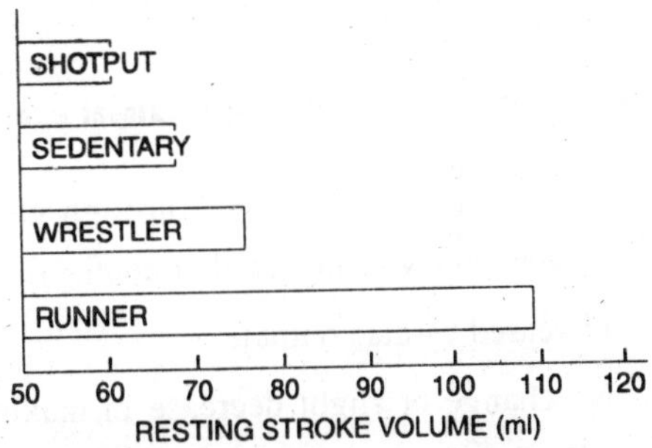

Fig. 15.7 : Diagrammatic representation of resting stroke volume in various sports and events

Cardiovascular changes during submaximal exercises

No change or slight decrease in cardiac output.

Increased stroke volume.

Increased ventricular cavity.

Greater amount of blood filling.

Decreased heart rate or bradycardia during submaximal exercise caused by a decreased sympathetic drive, which could have two origins (a) an intra-cardiac mechanim increased SV during Sub Max work, slight decrease of cardiac output. The need for higher heart rate through sympathetic stimulation is greatly reduced. (b) an extra cardiac mechanism — nervous impulses arising from the muscle and joints, descending impulses from the motor cortex, both can modify sympathetic stimulation to the heart. A reduced heart rate from this kind of modification means primary change is in the muscle, secondary training effect is on the heart.

Changes in muscle blood flow

Blood flow/kg of working muscles is lower in trained than in untrained individuals at submaximal exercise, this is compensated by a greater a-VO_2 differences **(Saltin, 1969)**. It may be related to the increased enzymatic activity for production of energy in the muscle. All the changes induced by training tend to reduce the relative stress imposed on oxygen transport and related systems.

Cardiovascular changes during maximal exercise

Increased stroke volume through cardiac hypertrophy & myocardial contractility.

Increased cardiac output.

No change or slight decrease in maximum heart rate.

An increased heart volume, a decreased sympathetic drive, no change in muscle blood flow.

Blood flow to the total working musculature is greater during maximal work following training. Increased blood flow is distributed over a larger muscle mass, thus making blood flow/kg of muscle mass constant. Improvement of peripheral hemodynamics by endurance training improve capillarization, mean increase in capillary area due to endurance training **(Brodal, 1977)**. Improved capillarization is by enlargement of existing capillaries, opening up of reserve capillaries **(Saltin et al, 1977)**. Improvement of peripheral hemodynamics by endurance training results in improving capillarization. Mean increase in capillary area of 36% due to endurance training was reported **(Schon et al, 1978)**. Improved Capillarization is by enlargement of existing capillaries, opening up of reserve capillaries.

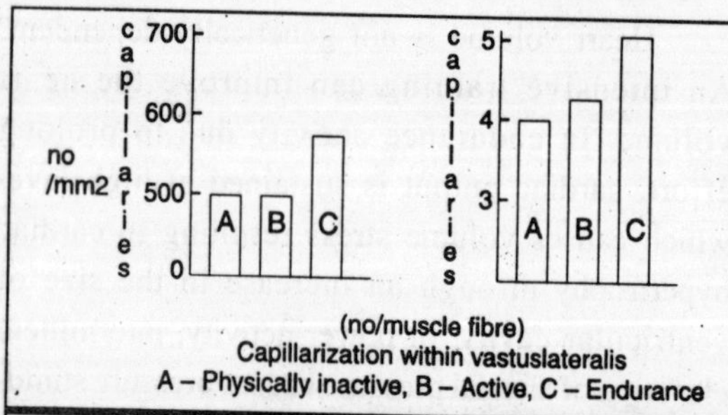

Fig. 15.8 : Diagrammatic representation of capillarization in Physically Inactive, Active and Endurance athletes

Collateral improvement

A more efficient intramuscular blood distribution. Blood flow characteristics are improved by endurance training with an improvement in the elasticity of the erythrocyte membrane which results an increase the ability of the erythrocytes to change their shape in the capillaries.

Changes in muscle fibre

Relative changes in red and white fibers : Increased aerobic capacity equal in both fibers. Increased glycolytic capacity greater in white fibers **(Gollnick et al, 1972)**.

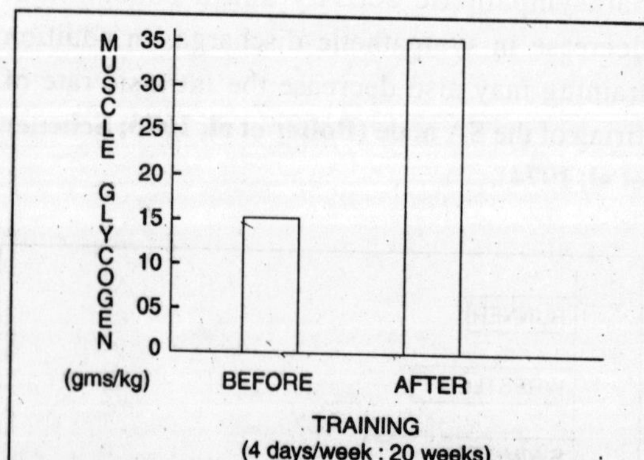

Fig. 15.9 : Effect of training on muscle glycogen

Human muscle normally contains 13-15 gms of glycogen/kg of muscle. After training this amount has been shown to increase as much as 2.5 times **(Gollnick et al, 1973)**.

Other changes

Changes in body composition, (i) A decrease in total body fat, (ii) No change or slight increase in lean body weight, (iii) A small decrease in total body weight. Changes in cholesterol and triglyceride levels. Regular exercise programs cause decrease in both cholesterol and triglyceride levels.

Training and aerobic capacity

No change or slight decrease in oxygen consumption at sub-maximal exercise. The decrease is due to an increase in mechanical efficiency. A decrease in O_2 consumption is most pronounced in comparisons of highly trained athletes and untrained individuals. The difference is also evident between good and average runners. At maximal effort, VO_2 max is increased. The increment is due to an increased oxygen delivery to the working muscles through an increased cardiac output and by an increased oxygen extraction from the blood by the skeletal muscles. The average improvement of 5-20% can be anticipated for college male and female student following 8-12 weeks of methodical training.

Training and anerobic threshold

Several studies have shown that, even when the VO_2 max is not much increased, significant improvement in anerobic threshold (AT) level is possible, provided the training schedule is administered at threshold. Significant improvement in VO_2 max may not be possible when the runner reaches a plateau. It is, therefore, suggested that more emphasis should be given to improve the AT level of athletes. During steady state exercise, sufficient oxygen is supplied to and utilized by the working muscles. In this condition lactic acid does not exceed resting values. However, if aerobic metabolism is insufficient, Anerobic Glycolysis contributes to the energy requirements and lactic acid is formed. The onset of this anaerobiosis normally occurs between 55% and 65% of the max VO_2 in healthy untrained subjects.

NEUROMUSCULAR ADAPTATION TO RESISTANCE TRAINING

Muscle strength is the maximum amount of force a muscle or a muscle group can generate (1-RM). Muscular power is the functional application of both strength and speed. Though two individual may have the same strength, if one requires less time than the other to move an identical load the same distance, the first individual has more power. Muscular endurance is the ability of your muscles to sustain repeated muscle actions or a single static action.

Table 7 : Strength, power and muscular endurance while performing the bench press

Component	Athlete a	Athlete b	Athlete c
Strength (a)	200 lb	400 lb	400 lb
Power (b)	200 lb lifted 2 ft in 0.5 sec	400 lb lifted 2 ft in 2 sec	400 lb lifted 2 ft in 1 sec
	or	or	or
	800 ft lb s-1	400 ft lb s-1	800 ft lb s-1
Muscular endurance (c)	10 rep. with 150 lb	10 rep. with 300 lb	5 rep. with 300 lb

Strength was determined by one repetition maximum.

Power was determined by performing the one arm test as explosively as possible. Power was calculated as the product of force (weight lifted) times distance lifted/time needed to complete the 1 RM.

Muscular endurance was determined by the greatest number of repetitions that could be performed using 75% of the 1 RM. Adopted from **(Wilmore, Costill 1988)**.

Strength gain in resistance training

Resistance training program can produce substantial strength gains — within 3-6 months you see from 25% to 100% improvement, sometime even more. What physiological adaptation occur that allow to exert greater level of strength?

Some evidence (**Gonyea et al, 1986; Larsson and Tasch 1986**) suggests that an increase in the no. of muscle fiber (Hyperplasia) might also be involved. Hypertrophy from resistance training appears to result from a net increase in muscle protein synthesis. During exercise, protein synthesis decreases while protein degradation

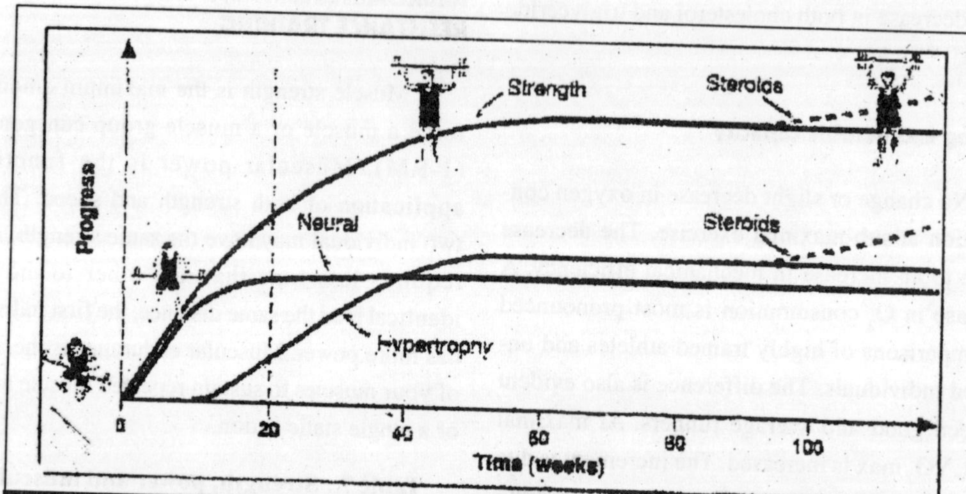

Fig. 15.10 : Neuromuscular adaptation during resistance training. Most training studies span only 8-20 weeks. Long term studies reveal that neural adaptation dominates early in training. Whereas ,most changes during later training phases are associated with muscle hypertrophy — Adopted from Sale (1983)

Neural adaptations always accompany the strength gains that result from resistance training, but hypertrophy might or might not be present. Neural mechanisms leading to strength gains can include recruitment of more motor units to act synchronously and decreases in autogenic inhibition from the 'Golgi tendon organs'. Transient muscle hypertrophy is the pumped up feeling you get immediately after an exercise bout. It results from edema and is short-lived. Chronic muscle hypertrophy occurs from repeated resistance training and reflects actual structural change in the muscle. Although most muscle hypertrophy probably results from an increase in the hypertrophy, it probably results from an increase in the size of individual muscle fiber (Muscle hypertrophy). This could be explained by more myofibril; more actin, myosin filament; more sarcoplasm; more connective tissue or any combination of these.

apparently increases. This pattern reverses during post exercise recovery period, when the muscles protein content is in a continual state of flux. Muscles will atrophy' meaning they decrease in size and strength, when they become inactive such as with injury or disuse. Strength decreases are most dramatic during the 1st week of immobilization averaging 3-4% a day. This is associated with the atrophy and with decreased neuromuscular activity of the immobilized muscle. Atrophy can be stopped by reducing the load such as maintenance program. One fiber type can take on characteristics of the opposite type in response to training, and evidence indicates that one fiber type might actually be converted to the other type as a result of cross- innervation or chronic stimulation.

DELAYED-ONSET MUSCLE SORENESS (DOMS)

Acute muscle soreness occurs late in an exercise bout and during the immediate recovery period. Muscle soreness results primarily from eccentric action and is associated with actual muscle damage. DOMS occurs a day or two after the exercise bout. Proposed cause of DOMS include structural change to muscle cells — Sarcolemma may be ruptured, allowing the cells contents to float freely between the other normal fibers. Disks pulled apart as a result of the force of eccentric action or stretching of the tightened muscle fibers, and inflammatory reactions within the muscles. Armstrong's proposed model of the sequence of events that cause DOMS include : elevation of plasma enzymes; myoglobinemia (presence of myoglobin in the blood) and abnormal muscle histology and ultrastructure.

The sequence of events are :

High tension in the contractile elastic system of muscle results in structural damage to the muscle and cell membrane. The cell membrane damage disturbs calcium homeostasis in the injured fiber, resulting in necrosis (cell death) that peaks about 48 hours after exercise. The products of macrophage activity and intracellular content (viz., Histamine, Kinin and K^+) accumulate outside the cell and stimulate the free nerve ending in the muscle. This process appears to be accentuated in eccentric exercise, in which large forces are distributed over relatively small cross-sectional areas of the muscle.

Recent comprehensive review provided much greater insight. The muscle damage sets up a chain of events that includes the release of intracellular protein and an increase in muscle protein turnover. The damage and repair process involves Ca^{++} ion, lysosome, connective tissue, free radicals energy sources, inflamatory reactions, and intracellular and myofibrillar proteins. The cause of damage and mechanism of repair is still obscure. Some evidence suggests that this process is an important step in muscle hypertrophy.

Muscle soreness can be prevented or minimized by — Reducing the eccentric component of muscle action during early training; Starting training at low intensity and gradually increasing it; Beginning with high intensity exhaustive bout, which will cause much soreness initially but will decrease further pain.

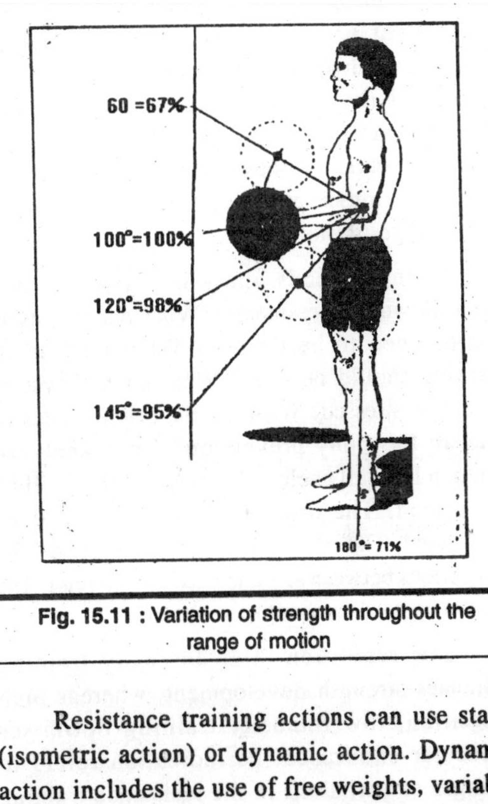

Fig. 15.11 : Variation of strength throughout the range of motion

Resistance training actions can use static (isometric action) or dynamic action. Dynamic action includes the use of free weights, variable resistance, isokinetic actions and pliometrics. With free weight (barbells and dumb-bells) the resistance or weight lifted remains constant throughout the dynamic range of movement 60° = 70%. In contrast, variable resistance involves varying the resistance in all attempts to match it to your strength curve 100° = 100%. Fig. 15.11, illustrate how your strength varies throughout the range of motion in a 120° = 98% two arm curl. Maximal strength production by elbow flexor occurs at approximately 140° = 95%. 100° in the range of movement, these muscles are weakest at 60° (Elbow fully flexed) and at 180° (Elbow fully extended).

With variable resistance device, the resistance is decreased in the weakest points in the range 180° = 71% of motion and increased in strongest point. The underlying theory is that the muscles can be more fully trained if they are forced to act at higher constant percentages of their capacity throughout each point in their range of movement. In isokinetic action, movement speed is held constant by the device — whether you apply very high force or an all-out maximal muscle action. The speed of movement does not vary using either electronics or hydraulics, the device can be preset to control the speed of movement (angular velocity) from 0° s^{-1} (Static action) up to 300° s^{-1} or higher. If properly motivated, the individual can contract the muscle at maximal force at all points in the range of motion.

Training needs analysis which include the following assessments : What major muscle groups need to be trained? What method of training should be used? What energy system should be stressed? What are the primary sites of concern for injury prevention? Once analyzed you can logically select the exercise that will be performed. The order in which they will be performed. The no. of sets in each exercise. The rest periods between sets and between exercise. The load to be used (amount of resistance).

Low repetition, high intensity training enhances strength development, whereas high repetition, low intensity training optimises muscular endurance. Periodization refers to changes or variations in the resistance training program that are implemented over the course of a distant period of time, such as a year. It is important to prevent overtraining or burnout. Typically, the goal is to decrease volume gradually while increasing the intensity.

A typical cycle has four phases :

Phase 1 — Muscular hypertrophy
Phase 2 — Strength
Phase 3 — Power
Phase 4 — Peak strength

Each of the components emphasize a different muscle fitness component.

Table 8 : Periodization Training for strength/ power sports using 2 cycles per year

Variable	Phase 1 Hypertrophy	Phase 2 Strength	Phase 3 Power	Phase 4 Peaking	Active Rest
Set	3-5	3-5	3-5	1-3	General activity
Repetition	8-20	2-6	2-3	1-3	or light
Intensity	low	high	high	very high	resistance
Duration	6 weeks	6 weeks	6 weeks	6 weeks	training 2 weeks

(Fleek and Kraemer, 1987)

Strength gains are highly specific to the speed of training and the movement patterns used in training. For maximum benefit, a resistance training program must include activities quite similar to those experienced by the athlete in actual performance.

Resistance training can benefit almost everyone, regardless of a person's gender, age or athletic movement. Many people believed that children would not benefit from resistance training based on the assumption that the hormonal changes associated with puberty age necessary for gaining muscle strength and mass. **Willmore and Costill (1994)** stated that children and adolescents can train safely with minimal risk of injury if appropriate safeguards are followed. Further, they can indeed gain both muscular strength and muscle mass.

Most athletes in most sports can benefit from resistance training if an appropriate program is designed for them. But to ensure that the program is working, performance should be assessed periodically and adjustments made to the training regime as needed.

EFFECTS OF STRENGTH TRAINING

Increase in Muscle Mass : Increase in muscle size via resistance training is due to Hypertrophy (increase in muscle fibre diameter due to an increase in the number and size of myofibril). Muscles also increase their size in response to strength training by Hyperplasia (increase in the number of muscle fiber).

CNS Changes : Increase the number of motor units recruited, alter motor neuron firing rates, enhance motor unit synchronization during particular movement pattern, and removal of neural inhibition. Early responses to strength training are the result of better innervation. Hypertrophy becomes the dominant factor after 3-4 weeks, strength training in elderly result largely in improving activations of muscle tissue with little hypertrophy.

Overload causes gain in muscular strength, when muscles work against greater resistance produce hypertrophy. Necessary stimulus for strength gain is approximately 20% of maximum voluntary contraction for 1 sec/day is the load required to prevent atrophy. 35% of MVC is the threshold value from which response began to occur. 35% to 100% MVC physiological changes include increase tension in muscle and connective tissue, gradual occlusion of blood flow, increased local temperature hypoxia and increased level of metabolic end products.

Effect of Strength Training is specific to the angle at which the greatest resistance is applied. **(Ikai 1973)** found that training at 100% MVC improved force but not velocity, training at 30 - 60% MVC improved both force and velocity.

METHODS FOR MEASUREMENT AND TRAINING OF STRENGTH

Isometric contraction (Static contraction); Strength improvement occurs only at one angle. 2/3rd MVC, 1 sec isometric contraction, 5 days/week, improvement 5%/week occlusion of vessel results in ischemia, which causes hypertrophy, increases tension.

Concentric isotonic contraction (Shortening); high repetition, low resistance training with weight causes volume stress — aerobic change results. No strength improvement. Muscle endurance improved. Eccentric isotonic contraction (Lengthening); Provides protection from injury to joint, ligament and cartilage. Fiber recruitment is less, heavier load is suggested for greater gains. Limitation — muscle soreness and local inflammation. Isokinetic contraction (Angular velocity of the limb segment is constant), Isotonic training with speed training increased maximal muscle torque (angular force production). Gain is made by change in the recruitment pattern of muscle fibers.

Gain in strength

Isokinetic	Isotonic	Isometric
35%	27.5%	9.4%

OVERTRAINING

Excessive training refers to training that is done with an unnecessarily high training volume, training intensity, or both. It leads to no additional improvements in conditioning or performance and can lead to chronic fatigue and decreased performance because of muscle glycogen depletion. Training volume can be increased by increasing the duration of frequency of training bouts. But numerous studies comparing athletes training with typical training volume to those training with twice the volume (training conducted once a day instead of twice a day) have shown no significant differences in improvement.

Training intensity can determine the specific adaptations that occur in response to the training stimulus. High-intensity, low-volume training can be tolerated only for brief periods, so, although it does increase muscle strength, aerobic capacity will not be improved. Conversely, low-intensity high-volume training stresses the oxygen transport and oxidative metabolism systems, causing greater gains in aerobic capacity. Training intensities of between 50% to 90% of VO_2 max produce marked improvement in aerobic capacity for most people.

Overtraining is attempting to do more work than you are physically capable of. Over-training leads to decreased performance capacity. The symptoms of overtraining syndrome are subjective, and many also accompany regular training, which makes prevention or diagnosis of overtraining syndrome difficult. Possible explanations for overtraining syndrome include changes in the functioning of the divisions of the autonomic nervous system, altered endocrine responses, and suppressed immune function. Signs looked at in hopes of being able to diagnose overtraining include, changes in blood levels of enzymes normally found inside the cells, increased oxygen consumption at a fixed rate of work as performance becomes less efficient, abnormal ECGs showing T wave inversions, and increased heart rate and blood lactate responses to a fixed rate of work.

Only heart-rate response can provide a somewhat reliable warning of overtraining. Overtraining syndrome is treated by a marked reduction in training intensity or complete rest. Prevention can best be accomplished by using cyclic training procedures that vary training intensity and, for endurance athletes, ensuring adequate carbohydrate intake to meet energy needs.

Many athletes decrease their training intensity prior to a competition to avoid reductions in strength, power, and performance capacity that accompany high-intensity training. This practice is called tapering. Muscle strength increases significantly during the tapering period. Less training is needed to maintain previous gains than was originally needed to attain them, so tapering does not lead to a loss of conditioning.

DETRAINING

Detraining refers to the cessation of regular physical training. The effects of stopping training are quite minor compared to those that result from immobilization. In general, the greater the gains during training, the greater the losses during detraining — simply because the well-trained person has more to lose than the untrained person. Detraining causes muscle atrophy, which is accompanied by losses in muscle strength and power. However, muscles require only minimal stimulation to retain these qualities during periods of reduced activity. Muscular endurance decreases after only 2 weeks of inactivity. Possible explanations for this are decreased oxidative enzyme activities, decreased muscle glycogen storage, disturbance of the acid-base balance, and decreased blood supply to the muscles.

Detraining losses in speed and agility are small, but flexibility is lost quickly. To avoid injury, athletes should engage in year-round flexibility training. With detraining, losses of cardiorespiratory endurance are much greater than losses of muscle strength, power, and endurance.

To maintain cardiorespiratory endurance, training must be conducted at least three times per week, and training intensity should be at least 70% of the regular training intensity.

RETRAINING

Retraining is the recovery of conditioning after a period of inactivity. It is affected by the person's fitness level and the duration and extent of the inactivity. The time needed for retaining can be reduced in cases of immobilization if the cast used allows some range of movement. Electrical stimulation of the muscles prevents the usual decrease in muscle oxidative capacity and can prevent muscle fiber atrophy. The earlier an individual can resume active motion after immobilization of inactivity, the quicker the recovery of muscle function.

WARM-UP

Engaging in some type of physical activity or warm-up prior to exercise is generally accepted as a valid procedure by the coaches, trainers and athletes at all levels of competition. The underlying belief is that this preliminary exercise aids the performer in preparing either physiologically or psychologically for an event and may reduce the chances of joint or muscular injury. The warm-up is generally classified into two categories although overlap often exists. These are general warm-up, involving calisthenics, stretching and general body movement or loosening up. Specific warm-up provides a skill rehearsal in the actual activity related to the specific neuromuscular action for which the participant is preparing.

General warming is related to physiological aspect specific to the technical aspect related to either the tasks involved in a particular training session and/or game, respectively.

Psychological aspect of warming-up

The period preceding a competition may be a time of extreme frustration for certain players and warming-up acts as suitable constructive outlet for players to overcome their anxiety and tension through the increasing level of readiness, concentration, confidence, determination, arousal level, etc.

Guideline for warming-up

Warm-up must include stretching and loosening up exercises alternating with more vigorous work out. It must comprise of movements common to the actions required for the task to take place. This helps to prepare specific groups and, at the same time, improves and sharpens nerve innervation. Exercises should not be done quickly and jerk type exercises should be avoided as these may cause damage. Do not hold breath when exercising but inhale and exhale deeply. Warming-up should avoid muscular strength or endurance building up activities and should not be limited to one body area only. The warming-up should end up to taper-off 10-15 min. before main activity, at least 5 min before the main task except for light stretching. This allows recovery from any temporary fatigue. Another important aspect to be taken into consideration by coaches and players is to give brisk warming-up after undertaking long distance journey by road, rail or air, this general warming-up helps to stretch their muscle and/or to keep up their flexibility of various joints.

Physiological Effects

Warm-up should improve performance due to subsequent increase in blood flow in the working muscle which results in augmentation of core temperature (**DeVries, 1974**).

There are six possible mechanism by which warm-up should improve performance : (i) increased speed of contraction and relaxation of the muscles; (ii) greater mechanical efficiency because of lowered viscous resistance within the muscles; (iii) facilitated oxygen utilization by the muscles because hemoglobin releases oxygen more rapidly in higher temperatures; (iv) The benefit of higher temperature during exercise lies in the fact that the metabolic process in the cell can proceed at a higher rate, since these processes are temperature-dependent. For each degree of temperature increase, the metabolic rate of the cell increases by about 13 percent. At the higher temperature, the exchange of oxygen from the blood to the tissues is also much more rapid. Temperature effects of myoglobin similar to that of hemoglobin; (v) Facilitated nerve transmission and muscle metabolism at higher temperatures, **Hill A.V. (1958)** found that the speed of contraction may be increased approximately 20% by raising the body temperature 2°C (35.6°F) and the speed of contraction diminished by a reduction in temperature of 10°C (50°F). A specific warm-up may also facilitate the recruitment of motor unit required in a subsequent all-out activity. The higher the muscle temperature (i.e., the heavier the preceding warm-up exercise), the better the performance, in accordance with this **Davies and Young (1982)**, observed that the peak power output during cycling and jumping was entirely related to muscle temperature, while heating the leg muscle was without effect on supramaximal twitch and titanic tension and maximum voluntary contraction, and (vi) increased blood flow through active tissues as the local vascular bed dilates with higher muscle temperatures. Through warming-up efficiency of muscular contraction increases to its optimum in alter of which poorer performance results.

Advantages of Warming-up

(a) The danger of injury is decreased as a result of the increase in muscle tone and the effect in the nervous system. (b) Warm-up increases the metabolic processes of body which helps to perform better during actual work-out. (c) Warm-up is concerned with the muscle ligaments and tissues of the joints. The mobility (Flexibility) of the joint increase through warming-up. (d) Warm-up related to particular activity increases necessary co-ordination by improving the cohesion among nerve impulse, motor-units and muscle groups.

Effects on performance

Physical performance is improved following warm-up (**Simonson et al, 1936; Asmussen and Boje, 1945**). Furthermore, the nerve messages travel faster at higher temperatures. At the temperature of the human body, which is much higher than that of a frog, our nerve messages go up to 8 times as fast as those of the frog (**Hill, 1927**). Thus, there is a very good reason for a person to keep the body temperature up as he or she does, even at considerable expense, in order to be able to move more quickly. This is also the reason why athletes have discovered that it pays to warm-up before athletic event. This warming-up may make a difference of 3 s in a 400-yard dash. The warming-up may profitably consist of rather vigorous exercise, such as running at rate of about 12 km/hr for 15 to 30 min just before the event (**Hogberg and Ljunggren, 1947**). In the case of ordinary exercise, a 5-min warm-up consisting of light to moderate exercise is usually adequate.

Hogberg and Ljunggren (1947) examined the effect of warm-up in form of running at moderate speed combined with calisthenics on the speed of running 100, 400, or 800 m in well-trained athletes. They compared this effect with the effect of heating the body passively in a sauna bath for a period of 20 min prior to the race and found that the beneficial effect of passively elevating the body temperature by such a bath was much less than that of elevating the body temperature by a warm-up through physical exercise. In the 100-m dash, the improvement after a proper warm-up was of the order of 0.5 to 0.6 s, corresponding to 3 to 4 percent, compared with the results without any warm-up. In the 400-m race, the improvement amounted to 1.5 to 3.0 s, corresponding to 3 to 6 percent. In the 800-m race, the improvement was 4 to 6 s, or 2.5 to 5.0 percent. Thus the percentage improvement was roughly the same at all distances examined. Similar results have been obtained in swimming (**Muido, 1946**).

With regard to the duration of the warm-up, **Hogberg and Ljunggren (1974)** observed better results after a 15-min one, but no further significant improvement occurred in the 100-m race when the warm-up was extended from 15 to 30 min. The authors observed no deterioration in performance attributable to fatigue as a consequence of rather vigorous warm-up. They recommend a warm-up period of 15 to 30 min at a relatively high rate of energy expenditure (in their experiments about 3.0 to 3.4 liter O_2 uptake min^{-1}, equivalent to running at a speed of 12 to 14 km hr^{-1}). The duration and intensity of warm-up should be adjusted according to the environmental temperature and amount of clothing. The higher the environmental temperature and the greater the amount of clothing, the sooner the desired body temperature of about 38.5°C is attained (muscle temperature 39°C or higher). Ideally, the rest period between warm-up and the start of the race should be no more than few minutes. In any case, no more than 15 min. After 45 minutes rest, the beneficial effect of the warm-up is abolished, at which time the muscle temperature has also returned to the pre warm-up levels. The use of warm clothing is recommended during warm-up, and this clothing should be worn until the athlete is ready to start the race.

Barnad et al (1973) report that strenuous exercise, without prior warm-up, induced abnormal ECG changes in 70% of their 44 normally asymptomatic subjects (aged from 21 to 52 years). Two minutes of jogging in place as a warm-up just prior to the exercise eliminated or reduced these abnormal ECG responses.

Warming-Down

Warming down has been proved to be an effective means of decreasing the effects on the musculo-skeletal system of the stimuli of training competition. Warm down or cool down means gradual drop-back of the body, chiefly somatically to a level where parasympathetic nervous system prevails. During the process of warm-down the waste in tissue and muscles are immediately removed. The metabolic products (viz. lactic acid) deposited during activity (vigorous) are reduced by slow jogging — active loosening and shaking of the extremities. Immediate cessation of activity causes delay as the circulation and respiration dropped down abruptly for the removal of metabolic waste products. A warm down period of 10-20 min should follow every workout or competition. Proper warm-down can also help for the preparation of next morning session or the next competition.

REFERENCE

Asmussen, E., and O. Böje (1945) : Body Temperature and Capacity for Work, ***Acta Physiologica Scandinavia*** 10 : 1.

Barnard, R. J., G. W. Gardner, N. V., Diaco, R. N., MacAlpin, and A. A. Kattus (1973). Cardiovascular responses to sudden strenuous exercise Heart Rate, Blood pressure, and ECG, ***Journal of Applied Physiology*** 34 : 833.

Bolter, C et al (1973) : Intrinsic rate and cholinergic sensitivity of isolated atria from trained and sedentary rats. Proc. Soc. Exp. Bidi, Med 144 : 364.

Brodal, P. et al (1976) Capillary supply of skeletal muscle fibers ih untrained and endurance trained men. ***Acta Physiologica Scandinavica*** (Suppl.) 440.

Costill, D. L., Daniel, J., Evans, W., Fink, W., Krahenbuhl, G and Saltin, B., (1976) Skeletal muscle enzyme and fiber composition in the male and female track athletes, ***Journal of Applied Physiology*** 40; 149-154.

Costill, D. L., Coyle, E. F., Fink, W. J., Lesmcs, G. R. & Witzmann, F. A. (1979) Adaptation in skeletal muslce following strength training. ***Journal of Applied Physiology***, Respiratory, environmental exercise physiology 46; 96-99.

Costill, D. L., Tomas, R., Robergs, R. A., Pascoe, D. D., Lambert, C. P., Barr, S. I. and Fink, W. J. (1991) Adaptation to swim training, influence of training volume, ***Medicine and Science in Sports and Exercise*** 23; 371-377.

Costill, D. L., (1985) Practical problems in exercise physiology research. ***Research Quarterly*** 56; 376-384.

Davies, C. T. M., and K. Young (1982) : Maximal Power Output in relation to the Contractile properties of the Triceps Surae in Man, ***Journal of Physiology*** 325 : 51.

DeVries, H. A. (1974) ***Physiology of Exercise for Physical Education and Athletics***, DuBugue Iowa, W. C. Brown.

Fleck, S. T. and Kraemer, W. J. (1987) Designing resistance training programs, Champaign IL, Human Kinetics.

Fox, E. L., et, at (1973) Intensity and distance of interval training programs and changes in aerobic power. Med. Sci. Sports 5; 1; 18-22.

Fox, E. L. and Mathews (1974) : ***Interval training : Conditioning for sports and general fitness***. Philadelphia, W. B. Saunders company.

Gollnick P et al (1972) Enzyme activity and fiber composition in skeletal muscle of untrained men, J Appl. Physiol 33, 312.

Gollnick P et (1973) Effect of training of enzyme activity and fibre composition of human skeletal muscle ***J. Appl. Physiol*** 34, 107.

Gonyea, W. L., Sale D. G., Gonyea, F. B. and Mikesky, A. (1986) Exercise induced increases in muscle fiber number : ***European Journal of Applied Physiology*** 55. 137-147.

Harmansen, L. and Wachtlova, M. (1971) Capillary density of skeletal muscle in well trained and untrained men. ***Journal of Applied Physiology*** 30; 8670-863.

Hill, A. V. (1927) : ***"Living Machinery,"*** Harcourt, Brace and World, Inc, New York.

Högberg, P. and O. Ljunggren (1947) : Uppvärmningens inverkan på löpprestationerna, ***Svensk IdrottB*** 40.

Ikai, Y. and Yabe (1969) Training effect of muscular endurance by means of voluntary and electrical stimulation. ***European Journal of Applied Physiology*** 28 : 55-60.

Ingler, F. (1979) Capillary supply and mitochondrial content of different skeletal muscle fiber types in untrained and endurance trained men : A histological and ultrastructural study. ***European Journal of Applied Physiology*** 40; 197-209.

Larsson, L. and Tasch, P. A. (1986) Motor unit, fiber density in extremely hypertrophied skeletal muscle in man : Electro physiological signs of muscle fiber hyperplasia — ***European Journal of Applied Physiology*** *55, 130-136.*

Saltin, B. et al (1977) Fiber types and metabolic potentials of skeletal muscles in sedentary man and endurance runners. ***Annal New York Academy of Science*** 301; 3.

Saltin, B. and Karlsson, J. (1971) : Muscle glycogen utilization during work of different intensities. In Pernow, B, nd Saltin, B. (eds), ***Mmuscle Metabolism During Exercise*** New York, Plenum Press pp 289-299.

Saltin, B., Hartley, L., Kilbom, Å. and Åstrand I, (1969) Physical training sedentary middle aged and older men II, Oxygen uptake, heart rate and blood lactate concentrations at submaximal and maximal exercise, ***Scandinavian Journal of Clinical lab Investigation*** 24 : 323-334.

Saltin, B. (1969) Physiological effects of physical conditioning. ***Medicine Science Sports*** 1; 50.

Scheuer, J. et al (1974) Experimental observations on the effects of physical training upon intrinsic cardiac physiology and biochemistry. ***American Journal of Cardiology*** 33 : 744.

Schön, F. A., Hollman, W., Liesen, H. and Waterioh, E. (1980) Elektronen-mikroskopische befunde an M. Vastus Lat. Von Untrainierten and Marathon laufern sowie ihre Beziehung zur relativen maximalev sauerstoffaufnane and laktatproducktion. Disch z sportmed 31 (12) 343.

Sharp, R. L., Costill, D. L., Fink, W. J. and Kind, D. S. (1986) Effects of eight weeks of bicycle ergometer sprint training on human muscle buffer capacity, ***International, Journal of Sports Medicine*** 7; 3-17.

Simonson, E., N. Teslenko, and M. Gorkin (1936) : Einfluss von Vorübugen auf die Liestung beim 100 m. Lauf, ***Arbeitsphysiology*** 9 : 152.

Wilmore, J. and Costill, D. (1988) Training for sports and activity Dubuque, la Wmc Brown.

16

ABSTRACTS

Secular trend in maximum aerobic and anerobic capacity of Indian national endurance sportsmen

G. L. Khanna, P. Majumdar, M. Mandal
NIS Scientific J. 1995, 4, 5-13

In most of the countries, irrespective of any game or event, performances of sports persons is increasing day by day. Whereas, in India, in most of sports a steady progress in the performance is not observed when compared to their international counterparts. Physiological parameters like aerobic and anerobic capacities play an important role in improving the performance. The present study was conducted on Indian middle and long distance runners, cyclists and swimmers while attending the National Camp at Sports Authority of India, Bangalore. The aim of the present study was to find out the trend in physiological parameters of Indian sports-persons in last one decade. The study is also aimed to compare the values with the trend of international counterparts. Cardiorespiratory parameters like oxygen consumption (VO_2), pulmonary ventilation (VE), heart rate (HR) were assessed in computerized EOS sprint (Jaeger and CO.). O_2 debt was calculated by standard method. Speed-HR- lactate relationship was derived by the measurement of response of HR and lactate in different speeds. In middle and long distance runners the study reveals that there is an increasing trend of VO_2 max of Indian middle and long distance runners. However, the present rate of increment is not comparable with the international counterparts. Amongst the swimmers no change is observed in 1982 and 1993 groups. From the study on the juniors it is observed that the present young swimmers of 12-13 yrs of age may not be able to attain the desired level of VO_2 max to achieve the high performance at international level. In case of cyclist a decreasing trend in VO_2 max and O_2 debt is observed — even the young junior cyclists have aerobic capacities of 63.7 ml/kg/min and they may not be able to achieve the desired level of VO_2 max. It is concluded that in case higher performance is to be achieved at the international level, the sports persons should be selected on the basis of physiological responses and trained scientifically from the young age.

Body composition and physique of Indian athletes

G. L. Khanna, P. Majumdar, T. Vrinda, M. Mandal
Exercise Physiology & its Training Application pb. Sports Authority of India, 1995, 19-21

The present study was carried out on 60 athletes of different events who attended the camp at SAI, Bangalore, in preparation for Asian Games

1994. The physical characteristics of the subjects including age, weight, body fat%, lean body mass and somatotype were measured. The results indicate that long distance, middle distance and throwers have somatotype rating of 1.42 -2.15 - 4.12; 1.68 - 2.90 - 3.31; 2.95 -4.79 - 1.05, respectively. The long distance runners of Indian athletes are slightly leaner than the Olympic athletes. But the Olympic athletes have more mesomorphic structure rather than ectomorphic. In middle distance running Olympic athletes seems to be more mesomorphic as compared to Indian athletes. Whereas, in throwers, Olympic athletes are more mesomorphic in structure than the Indian athletes and ectomorphic component is comparable. From this study it can be concluded that Indian athletes are lacking in mesomorphic component. We should select the athletes on the basis of physical characteristics with more muscular physique for middle and long distance runners.

A comparative study of physiological profile of Indian national vs Cuban Olympic boxers

G. L. Khanna, P. Majumdar, M. Saha

J. of Sport Sci. & Phys. Edu. 1994, 6, (1) 13-21

The present study was conducted to compare the world level Cuban boxers with Indian boxers to find the physical and functional abilities which contribute to the success of Cuban boxers. The study was conducted on 12 Cuban and 14 Indian boxers preparing for international competition at Bangalore. Body fat and physique were calculated by standard methods. Cardiorespiratory parameters including VO_2, VCO_2, VE, Breathing equivalent were recorded every 30 seconds on a computerized Ergopneumotest during exercise and recovery O_2 debt was computed from the recovery responses of O_2 consumption. The study revealed that the Cuban boxers are taller. It gives them advantage over the opponent during competition. There is optimum requirement of developing the mesomorphic components — beyond that it may not play a significant role in improving the performance. Body fat should not exceed 10%, 12% and 15% in lower, middle and heavy weight category, respectively. The aerobic and anerobic development of the boxers should be optimum. The most important aspect, that is, recovery, should be faster and the boxers should have better cardiorespiratory adaptation to submaximal load. The cardiorespiratory adaptation with technical superiority can determine the success in the competition.

Effect of six weeks' conditioning programme on Submaximal and Maximal cardiorespiratory variables in national badminton players

G. L. Khanna, P. Majumdar, M. Mandal, M. Saha

Ind. J. of Sport Sc. & Phys. Edu. 1994 (2) : 199-126

The present study was conducted on seventeen National Badminton players to find out the effect of six weeks' conditioning programme on submaximal and maximal cardiorespiratory responses during graded exercise on treadmill. The study was also aimed to observe whether the adaptation in maximum parameters can reflect the change in submaximal cardiorespiratory parameters. Heart rate, VO_2, VCO_2 were monitored during graded exercises with the help of EOS sprint (Jaeger & Co.) at an interval of 30 seconds. Anerobic threshold was determined by VE-VO_2 relationship. The study revealed that 6 weeks of training resulted in significant change in heart rate at submaximal speed of treadmill. Ventilatory threshold (%), VO_2 and VE at ventilatory threshold did not change significantly. Heart rate at ventilatory threshold was higher after six weeks training. Present study revealed that maximum aerobic capacity does not change with training in highly trained badminton players. However, it leads to adaptation and changes at sub-maximal heart rate.

Physiological effect of three months' training on Indian national volleyballer

G. L. Khanna, M. Saha, P. Majumdar

Ind. J. Sports Sc. & Phys Edu. 1993, 5 (2) 67-73

Ten Indian National volleyballers attending a 3 months' preparatory camp at Sports Authority of India prior to International competition were tested for anthropometric and physiological test to determine the effect of 3 months of training. They were trained by an Internal Cuban Coach. Training included two sessions for endurance, two sessions of weight training, 3 sessions for speed training and 5 sessions for tactical and technique training. Body fat, somatotype, VO_2 max, VE max, O_2 pulse, breathing equivalent, O_2 debt were determined by standard methods. Lung function tests were monitored by flowmate. The submaximal heart rate at 10 to 12 km/hr were also compared before and after training. Statistical analysis revealed that three months of training significantly improves Lean body mass, VO_2 max, O_2 pulse and forced vital capacity. Heart rate at 10 km and 12 km speed decreased significantly. However, O_2 consumption at both the speeds did not significantly change. It shows that three months' training significantly adapts the cardiorespiratory system. However, efficiency of metabolism is not affected. It indicates that longer time is required to have cellular level adaptations since it involves changes at the enzymatic level.

Effect of high altitude training on morpho-physiological parameters of middle and long-distance runners

G. L. Khanna, P. Majumdar, M. Mandal

Ind. Jr. Physiol. & Allied Sci. 1996 (Accepted)

The aim of the present study was to find out the effect of four weeks of training camp (TC-1) held at 2,000 meter altitude followed by a training camp at sea level without competition and to find out the effect of six weeks of training camp (TC-2) held at the same place followed by competition at sea level. Maximum oxygen consumption (VO_2 max), oxygen debt (O_2 debt) and maximum heart rate (MHR) were measured during graded exercise on treadmill. Blood hemoglobin was also estimated. The results revealed that after four weeks of altitude training VO_2 max improved significantly in both male and female athletes. There was no significant change in body fat and lean body mass in male athletes, whereas, in case of female athletes, body fat decreased significantly. MHR was not significantly changed in either male or female. The effect of six weeks of training camp revealed that no significant change was observed in VO_2 max and O_2 debt in either male or female athletes. Body fat decreased significantly and lean body mass improved significantly in case of male athletes. But in case of female athletes there was no significant change in body fat and lean body mass. From this study it can be concluded that the effectiveness of the altitude training depends on the magnitude of the training stress and the purpose of the training.

Physiological analysis to quantify Training load in badminton

P. Majumdar, G. L. Khanna, V. Malik, S. Sachdeva, Md. Arif, M. Mandal.

British Journal of Sports Medicine, December 1997, Vol. 31, Number 4 pp. 342-345

To estimate the training load of a specific on-court training regimes based on the magnitude of variation of suitable physiological and biochemical variables viz., heat rate-lactate response and the level of urea, uric acid and creatine phosphokinase which can estimate the effectiveness of this training structure when compared to the physiological demand of the match play objectively. In 35 single's games (n = 6), heart rate and blood lactate were analyzed by heart rate monitor and lactate analyzer, respectively. On-court technical training routines consisted of three sets of 'shadow play' and two sets of 'multishuttle' work. The training load was estimated by measuring serum urea, uric acid and creatine phosphokinase in the morning following the training days (from vein) by Hitachi UV-2000 spectrophotometer, using Boehringer Mannheim reagents and compared with off-season resting values. Analysis of the on court training regimes revealed high lactate values of 8-10.5 mmol,l^{-1} in different phases. The high percentage (82-100%) of maximum heart rate depicts a considerable stress on the cardiovascular system. Biochemical variables indicate that urea, uric acid and CPK activity increased significantly from 29.5 ± 4.5 mgs% to 32.9 ± 5.0 mgs%, 3.9 ± 0.6 to 5.6 ± 4.0 mgs% and 312 ± 211.8 to 363 ± 216.4 IU.1^{-1}, respectively, which may be due to intense training. The magnitude of training load may be proper to avoid overtraining. Intense workouts can interfere coordination capacity that is very important in sports requiring highly technical skill such as Badminton.

A study of physiological responses during match on Indian national kabaddi players

G. L. Khanna, P. Majumdar, V. Malik, T. Vrinda, M. Mandal

British Journal of Sports Medicine 1996; 30 : 232-235

The present study was conducted with an aim to study the physiological demand of kabaddi match as well as to find out the physical and physiological profile of top level kabaddi players. Sixteen players were investigated to find out the physiological parameters which includes maximum aerobic capacity (VO_2 max), maximum ventilation (V_E max), O_2 pulse, respiratory equivalent (RE), maximum heart rate and O_2 debt. These parameters were studied with the help of EOS sprint (Jaeger & Co., Germany) during a graded exercise protocol on treadmill. Oxygen debt (O_2 debt) was computed from the recovery oxygen consumption (VO_2). Somatotype of the players was calculated by Health and Carter method. Heart rate was monitored during selection trial match with the sport tester (PE 3000) on eight players who represented India in the Asian Games in 1994 and won the gold medal. From the playing heart rate VO_2 was computed through HR-VO_2 regression equation. Maximum lactate was evaluated from the blood samples collected at the end of the match by Analox instrument (U.K.). The results revealed that the average heart rate and oxygen consumption during the match were 146.5 ± 9.25 beats. min^{-1} and 2.25 ± 0.59 l. min^{-1}, respectively. During raiding the maximum heart rate attained varied from 162.4 ± 11.3 to 177.4 ± 4.2 beats. min^{-1}. It is observed that out of 40 minutes of match play a raider has to go for raid for 8.13 ± 2.03 times. The average time per raid was 20.8 ± 6.26 seconds. The total time spent on raiding will be around 169 seconds. The match heart rate and oxygen consumption was 72.3 to 83.3% of the maximum heart rate and 43.5 to 70.5% of the maximum oxygen consumption (VO_2 max), respectively. During raiding the player does not take any breath thereby indicating the dominance of the energy sources during raiding will be anerobic. The heart rate of the players remain below the threshold level during catching, holding and in-between raiding. Maximum lactate at the end of the match was found to be 6.13 ± 2.53 mmol.1^{-1}. Endomorphic-mesomorph physique (2.68-4.71-1.83) with body fat below 13%, VO_2 max of 48 ml.$kg.^{-1}$ $min.^{-1}$ and O_2 debt of 70 ml/kg. will be satisfactory for a kabaddi player.

Key words: Kabaddi, VO_2 max, O_2 debt, somatotype, anerobic threshold.

Assessment of playing heart rate and fractional oxygen utilization in hockey as determining factor in game planning

G. L. Khanna, P. Majumdar, T. Vrinda, M. Mandal
International Sci. Sports Congress 1996, 67 (Abstract)

The present study was carried out to determine the physiological stress during the hockey game with an aim to economize the energy expenditure and to introduce the concept of movement economy in total hockey to best utilize the fitness component for performance in the team game. The study was done on 13 National women hockey players attending a National camp in preparation for Asian Games 1994. Cardiorespiratory parameters were evaluated with the help of computerized Oxycon System (Jaeger & Co.). Regression equation of VO_2 and heart rate was computed. Heart rate in the actual game was measured with the help of Sport tester (PE-3000, Finland). Blood lactate at the end of the game was analyzed with the help of a standardized Automatic Lactate Analyzer (Analox Instrument Ltd.). The mean energy expenditure of women hockey players ranges from 34.6 to 50 KJ/min. There was no correlation observed between VO_2 max and energy expenditure. The game heart rate of right-in and left-in players was 183 and 184 bpm, respectively (88.4% and 92.9% of maximum heart rate, respectively), whereas, right-out and left-out players attained the game heart rate of 160 and 161 bpm, respectively (79.2% and 83.3% of maximum heart rate respectively). The right-in player played at 80% of VO_2 max and right-out player at 60.5% of VO_2 max. Left-back and right-back played the match at 85.2% and 69% of VO_2 max, respectively. The stress was highest on the left-in and right-in players (86% and 80% of VO_2 max, respectively). Even the center half has played at 67.2% of VO_2 max. Keeping in view the position-wise percentage utilization in the match the game planning can be done by the coach to utilize all the players to their best ability and avoid overstress to a particular positional player so as to maintain the peak performance throughout the game.

Analysis of training segment of national badminton players

P. Majumdar, G. L. Khanna, M. Mandal, A.K. Ghosh
Proc. 81st Ind. Cong. Part IV: Discussions 1994, 121

A study was conducted on eighteen male National Badminton players attending a Camp at SAI, South Center, Bangalore, in preparation for World Badminton Championship to assess the physiological profile in the laboratory and to monitor the training intensity while administering specific intensity workout on Badminton court. Oxygen consumption, CO_2 output, O_2 pulse, breathing equivalent, RQ were monitored during graded exercise on treadmill. The parameters were assessed by computerized EOS sprint (Jaeger and Co.) O_2 debt was evaluated from recovery O_2 consumption. The training load was identified by measuring urea, uric acid, CP kinase before and after the trainng of 60 to 80 minutes. The biochemical parameters were analyzed with the help of spectrophotometer (Hitachi, Japan). The training consisted of 5 segments in which different intensity efforts were imposed. The total workout of 60-80 minutes; work rest interval was 1:1 with varied repetitions from 5 to 7 in each segment. Lactic acid was measured at the end of each segment from the finger tip and was analyzed with Analox lactate analyzed (U.K.). The mean VO_2 max, O_2 debt, O_2 Pulse Breathing Equivalent and RQ were 3.57 ± O.52 1/min, 3.2 ± 0.90 1, 19.47 ± 3.07 ml/beat and 34.91 ± 5.34 1/1 of O_2, 1.12 ± 0.31, respectively. The urea level increased significantly from 29.5 ± 4.56 mgs% to 32.9 5.03 mgs% ($p < 0.05$). Uric acid level increased from 3.9

± 0.66 to 5.56 ± 0.94 mgs% ($p < 0.01$). CP Kinase did not reveal any significant changes in male after training. The result indicates that due to depletion of muscle glycogen and protein catabolism for supplying the required energy, the serum urea level is increased significantly. Since the demand of the game is not that intense as to cause a considerable reduction in muscle work capacity by fatigue and efflux of the enzyme CPK does not occur from the muscle. Segmental analysis of lactate revealed that mean lactate increased from Ist to IIIrd segment (7.07 ± 2.5 to 9.14.1 mmol/1) and thereafter it decreased in the 4th to 5th segment to 7.78 ± 2.53 and 6.28 ± 1.73 mmol/1), respectively indicating that the anerobic metabolism increases from 1st to IIIrd segments and, thereafter, due to the accumulation of lactate, the players are unable to withstand more muscular stress imposed through high intensity effort subsequently in Phase 4 to 5. The study concluded with the suggestion that strength training may be enhanced to develop muscular stength and intensive interval training may be administered to improve peak lactate tolerance to withstand the demand of the game. Adequate carbohydrate reserve may be ensured before exhaustive workout.

A study of physiological stress in different positional players in a hockey match

G. L. Khanna, P. Majumdar, Viney Malik, M. Mandal

Proc. 81st Ind. Sc. Cong. Part IV: Discussions, 1994, 199

The present study was conducted on 13 female National players attending camp at SAI, Bangalore, for preparation of Asia Cup 1993. The aim of the present study was to analyse physiological response during actual match condition at different positions and to identify the cardiovascular stress during match play. The study was also aimed to determine the influence of fitness determinant on the stress during match. The physiological parameters namely maximum aerobic capacity, Oxygen debt were measured in graded exercise protocol on treadmill (EOS Sprint, Germany). Heart rate was measured during the match with the computerized sport tester PE 3000 system. Heart Rate-Oxygen consumption regression was formulated and from there oxygen consumption was measured during actual match play. Fractional utilization of oxygen (% VO_2/VO_2 max) in relation to their maximum aerobic capacity was computed. Mean maximum aerobic capacity of Back, Half-back and Forwards were 46, 50.8, 53.9 ml/kg/min, respectively. A significant difference was observed between back and half-back and also between forwards and back. It may be due to low relative VO_2 max in half-back. The mean heart rate of forward and back line were at the same range (152-183 bpm and 158-181 bpm) during match condition. The backline played at lower heart rate range 9,141-174 bpm). The difference was found statistically significant amongst the three positions at 18th and 27th minutes and the first half and 3rd, 6th and 18th minutes of the second half. Similarly oxygen consumption and fractional utilization of oxygen were significantly higher in the half-back and forward line at the same time. Peak level of fractional utilization of oxygen amongst forward, half-back and back line were 84.7, 81.3 and 68.0%, respectively. Comparison of cardiac cost between first and second-half amongst various positions revealed that cardiac cost of half-backs were significantly lower ($p < 0.05$) in second-half compared to the first half. The study concluded that the strategy of the game should be planned in such a way that the stress of various positions should be equal and fitness level of half-backs should be improved, so that they can withstand the load till the completion of the match at the same pace.

Physiological demand of different positional players in women hockey

G. L. Khanna, P. Majumdar, Viney Malik, M. Mandal

NIS Sci. J. No. 1 : 5-14, 1995

The present study was conducted on 13 female National hockey players attending the camp at SAI, Bangalore, for preparation of Asian Games 1994. The aim of the present study was to analyze the physiological response during actual match condition at match play. The study was also aimed to determine the influence of fitness determinant on the stress during match. The physiological parameters, namely, maximum aerobic capacity, oxygen debt were measured in graded exercise protocol on treadmill (EOS Sprint, Germany). Heart rate was measured during the match with the computerized Sport Tester (PE-3000 system, Finland). Heart rate-Oxygen consumption regression was formulated and from there oxygen consumption was measured during actual match play. Fractional utilization of oxygen (percentage of VO_2 max) in relation to their maximum aerobic capacity was computed. Blood lactate was analyzed in a standardized automatic lactate analyzer (Analox Instruments Ltd. , UK.) Mean values of maximum aerobic capacity of full-back, half-back and forwards were 45, 50.91 and 53.88 ml/kg/min, respectively. A significant difference was observed between full-back and half-back and also between forward and full-back. The mean heart rate of forward and half-back was in the same range (152-183 bpm and 158-181 bpm) during match. The full-back played at lower heart rate range (141-174 bpm). The difference was found statistically significant amongst the three positions 18th and 27th minutes of the first half and 3rd, 6th and 18th minutes of the second-half. Similarly, oxygen consumption and fractional utilization of oxygen were significantly higher in the half-back and forward line at the same time. Peak level of fractional utilization of oxygen amongst forward, half-back and full-back were 84, 7, 81.3 and 68%, respectively. Comparison of sum of the heart beat between first and second-half amongst various position revealed that sum of the heart beat of half-back was significantly lower ($p < 0.05$) in the second-half as compared to the first-half. The mean value of blood lactate after the match was found to be 3.65 mmol/1/. The study concluded that the women's hockey is a stressful game, the training emphasis should be given depending on the physiological demand of different positional players.

Heart rate and blood lactate response in competitive badminton

A .K. Ghsoh, P. Majumdar, A. Goswami, A. Ahuja, and T. P. S. Puri

Annals of Sports Medicine, 1990, A6942-24-27

Ten junior National level (13-14 years of age) female badminton players having 3-6 years of training were studied to investigate the demands of the game on heart rate and blood lactate during competition. The mean VO_2 max and the anerobic threshold level were 48.3 ml/kg/min and 66.3% of the VO_2 max. Game analysis revealed that heart rates were higher in the second and third games than in the first game, whereas no difference was found in blood lactate concentration. Anerobic threshold heart rate and total duration of the game indicated on anerobic aerobic time domain ratio of 3 : 1. We conclude that junior national level female badminton players attained optimum aerobic capacity and anerobic threshold levels that could be improved later through further training and dissimilar strain on the cardiovascular and anerobic metabolic systems is possible due to the intermittent nature of the game.

Key Words: Badminton — Heart rate — Blood lactate.

Comparative study of iron status and lipid profile in elite endurance and strength trained athletes

G. L. Khanna, P. Majumdar, P. R. Lal, M. Mandal
International Pre-Olympic Sci. Congress, USA, 1996, 124 (Abstract)

The present study was conducted to determine the iron status and lipid profile of strength trained and endurance trained sports persons. Ferritin, Iron, Total Iron Binding Capacity (TIBC) and hemoglobin level were studied on 31 elite female middle and long distance runners (MLD) and weight lifters (WLT). Cholesterol, Triglycerides, HDL Cholesterol, Very low density lipoprotein (VLDL) and Low density lipoprotein (LDL) were tested on 212 middle and long distance runners and weight lifters. All the biochemical parameters were analyzed using Boehringer Manneheim kits. These groups had an experience of 4 to 7 years of training in their respective discipline. The results indicated that the iron status, i.e., ferritin, iron, TIBC and transferrin, were higher in WLT group; however, it was not significantly different from MLD group. It may indicate that the variation in the training may not change the iron status of the sports persons. Both the groups had low level of serum ferritin (MLD = 22.6 ng/ml, WLT = 34.4 ng/ml). Total cholesterol was not significantly different between two groups (WLT = 177.1 mgs%, MLD = 173.8 mgs%). However, significantly higher values of triglycerides were found in WLT group (85.6 mgs%) as compared to MLD group (69 mgs%). Similarly, HDL level was significantly higher in MLD group ($p < 0.01$). VLDL, LDL and Cholesterol/HDL ratio were significantly lower in MLD group. Body fat percentage and endomorphy components were significantly higher in WLT group ($p < 0.01$). Fat intake was also significantly higher ($p < 0.01$) in WLT group. The difference in the body composition, fat intake and type of training can make the significant difference in triglycerides. The difference in lipoprotein between WLT & MLD group may be due to combination of above-mentioned factors as well as the difference in the ergogenic aid taken during the training process.

Relationship of maximum aerobic capacity and serum iron status in relation to dietary iron intake of women hockey players

G. L. Khanna, P. Majumdar, P. R. Lal, M. Mandal
J. of Strength and Conditioning (Communicated)

Being the most important trace element, iron plays the key role in many biological reactions like formation of hemoglobin, myoglobin and cytochrome-c. The present study was conducted on 19 women hockey players attending National Camp at Sports Authority of India, Bangalore, in preparation for international competition with an aim to determine the relationship between the iron status and aerobic performance. Blood hemoglobin was determined by spectrophotometric analysis of cyanomethemoglobin. Serum ferritin was determined by enzyme immunoassay. Serum iron and transferrin were determined by spectrophotometric method. The subjects' dietary intake was measured using the 24 hrs recall method and the average daily iron, vitamin C and fiber intake were calculated using the Indian food value tables. Oxygen consumption was measured during graded exercise on treadmill with the help of computerized Oxycon champion (Jaeger & Co.). The results indicate that mean level of hemoglobin of the inmates was satisfactory. Only 5.3% of the total players had below 12 gms% hemoglobin level. The ferritin level ranged from 14.2 to 73.6 ng/ml with a mean value of 40.03 ng/ml. Dietary deficiency of iron, vitamin C and fiber intake was not influencing towards low ferritin level. The low level of serum ferritin does not affect transferrin level. The study revealed that there is no significant relationship between serum ferritin and aerobic performance but serum ferritin has significant correlation with serum iron. It is found that as long as the serum iron level is in the normal limit hemoglobin level is not affected. It can be concluded that intensive training may lead to more hemolysis and reduction in serum ferritin level. The dietary intake of iron for the women hockey player should be kept high to prevent manifest anemia.

Key words : Aerobic performance, Serum ferritin, Transferrin, Hemoglobin.

Effect of carbohydrate drink on endurance performance and recovery of sports persons

G. L. Khanna, P. Majumdar, M. Mandal
Ind. J. Sports. Sci. & Phys. Ed. 1997 (in press).

The present study was conducted with a view to find out the effect of supplementation of carbohydrate drink on submaximal endurance performance. It was also aimed to find out the effect on serum glucose and lactate level during exercise as well as during recovery. The study was conducted on eight sports-persons who are undergoing diploma course in coaching. Submaximal endurance performance was evaluated by making them run on the treadmill at 70% of their VO_2 max. VO_2 max was measured during graded exercise protocol with the help of Oxycon Champion (Jaeger & Co., Germany). 5% of carbohydrate solution was supplemented after every 15 minutes during exercise and 12.5% during recovery period at an interval of 10 minutes. Blood samples were collected during exercise and recovery period at an interval of 10 minutes. Blood glucose was evaluated on Hitachi U2000 spectrophotometer using Boehringer Manneheim Kit. Blood lactate was analyzed using Analox lactate analyzer (U.K.). The results revealed that there was a significant improvement (51%) in submaximal endurance time (62.3 minutes without carbohydrate and 94.3 minutes with carbohydrate). There was no significant difference in heart rate and lactate values with or without carboplus supplementation. Mean value of lactate during recovery was lower at the end of 10th and 20th minutes after carbohydrate supplementation indicating lactate removal was faster with carboplus supplementation. With the supplementation of carbohydrate the serum glucose level remains at higher level during exercise and recovery period though the difference was not significant. The present study concludes that carbohydrate supplementation during exercise improves endurance performance and keeps the lactate at lower level and glucose level remains at steady level for prolonged duration. During recovery lactate removal was faster and glucose level remains at higher level.

Key words : Blood glucose, Blood lactate, Heart rate, Submaximal load.

Comparison of serum ferritin, blood hemoglobin and VO_2 max between elite women hockey players and middle and long distance runners

Viney Malik, G. L. Khanna, P. Majumdar, M. Mandal
International Scientific Sports Congress, Bangalore, India 1996, 76 (Abstract)

The present study was conducted with a view to determine the influence of activity on serum ferritin, blood hemoglobin and VO_2 max in women hockey players (Group I) and middle and long distance runners (Group II). Both the groups were under training in preparations for 1994 Asian Games. Aerobic capacity was determined with the help of EOS sprint (Jaeger and Co., Germany). Serum Ferritin was estimated by enzyme-immunoassay using a commercial kit (Boehringer Manneheim GmbH Diagnostic, Germany). Blood hemoglobin concentration was determined within two hours from sampling. This method is based on the spectrophotometric analysis of cyanmet hemoglobin. Mean blood hemoglobin concentration was higher in Group II (14.83 gms%) as compared to Group I (12.77 gms%), whereas there was no difference in the mean serum ferritin in the two groups (Group I 56.29 ng/ml and Group II 59.50 ng/mol). The VO_2 max in Group II (54.86 ml/kg/min) was higher as compared to Group I (42.92 ml/kg/min). The study concludes that different activities does not influence the level of serum ferritin and the lower level of blood haemoglobin in Group I may not be only due to the low level of serum ferritin. The hemoglobin level can be one of the determinants of the aerobic capacity since long distance runners had higher VO_2 max and higher hemoglobin level as compared to women hockey players.

Physiological profile of 10-16 year talented children

G. L. Khanna, P. Majumdar, M. Saha, M. Mandal
NIS. Sci. J. 1996 (Accepted).

The present study was carried out with an aim to assess the cross-sectional development pattern of children (10 - 16 years) under training. The study is also aimed to frame physiological norms. This study was conducted on 777 children of 10-16 years of age group belonging to various schemes (NSTC, SPDA) of SAI. The morphophysiological parameters studied include somatotype, height, weight, body fat, lean body mass, back strength, aerobic anerobic capacity and recovery heart rate. Somatotype was calculated by using Heath and Carter method. Body fat % was calculated from skinfold thickness measured with Harpenden skinflod caliper at four different sites namely biceps, triceps, subscapular and suprailiac. For the calculation of the body fat percentage Durnin & Rehman and Siri formulae were used. Back strength was measured by back dynamometer. The other physiological parameters like aerobic-anerobic capacity and recovery heart rate were measured with computerized EOS sprint (Jaeger & Co., Germany). The results indicate that aerobic capacity in 10 years' children was 1.65 l/min. It increased to 3.10 l/min in 16 years age group. A significant increment was observed from 10-11, 11-12, 12-13, 13-14 and 14-15 years. Anerobic capacity at the age of 10 years was 1.38 l. it increased to 3.78 l at the age of 16 years. Mean recovery heart rate varied from 172.2 to 175.6. No significant variations were observed amongst the age group. Mean back strength varied from 57.7 kgs. to 109.2 kgs. Peak gain is observed from 14-15 years age group (10.1 kgs.). Mean body weight of 10 years children was 31.7 kgs. It increased up to 53.3 kgs. at the age of 16 years. The maximal gain occurred from 14-15 years of age (4.01 kgs.). The average height in children of 10 years age group was 144.10 cms. and 166.84 cms. in case of 16 years age group. Average gain in the height is 3.8 cms/year. Lean body mass increased from 27.46 kgs. in 10 years age group to 45.3 kgs. at 16 years of age. Maximum gain was observed from 13-14 years. Average body fat of 10-16 years children varied from 12.89% to 14.48%. No significant difference was found within the age group. Average somatotype of all the age group children was mesomorphic ectomorph. Mesomorphic component varied from 2.77 to 3.05. The present morphophysiological study will have much wider application. These normative data will help in talent selection and growth and development of age group children. This study will also help in assessment of effect of training of the talented children.

Anthropometric characteristics and motor function of 8-12 years' children in relation to auxological changes

P. Majumdar, G. L. Khanna, M. Mandal
Journal of Physical Education and Sports Sciences, 1996 (Accepted)

A research programme was conducted in the year 1990 on children volunteered for National Sports Talent Contest. The morphological characteristics viz., height, weight, viz. 30 mtr. run, broad jump, coordination ability, balance test, 6 × 10 mtr. run, 800 mtr. run, vertical jump and ball throw were assessed on 519 boys and 207 girls. The purpose of the study was to identify the growth and development of active boys and girls who participated in the contest of various age block and to estimate the influence on anthropometric variables on motor function. Suitable norms was constituted which can act as a tool for future selection. Test results indicate that highest weight gain achieved at the age of 10 years for both boys and girls. Maximum height gain observed at the age of 10 years for boys and 11 years for girls. Highest fat % was recorded at the age of 9 and 10 years for boys and girls, respectively, and after 10-12 years the body fat percentage remain stable. No significant sex difference was observed in somatotype. In motor function test boys and girls of 10 -12 years age group proved to be significantly different when compared to 8 and 9 years of age in ball throw, vertical jump and broad jump. This may be due to the gain in strength and neural maturation. In 800 mtr. run, balancing test and agility (6 × 10 mtrs.) no significant difference observed among the group of 8-12 years. Sex difference was observed in morphological and motor function test, the difference may be due to increased estrogen level which promotes greater fat deposition of girls. Correlation matrix revealed that gain in strength, speed and power is associated with stature. Regression equation was also formulated to establish morphological relationship with certain motor functions which enable the evaluator to predict/estimate the relative motor potentiality. Percentile distribution was laid which may be used as a frame of reference for rating the fitness level and development of 8-12 years children. It will be helpful for selection of talent and monitoring the growth and development.

Heart rate and blood lactate response in field hockey players

A. K. Ghosh, A. Goswami, P. Majumdar & D. N. Mathur

Indian J. Med. Res. [B] 94, October, 1991, pp. 351-356

The heart rate and blood lactate were studied in field hockey players (25 juniors and 29 seniors) as well as the blood lactate response in training to assess the anerobic demand of the game and the adaptability of the players to anerobic metabolism, respectively. The mean VO_2 max of the junior and senior players were 3.32 l/min (54.4 ml/kg/min) and 3.28 l/min (53.8 ml/kg/min), respectively. Blood lactate level after warm-up, training and the game were 2.1, 7.4 and 4.2 mmol/1, respectively for the juniors and 2.6, 7.7 and 5.6 mmol/1, for the seniors. The aerobic capacity (VO_2 max) of the juniors did not differ from their senior counterparts, indicating a similar adaptability to aerobic metabolism. However, the Indian players revealed a lower VO_2 max than their international counterparts. Similar lactate levels in juniors and seniors after training indicated a similar adaptability to the anerobic metabolism also. The higher blood lactate level in seniors after the game reflected that they played with greater intensity than the juniors due to more experience, better motivation and skill.

Sex differentiation in the physiological variables of Indian road cyclist at anerobic threshold level

A. K. Ghosh, P. Majumdar, G. L. Khanna and D. N. Mathur

Proc. 74th Ind. Sc. Cong. Part III : (Abstract), 1987, p. 34

In long distance continuous events, the determination of an anerobic threshold (AT) variables is gaining more importance day by day than the maximum aerobic capacity (VO_2 max). Hence the laudable objective of the present study was to assess the cardiorespiratory variables of Indian male and female road cyclists. AT level including the sex differentiation. The investigation materials of the present study consisted of 11 male and 9 female road cyclists. The subjects were administered a graded protocol of exercise on a bicycle ergometer. The initial load was 1 watt/kg and the increment was at the rate of 1 watt/kg after every two minute till exhaustion. The pedalling frequency was kept initially at 50 rpm and the same was increased at a rate of 10 rpm with each load increment. The AT level was determined from the deviation point of VE-VO_2 relationship. The physiological variables like heart rate (HR), ventilation (VE), Oxygen pulse (O_2-P), breathing equivalent (BE) were recorded on a computerized ergopneumotest at every 30 seconds interval. The results revealed that the mean VO_2 max, O_2-P, and BE at maximal work differed significantly between male and female road cyclists. However, the mean maximum heart rate in both the cases did not differ. The sex differentiation in the cardiorespiratory fitness has also been reported in the literature. The VO_2 and O_2-P of the female road cyclists at AT level were significantly lower ($p < 00.1$) than their male counterparts, while the percentage VO_2 max at the same point did not exhibit any significant difference. The mean BE in female road cyclists at AT level was significantly higher ($p > 0.01$) than the male cyclists which denoted a lower respiratory efficiency of female cyclists at AT level. At this point no significant difference existed between the heart rate of both the groups. Hence the present study concluded that the cardiorespiratory variables of both male and female cyclists at maximum level and at AT level differed significantly whereas, no difference was observed in the percentage VO_2 max at anerobic threshold point.

Aerobic-anerobic transition level of Indian middle and long distance runners

A. K. Ghosh, P. Majumdar, A. Goswami & G. L. Khanna

Indian J. Med. Res. 88, October 1988, pp. 371-375

A study was carried out on 23 elite Indian runners (12 middle distance and 11 long distance runners) to assess the aerobic-anerobic threshold level and also to compare them with international counterparts to enable the coaches and sports medicine specialists in using the anerobic threshold (AT) concept more efficiently as a training tool in endurance events. The cardio-respiratory variables at maximum effort were determined during a graded protocol of running on treadmill, starting from 10 km/h and increasing every 2 min at the rate of 2 km/h till exhaustion. The At was considered from the ventilatory threshold (VT) measured by non-invasive gas exchange method. The maximum aerobic capacity of Indian middle and long distance runners found to be 62.0 and 68.1 ml/kg/min, respectively, were significantly lower than those of their international counterparts. The mean VO_2 of the Indian middle distance runners at AT level was 49.9 ml/kg/min as compared to 58.0 ml/kg/mim of the world class runners. The long distance runners also exhibited a lower VO_2 at AT level as compared to international runners. It is concluded that, as the AT level is a well established determinant in distance running performance and significant improvement of maximum aerobic capacity (VO_2 max) may not be possible if the runners reach a plateau, more emphasis should be given to improve AT level of Indian distance runners.

Assessment of aerobic, anerobic capacity and aerobic to anerobic transition point of handball players

G. L. Khanna, P. Majumdar, A. K. Ghosh and D. N. Mathur

Proc. 74th Ind. Sc. Cong. Part III : (Abstract), 1987, p. 35

Physiological evaluation of sportsmen is of utmost importance, since these help the coaches and trainees in improving the performance by monitoring the daily training schedule. The aim of the present study was to assess the physiological capacities (Aerobic and anerobic capacities) and the anerobic threshold variables of national handball players and also to compare them with their international counterparts. Cardiorespiratory variables of 17 handball players which included VO_2 max, VE max, O_2-P, Breathing equivalent (BE) and heart rate were studied during graded protocol of exercise on a bicycle ergometer. The initial load administered in each case was 1 watt/kg after every two minute till exertion. The above-mentioned variables were recorded on Erich Jaeger's ergopneumotest (FRG) continuously at every 30 seconds. Recovery was taken for 15 minutes after exhaustive exercise to calculate oxygen debt which reflect anerobic capacity. The deviating point of VE-VO_2 relationship was considered as anerobic threshold level. Mean values of VO_2 max, VE max, O_2-P, BE and HR max and O_2 debt were 3.891 l/min. 958.91 ml/kg/min, 113.4411/min, 22.1 ml/beat, 31.17 l/l of O_2, 176.6 bpm and 4.471, respectively. The mean AT level have been determined and discussed. The results indicates that aerobic performance of Handball players is comparable to those of other international counterparts. However, aerobic capacity is observed to be low for playing Handball since the major part (80%) of the energy in Handball is released from anerobic sources. The date on anerobic threshold level of Handball players are lacking in the literature. However, it is comparable to that of the top Indian badminton players.

Specific training and its effect on VO_2 max and ventilatory threshold of badminton players

A. Ahuja, A. K. Ghosh, A. Goswami, P. Majumdar, G. L. Khanna, P. Bhandari & T. P. S. Puri

Jakarta Coaching Seminar, 1989

The objective of the present study was to investigate the intensity of a specific training programme in badminton and the effect of short term (3 weeks) training programme dominated by specific training on the VO_2 max and ventilatory threshold of badminton players. Five female badminton players volunteered as subjects. Pre-and post-test of VO_2 max was evaluated on automatic analyzer. The training schedule contained basic speed work, basic endurance activity and specific training on the court. The study concludes that the intensity of a specific training on the court for badminton is 78-90% of the maximum heart rate. It was also found that the three weeks training schedule dominated by specific type of training on the badminton court is enable to alter the VO_2 max.

Aerobic-anerobic demand in competitive badminton

A. K. Ghosh, A. Goswami, P. Majumdar, G. L. Khanna, A. Ahuja, P. K. Bhandari, T. P. S. Puri

The aim of the present study was to investigate the aerobic-anerobic dominance in competitive badminton from heart rate. Ten Indian female badminton players (14-16 yrs age) who have represented the junior National level competitions with an experience of 3-6 yrs training, participated in the present study as investigation subjects. The study was conducted in a precompetition training camp held at NIS, Patiala. The maximum aerobic capacity of the players was determined in the laboratory administering a graded running protocol on treadmill till volitional exhaustion. The heart rate (HR), VO_2, VCO_2 and VE were monitored continuously on Ergopneumotest (FRG). The anerobic threshold level of each player was calculated by a non-invasive gas exchange method. The HR at this level was considered as anerobic threshold HR. In the second phase of investigation, the hr was measured continuously at every 5 sec interval by a sports tester system (Polar Electro, Finland), in a selection trial under actual conditions of competitive badminton. The mean height, weight and VO_2 max of the players were 163 cm, 48.3 kg and 2.32 l/min (48.6 ml/kg/min), respectively. Continuous heart rate and time monitoring in 25 matches, revealed that in the 1st (n = 25), 2nd (n = 25) and 3rd (n = 11) game, the mean heart rates were 159.5, 170.6, 179.4 bpm, while the durations were 10.8, 9.2 and 10.2 min, respectively. From the heart rate and time, taken in a game, it was observed that in the 1st game, the heart rate crossed the anerobic threshold.

REFERENCE

Adams, R. P. and H. G. Welch (1980) : Oxygen uptake, acid-base status, and performance with varied inspired oxygen fractions. ***Journal of Applied Physiology*** 49 : 863-868.

Ahlberg, A., Weatherwax, RS., Deady, M. et al. (1986) : Effects of phosphate loading on cycle ergometer performance [abstract]. ***Medicine Science in Sports Exercise*** 18 : S11.

Ahlberg, G., Felig, P., Hagenfeldt, L, et al, (1974) : Substrate turnover during prolonged exercise in man. ***Journal of Clinical Investigation*** 53 : 1080-90.

Alen, M., Pakarinen, A and Hakkinen, K. (1993) : Effects of prolonged training on serum thyrotropin and thyroid hormone. In elite strength athletes, ***Journal of Sports Science*** 11 : 493-97.

Anderson, O. (1993) Creatine propels British athletes to Olympic gold medals : is creatine the one true ergogenic aid? ***Running Research News*** 9 : 1-5.

Arenas, Ricoy JR, Encinas, AR. et al, (1991) Carnitine in muscle, serum, and urine of nonprofessional athletes : effects of physical exercise, training, and L-carnitine administration. ***Muscle Nerve*** 14 : 598-604.

Armstrong, R (1979) ***Biochemistry*** : Energy liberation and use in sports Medicine and physiology, ed R Strauss, Philadelphia WB Saunders.

Asmussen and Mazin, (1978)[b] : Recuperation after muscular fatigue by "diverting activities". ***European Journal of Applied Physiology*** 38 : 1-7.

Asmussen, E., and O. Boje. (1945) : Body Temperature and Capacity for Work, ***Acta Physiologica Scandinavia*** 10 : 1.

Asmussen and Mazin, (1978)[a] : A central nervous component in local muscle fatigue. ***European Journal of Applied Physiology*** 38 : 9-15.

Asterita, M. (1985) : ***Physiology of Stress***, New York Human Sciences Press.

Astrand, P. and Rodahl, K. (1986) : ***Text Book of Work Physiology***, New York McGraw Hill.

Astrup, A., Toubro, S., Cannon, S. et al, (1990) Caffeine : a double blind, placebo-controlled study of its thermogenic, metabolic and cardiovascular effects in healthy volunteers, ***American Journal of Clinical Nutrition*** 51 : 759-67.

Bachman, J. C., and Harvath, S. M. (1968) : Pulmonary function changes which accompany athletic training programs. ***Research. Quarterly*** 39 : 235-242.

Bagbay, G., B. Sembrowich and P. Gollnick. (1972) : Myosin ATP are and fiber type composition from trained and untrained rat skeletal muscle, ***Journal of Applied Physiology*** 223 : 1415-17.

Bak, J. E. and Padersen, O. (1990) : Exercise enhanced activation of glycogen synthase in human skeletal muscle. ***American Journal of Physiology*** 258 : E957-E963.

Baker, H., Frank, O., DeAngelis, B. et al, (1992) : Absorption and excretion of L-carnitine during single or multiple dosing in humans. ***International Journal of Vitamin and Nutritional Research*** 63 : 22-6.

Baldwin, K. et al, (1972) : Respiratory capacity of white, med and intermediate muscle : Adaptive response to exercise, ***Journal of Applied Physiology*** 222 : 373-78.

Balsom, PD., Ekblom, B., Soderlund, K. et al, (1993) : Creatine supplementation and dynamic high-intensity intermittent exercise. ***Scandinavian Journal of Medicine Science Sports*** 3 : 143-9.

Balsom, PD., Harridge, SDR., Soderlund, K. et al, (1993) : Creatine supplementation *per se* does not enhance endurance exercise performance. ***Acta Physiologica Scandinavica*** 149 : 521-3.

Banerjee, P. K., Ghatterjee, S .P., Chatterjee and Maitra, S. R. (1974) : Aerobic capacity in Bengali young men trained and untrained. ***Indian Journal of Physiology & Allied Sciences*** 28 : 91.

Banerjee, P. K., Chatterjee, S. P., and Maitra, S. R. (1969) : Changes in concentration of serum protein fractions in response to treadmill runners. ***Indian Journal of Physiology & Allied Sciences*** 23 : 26-30.

Banerjee, S., and Sen, R. N. (1955) : Determination of the surface of the body of Indians. ***Journal of Applied Physiology*** 7 : 585-88.

Bhardwaj, KH., Malhotra, M. S., and Srivastava, K. K. (1972a) : Body composition changes in the plains on descend from high altitude. ***Human Biology*** 46 : 41-56.

Bhardwaj, S., Singh, A. P. and Malhotra, M. S. (1973b) : Body composition of the high altitude natives of Ladakh. A comparison with sea level residents. ***Human Biology*** 45 : 423-434, 1973.

Brahmachari, H. D., Malhotra, M. S., and Joseph, S. (1972a) : Carbohydrate metabolism under environmental stess. Part II : Glucose tolerance under heat, cold and hypoxic stress. ***Indian Journal of Experimental Biology*** 10 : 272-273, 1972.

Brahmachari, H. D., Malhotra, M. S., and Joseph S. (1972b) : Effect of stay at high altitude on the serum proteins of man. ***Indian Journal of Physiology & Pharmacology*** 17 : 365-369.

Banerjee, S. and Sen, R. N. (1958) : Body composition of Indians and its relation to basal metabolic rate. ***Journal of Applied Physiology*** 12 : 29-33.

Banerjee, P. K., Chatterjee, S., and Maitra, S. R. (1969) : Changes in concentration of serum protein fractions in response to treadmill runners. ***Indian Journal of Physiology & Allied Sciences*** 23 : 26-30.

Barnard, R. J., G. W. Gardner, N. V., Diaco, R. N., MacAlpin, and A.A. Kattus (1973) : Cardiovascular responses to sudden strenuous exercise-Heart Rate, Blood pressure, and ECG, ***Journal of Applied Physiology*** 34 : 833.

Barnard, R. and Foss, M. (1969) Oxygen debt : Effect of beta adrenanil blockade and on lactacid and alactacid components, ***Journal of Applied Physiology*** 27 : 813-16.

Barnett, C., Costill, D., Vukovich, K. et al, (1994) : Effect of L-carnitine supplementation on muscle and blood carnitine content and lactate accumulation during high-intensity sprint cycling. ***International Journal of Sport Nutrition*** 280-8.

Bautellier, U. et al, (1984) : After effect of chronic hypoxia on oxygen kinetics and on oxygen deficit and debt. ***European Journal of Applied Physiology*** 53 : 87-91.

Bergstrom, J. (1962) : Muscle electrolytes in man. Scandinavian, ***Journal of Clinical Investigation*** 14 (Supply.), 1-100.

Bergstrom J., Hermansen L., Hultman E. and Saltin B. (1967) : Diet, muscle glycogen and physical performance. ***Acta Physiologica Scandinavica*** 71 : 140-150.

Bevegard, S., Holmgren, A. and Jonsson, B. (1963) : Circulatory studies in well trained athletes at rest and during heavy exercise with special reference to stroke volume and the influence of body position. ***Acta Physiological Scandinavia*** 57 : 26-50.

Bigland-Ritchie, B., Dawson, N. J., Johansson, R. S., Leppold, OCJ. (1986) : Reflex origin for the slowing of motoneurone firing rates in fatigue of human voluntary contraction. ***Journal of Physiology*** Lond 379 : 451-459.

Bigland-Ritchie, (1981) : EMG and fatigue of human voluntary and stimulated contractions. In ***Human Muscle Fatigue : Physiological Mechanisms*** 130-56. London: Pitman Medical.

Bigland-Ritchie, B., Jones, D. A. Hoods, J. J. (1979) : Excitation frequency and muscle fatigue : Electrical responses during human voluntary and stimulated contractions. ***Experimental. Neurology*** 64 : 414-427.

Bird, SR., Wiles, J., Robbins, J. (1995) : The effect of sodium bicarbonate ingestion on 1500m racing time. ***Journal of Sports Science*** 13 : 399-403.

Bjorkman, O., Sahlin, K., Hagenfeidf, L., Wahren, J. (1984) : Influence of glucose and fructose ingestion on the capacity for long term exercise in well trained men. ***Clinical Physiology*** 4 : 483-494.

Blom, PCS., Costill, DL., Vpllestad, NK. (1987)[a] : Exhaustive running: inappropriate as a stimulus of muscle glycogen compensation, ***Medicine & Science in Sports and Exercise*** 19 : 398-403.

Blom, PCS. Hostmark, AT., Voage, O., Kardel, K., Maehlum, S. (1987)[b] : Effect of different sugar diet on the rate of muscle glycogen synthesis. ***Medicine & Science in Sports and Exercise*** 19 : 491-496.

Blomstrand, E., Andersson, S., Hassmen, P. et al, (1995) : Effect of branched chain amino acid and carbohydrate supplementation on the exercise induced change in plasma and muscle concentration of amino acid in human subject. ***Acta Physiological Scandinavica*** 153 : 87-96.

Bolter, C. et al, (1973) : Intrinsic rate and cholinergic sensitivity of isolated atria from trained and sedentary rates. ***Proc. Society Experimental. Biology Medicine*** 144 : 364.

Bonen, A. (1976) : Effect of exercise on excretion rates of urinary free cortisol, ***Journal of Applied Physiology*** 40 : 155-158.

Brass, EP., Hiatt, WR., Minierview (1994) : Carnitine metabolism during exercise. ***Life Science*** 54 : 1383-93.

Brazy, P., Mandel, L. (1986) : Does availability of inorganic phosphate regulate cellular oxidative metabolism? ***News in Physiological Sciences*** 1 : 100-2.

Breale, D., Stager, JM., Berchue, WF. et al, (1998) : Phosphate supplementation, cardiovascular function, and exercise performance in humans. ***Journal of Applied Physiology*** 65 : 1821-6.

Brengelmann, G. (1983) : Circulatory adjustments to exercise and heart stress, ***Annual Review of Physiology*** 45 : 191-212.

Broberg, S., and Saltin, K. (1989) : Adenine nucleotide degradation in human skeletal muscle during prolonged exercise, ***Journal of Applied Physiology*** 76 : 116-22.

Brodal, P. et al, (1976) : Capillary supply of skeletal muscle fibers in untrained and endurance trained men. ***Acta Physiologica Scandinavica*** (Suppl.) 440.

Brooks, G. A. (1986) : The lactate shuttle during exercise and recovery, ***Medicine and Science in Sports and Exercise*** 18 : 360-8.

Brooks, G. A., and Fahey, T. (1984) : ***Exercise Physiology*** : Human Bioenergetics and its Application. New York: John Wiley & Sons.

Brooks, G., and Fahey, T. (1987) : ***Fundamentals of Human Performance*** New York: John Wiley and Sons.

Brooks, G. et al, (1971) : Temperature Skeletal muscle, mitochondrial functions and oxygen debt, ***American Journal of Physiology*** 220 : 1053-59.

Brooks, G. A. (1994) : Basic exercise physiology, ***American College of Sports Medicine 40th Anniversary Lectures, Indianapolis***, American College of Sports Medicine.

Brooks, G. (1986) : Lactate production under fully aerobic conditions. The lactate shuttle during rest and exercise. ***Federation Proceedings*** 45 : 2924-29.

Brouns, F. Saris, WHM., Stroecken, J., Beckers, E., Thijssen, Rehrer, N. J. and Ten, Hoor, F. (1989) : Eating, drinking and cycling. A controlled tour de France simulation study. Part II. Effect of diet manipulation. ***International Journal of Sports Medicine*** 10 : S41-S48.

Bucci, LR. (1989) : Nutritional ergogenic aids. in: Hickson, JF., Wolinsky, I. editors. ***Nutrition in Exercise and Sports***. Boca Raton; CRC press: 107-84.

Burke, L., Collie,r G., Hargreaves, M. (1991) : Effect of glycemia index on muscle glycogen resynthesis following exhaustive exercise. Submitted for publication.

Buskirk, E. R., Kollias, J., Picon, Reatigue, E. and others (1966) : Physiology and performance of track athletes at various altitude in the United States and Peru. In Goddard R.F. editor : ***The Effects of Altitude on Physical Performance***. Chicago, The athletic institute.

Burkitch, E. R. (1992): from Harvard to Minnesota : Keys to our history, ***Exercise Sports Science Review*** 20 : 1-26.

Cade, R., Conte, M., Zauner, C. et al, (1984) : Effects of phosphate loading on 2, 3-diphosphoglycerate and maximal oxygen uptake. ***Medicine Science in Sports Exercise*** 16 : 263-8.

Carey, C. R. et al, (1955) : Effect of skin diving on lung volummes. ***Journal of Applied Physiology*** 8 : 519-527.

Carlsten, A. & Grimby, G. (1966) : ***The Circulatory Response to Muscular Exercise in Man***, Springfield I L, Charles C Thomas.

Cerretelli, P., Marconi, C. L. (1990) : Camitine supplementation in humans. The effects on physical performance. ***International Journal of Sports Medicine*** 11 : 1-14.

Cerretelli, P. et al, (1977) : Oxygen uptake transients at the onset and offset of arm and leg work. ***Respiration Physiology*** 30 : 81-97.

Chapman, C. B. (1990) : The long reach of Harvard's fatigue laboratory: 1926-1947, ***Perspect Biol Med*** 34 : 17-33.

Chapman, C. B., and J. H. Mitchell (1965) : The physiology of exercise, ***Scientific American*** 212 : 88-96.

Chatterjee, S., Chatterjee, P., and Maitra, S. R. (1978) : Effect of graded workload on the heart of different age groups. ***Digest, ESWBME***, New Delhi pp126.

Clancy, L. J., Critchley, J. A. J. H., Leitch, A. G. and others (1975) : Arterial catecholamine in hypoxic exercise in man, ***Clinical Science Molecular Medicine*** 49 : 503.

Clarkson, P. M. (1993) : Nutritional ergogenic aids: caffeine. ***International Journal of Sports Nutrition*** 3 : 103-11.

Clarkson, P. M. (1992) : Nutritional ergogenic aids: carnitine. ***International Journal of Sport Nutrition*** 2 : 185-90.

Clarkson, P. M. (1991) : Minerals: exercise performance and supplementation in athletes. ***Journal of Sports Science*** 9 : 91-116.

Coggan, A. R., Coyle, E. F. (1987) : Reversal of fatigue during prolonged exercise by carbohydrate infusion or ingestion; ***Journal of Applied Physiology*** 63 : 2388-2395.

Conlee, R. K. (1991) : Amphetamine, caffeine, and cocaine. In Lamb, DR, Williams, MH, editors. ***Ergogenics : Enhancement of Performance in Exercise and Sports***. Vol. 4. Perspective of exercise science and sports Medicine. Dubuque: Brown and Benchmark 285-325.

Coombes, J., McNaughton, L. R. (1993) : Effects of bicarbonate ingestion on leg strength and power during isokinetic knee flexion and extension. ***Journal of Strength and Conditioning Research*** 7 : 241-9.

Cooper, D. M., Wasserman, D. H., Vranic, M., and Wasserman, K. (1986) : Glucose turnover in response to exercise during high and low — F102 breathing man. ***American Journal of Physiology*** 251 : E209-214.

Cooper, K. H. (1968) ***: Aerobic***, New York : Evans.

Costill, D. L., Hargreaves, M. (1992) : Carbohydrate nutrition and fatigue. ***Sports Medicine*** 13 : 86-92.

Costill D.L., Pascoe, D. D., Fink, W. J., Robergs, R. A., Barr, S. I. and Pearson, D. (1990) : Impaired muscle glycogen resynthesis after eccentric exercise. ***Journal of Applied Physiology*** 69 : 46-50.

Costill, D. L. (1988) : Carbohydrates for exercise: dietary demands for optimal performance. ***International Journal of Sports Medicine*** 9 : 1-18.

Costill, D. L., Coyle, E. F., Fink, W. J., Lesmcs, G. R., & Witzmann, F. A. (1979) : Adaptation in skeletal muscle following strength training. ***Journal of Applied Physiology***, Respiratory, environmental exercise physiology 46 : 96-99.

Costill, D. L., Pascoe, D. D., Fink, W. J., Robergs, R. A., Barr, S. I. et al, (1990) : Impaired muscle glycogen resynthesis after eccentric exercise. ***Journal of Applied Physiology*** 69 : 46-50.

Costill, D. L., Thomas, R., Robergs, R. A., Pascoe, D. D., Lambert, C. P., Barr, S. I., and Fink, W. J. (1991) : Adaptation to swim training, influence of training volume, ***Medicine and Science in Sports and Exercise*** 23 : 371-377.

Costill, D. L., Daniel, J., Evans, W., Fink, W., Krahenbuhl, G., and Saltin, B. (1976) : Skeletal muscle enzyme and fiber composition in the male and female tract athletes, ***Journal of Applied Physiology*** 40 : 149-154.

Costill, D. L. (1985) : Practical problems in exercise physiology research. ***Research Quarterly*** 56 : 376-384.

Costill, D. L., Fink, W. L., and Pollock, M. L. (1976) : Muscle fibre composition and enzyme activities of elite distance runners, ***Medicine & Science in Sport*** 8 . 96-100.

Costill, D. L., Coyle, E., Dalsky, G., Evans, W., Fink, W., and Hopes, D. (1977) : Effect of elevated plasma FFA and insulin on muscle glycogen usage during exercise. ***Journal of Applied Physiology*** 43 : 695-9.

Costill, D. L., and Hargreaves, M. (1992) : Carbohydrate Nutrition and fatigue. ***Sports Medicine*** 13(2) : 86-92.

Costill, D. L. (1986) : ***Inside Running, Basics of Sports Physiology***, P (178) : Indianapolis. Benchmark press.

Coyle, E. F., Coggan, A. R., Hemmert, M. K., Lowe, R. C., Walters, T. J. (1985) : Substrate usuage during prolonged exercise following a pre exercise meal. ***Journal of Applied Physiology*** 59 : 429-433.

Craig, A. H., Park, S. H., and Roemmich, J. N. (1990) : Changes in protein nutritional status of adolescent wrestlers. ***Medicine and Science in Sports and Exercise*** 22 : 599-604.

Crawford, M. H., Petru, M. A., and Rabinowitz, C. (1985) : Effect of isotonic exercise training on left ventricular volume during upright exercise. ***Circulation*** 72 : 1237-1243.

Dahlstrom, M. E., Jansson, E., Nordevang, E., and Kijser, L. (1990) : Discrepancy between estimated energy intake and requirement in female dancer, ***Clinical Physiology*** 10 : 11-25.

Das, S. K., Chatterjee, S., Chatterjee, P., and Maitra, S. R. (1968) : Studies on some aspects of respiration and metabolism in dog under pentothal sodium anaesthesia. ***Indian Journal of Physiology & Allied Sciences*** 22 : 70.

Davies, C. T. M., and K. Young (1982) : Maximal Power Output in relation to the Contractile properties of the Triceps Surae in Man, ***Journal of Physiology*** 325 : 51.

Davis, J. M. (1995) : Central and peripheral factors in fatigue. ***Journal of Sports Science*** 13 : S49-S53.

Davis, J. M. (1995) : Carbohydrates branched-chain amino acids, and endurance: the central fatigue hypothesis. ***International Journal of Sport Nutrition*** 5 Suupl. : S29-S38.

Davis, C. T. M., and Thompson, M. W. (1979) : Aerobic performance of female and male ultramarathon athletes. European, ***Journal of Applied Physiology*** 41 : 233-45.

Decombaz, J., Deriaz, O., Acheson, K. et al, (1993) : Effect of L-carnitine on submaximal exercise metabolism after depletion of muscle glycogen. ***Medicine and Science in Sports and Exercise*** 25 : 733-40.

Dejours, P. : Control of respiration in muscular exercise. (1964) : In. (W. Fenn, ed) Handbook of physiology, section 3. Washington : ***American Physiological Society.***

DeVries, H. A. (1974) : ***Physiology of Exercise for Physical Education and Athletics***, DuBugue Iowa, W.C. Brown.

Dey, S. K., Khanna, G. L., and Batra, M. (1991) : Morphological and physiological study on Indian National Kabaddi player, ***Indian Journal of Physiology & Allied Sciences*** 45 (4) : 30-31.

Dey, S. K., Khanna, G. L., Batra, M. (1993) : Morphological and physiological studies on Indian National Kabaddi players. ***British Journal of Sports Medicine*** 27 (9) 237-41.

Dhinney, S. D., Bistrain, B. R., Evans, W. J. et al, (1983) : The human metabolic response to chronic ketosis without caloric restriction: preservation of submaximal exercise capacity with reduced carbohydrate oxidation. ***Metabolism*** 769-76.

Dill D.B., and Adams W.C. (1971) : Maximal oxygen uptake at sea level and at 3,090 in altitude in high school champion runners. ***Journal of Applied Physiology*** 30 : 854.

Dill, D. B. (1985) : ***The Hot Life of Man and Beast.*** Springfield, I. L. Charles C Thomas.

Dill, D. B., H. T. Edwards, and J. H. Talbot, (1932) : Alkalosis and the capacity for work. ***Journal of Biological Chemistry*** 97 : LVII-LIX.

Dill, D. B. (1938) : ***Life Heat and Altitude.*** Cambridge, MA Harvard University press.

Dodd, S. et al, (1988) : Effects of beta blockade on ventilation and gas exchange during the rest to work transition. ***Aviation Space and Environmental Medicine*** 59 : 255-58.

Donovan, C. and G. Brooks (1983) : Endurance training effects lactate clearance not lactate production. ***American Journal of Physiology*** 244 : E83-E92.

Dowson, M. J., Smith, S., and Wilkie, D. R. (1986) : The ($H_2PO_4^{-1}$) may determine cross bridge cycling rate and force production in living fatiguing muscle, ***Biophysics Journal*** 49 : 268a.

Drinkwater, B. L., Bruemmer, B. and Chesnut, C. H. (1990) : Menstrual history as a determinant of current bone density in young athletes, ***Journal of American Medical Association*** 236 : 545-8.

Drinkwater, B. L., Folinsbee, L. J., Bedi, T. F. and others (1979) : Response of women mountaineers to maximal exercise during hypoxia. ***Aviation Space Environment Medicine*** 50 : 657.

Duffin, J. (1994) : Neural drives to breathing during exercise. ***Canadian Journal of Applied Physiology*** 19 : 289-304.

Duffy, D. J., Conlee, R. K. effect of phosphate loading on leg power and high intensity treadmill exercise, (1986) : ***Medicine and Science in Sports and Exercise*** 18 : 674-677.

Dyck, D. J., Pitman, C. T., Heigenhauser, GJF. et al, (1993) : Regulation of fat carbohydrate interaction in skeletal muscle during intense aerobic cycling, ***American Journal of Physiology*** 265 : E852-9.

Earnest, C. P., Snell, P. G., RodriguezR. et al, (1995) : The effect of creatine monohydrate ingestion on anaerobic power indices, muscular strength, and body composition. ***Acta Physiologica Scandinavica*** 153 : 207-9.

Ebashi, S. (1976) : Excitation-contraction coupling, ***Annual Review of Physiology*** 38 : 293-309.

Edstrom, L. and Grimby, L. (1986) : Effect of exercise on a motor unit muscle and nerve, ***International Journal of Sports Medicine*** 9 : 104-26.

Edwards, R. H. T., Hill, D. K., Jones, D. A., Merton, P. A. (1977) : Fatigue of long duration in human skeletal muscle after exercise. ***Journal of Physiology*** London 272 : 769-778.

Edwards, R. H. T. (1981) : Human muscle function and fatigue; in Porter (ed) : ***Human muscle fatigue : Physiological Mechanisms*** pp 1-18 (Pitman, London).

Edwards, R. H. T. (1983) : Biochemical basis of fatigue in exercise performance: catastrophe theory of muscular fatigue. ***In Biochemistry of Exercise eds***. H. Kunttage, J. Vogal, and J. Poortmans. Champaign IL Human Kinetics.

Ekblom, B. and Hermansen, L. (1968) : Cardiac output in athletes, ***Journal of Applied Physiology*** 25 : 619-625.

Ekblom, B., Astrand, P., Saltin, B., Stenberg, J. and Walstrom, B. (1968) : Effect of training on circulatory response to exercise, ***Journal of Applied Physiology*** 24 (4) : 518-528.

Erp-Boart, A. M. J., Van Saris, W. H. M., Blnkhors,t R. A., Vas, J. A. and Elvers, J. W. H. (1989) : Nation wide survey on nutritional habits in elite athletes, Part 1 : Energy, Carbohydrate, protein and fat intake, ***International Journal of Sports Medicine*** 10 : S3-S10.

Essen, B. and L. Kayser. (1978) : Regulation of glycolysis in intermittent exercise in man, ***Journal of Physiology*** (London) 231-56.

Euler, U.S., Von. (1969) : Sympatho-adrenal activity and physical exercise. ***Biochemistry of Exercise, Medicine and Sports,***, 3rd ed, J.R., Poortman, 170-81, New York, Karger, Basal.

Faber, M., Spinnler-Benade S-J., Daubitzer ,A. (1990) : Dietary intake, anthropometric measurements and plasma lipid levels in throwing field athletes. ***International Journal of Sports Medicine*** 10 : 140-145.

Favier, R. et al, : Ventilatory and circulatory transients during exercise (1983) : New arguments for a neurohumoral theory. ***Journal of Applied Physiology*** 54 : 647-653.

Fenn, W. O. and H. Rahn eds (1964) : ***Handbook of Physiology : Respiration***, Vol. 1, American physiology society, Washington, D. C.

Fetg, P. and Wahren, J. (1975) : Fuel homeostasis in exercise, ***New England Journal of Medicine*** 293 : 1078-84.

Fetig, P., Cherif, A., Minagawa, A. and Wahren, J. (1982) : Hypoglycemia during prolonged exercise in normal men, ***New England Journal of Medicine*** 306 : 895-900.

Fitts, R. H., and J. O. Holloszy (1976) : Lactate and contractile force in frog muscle during development of fatigue and recovery. ***American Journal of Physiology*** 231 : 430-33.

Fitts, R. H., Kim, D. H., Witzmann, F. A. (1976) : The development of fatigue during high intensity endurance exercise in Nagle (ed) : ***Exercise in Health and Disease***, pp 118-135 (Thomas Springfield).

Fleck, S. T. and Kraemer, W. J. (1987) Designing resistance training programs, Champaign IL, Human Kinetics.

Fleckenstein, J. L., Watamull, D., McIntire, D. D. et al, (1993) : Muscle Proton T2 relaxation times during work and during repetitive voluntary exercise, ***Journal of Applied Physiology*** 74 (60) : 2855-2859.

Fluco, C. S., Rock, P. B., Trad, L. A. (1994) : Effect of caffeine on submaximal exercise performance at altitude. ***Aviation Space Environmental Medicine*** 65 : 539-45.

Fox, E., Bartels, R., Billings, C., O'Brien, R., Bason, R. and Mathews, D. (1975) : Frequency and duration of interval training programs and changes in aerobic power. ***Journal of Applied Physiology*** 38 (3) 481-484.

Fox, E. (1987) : Human Physiology, Dubuque Ia: Wm C. Brown Guyton, a (1986) : ***Test Book of Medical Physiology***, Philadelphia WB Saunder company.

Fox, E., and Costill, D. (1972) : Estimated cardiorespiratory responses during marathon running. ***Arch. Environment and Health*** 24 : 315-324.

Fox, E., Barteis, R., Billings, C., Mathews, D., Bason, R., and Webb, W. (1973) : Intensity and distance of interval training programs and changes in aerobic power, ***Medicine and Science in Sports*** 5 (1) : 18-22.

Fox, E. (1987) : ***Human Physiology***. Dubuque, Ia : Wm C Brown.

Hole, J. (1987) : ***Human Anatomy and Physiology***, Dubuque, Ia Wm C Brown.

Fox, E. L. and Mathews (1974) : ***Interval training : Conditioning for Sports and General Fitness***. Philadelphia, W. B. Saunders company.

Favier, R. et al, : Ventilatory and circulatory transients during exercise (1983) : New arguments for a neurohumoral theory. ***Journal of Applied Physiology*** 54 : 647-653.

Fox, E. (1996) : ***Human Physiology***, Dubugue Ia, Wm C Brown.

Frick, M., Kowttiner, A. and Sarayas, S. (1963) : Effects of physical training on circulation at rest and during exercise, ***American Journal of Cardiology*** 12 : 142-147.

Frisancho, A. R. (1979) : ***Human Adaptation: a Functional Interpretation***, St. Louis. The C. V. Mosby. Co.

Fuchs, F., V. Reddy and F.,N. Briggs. (1970) : The interaction of cations with the calcium-binding site of troponin. ***Biochemistry Biophysics***. *Acta* 221 : 407-9.

Gaesser, G., and Brooks, G. (1984) : Metabolic bases of excess post exercise oxygen consumption: A review. ***Medicine and Science in Sport and Exercise*** 16 : 29-43.

Ganong, W. F. (1979) : ***Review of Medical Physiology***, Los Affas CA Lange Medical Publications.

Ghosh, A. K., Ahuja, A., Khanna, G. L. (1985e) : Physical and physiological determinants of fitness in Indian football players. Paper presented at ***OCA Sports Medicine Symposium Baharainj*** 10-12 April 1985.

Ghosh, A. K., Ahuja, A., Khanna, G. L. (1986b) : Intercorrelation of Physical and Physiological parameters of National soccer players. ***Proc. Asian Games Conference***. Seoul, Korea.

Ghosh, A. K., Ahuja, A., Khanna, G. L. (1987c) : Physiological variables Indian National badminton players at anaerobic threshold level ***World Badminton*** 15 (4) : 36.

Ghosh, A. K., Majumdar, P., Goswami, A., Khanna, G. L. (1988a) : Aerobic — Anaerobic transition level of Indian middle and long distance runners, ***Indian Journal of Medical Research*** 1988, pp 371-375.

Ghosh, A. K., Ahuja, A., Khanna, G. L. (1985d) ; Physical and physiological variables of Indian National soccer players, ***3rd World Congress of Medical Aspects of soccer — USOC Sports Medicine Division***, Colorado USA.

Ghosh, A. K., Majumdar, P., Goswami, A. and Khanna, G. L. (1988b) : Aerobic-anaerobic transition level of Indian middle and long distance runners. ***Indian Journal of Medical Research*** 88 : 371-375.

Ghosh, A. K., Ahuja, A. and Goswami, A. (1991b) : Physical and physiological profile of Indian National Women hockey players. ***NIS Scientific Journal*** 14, 4, 1-9.

Ghosh, A. K., Ahuja, A. and Goswami, A. Heart rate and blood lactate response in amateur competitive boxing. ***Indian Journal of Medical Research*** 102, 10. 179-183, 1995.

Ghosh, A. K., Goswami, A. and Ahuja, A. (1993) : Evaluation of sports specific training program in badminton players. ***Indian Journal of Medical Research*** 98[B], 10, 232-236.

Ghosh, A. K., Majumdar, P., Goswami, A., Ahuja, A. and Puri, T. P. S. (1990b) : Heart rate and blood lactate response in competitive badminton. ***Annals of Sports Medicine*** (USA), 5, 85-88.

Ghosh, A. K., Khanna, G. L., Ahuja, A., Kaul, T. K. (1986d) : Cardiorespiratory fitness of Silent Cricketers in India. **XX III *FIMS World Congress on Sports Medicine*** 1986.

Ghosh, A. K., Ahuja, A., Khanna, G. L. (1985f) : Physiological status of Indian National Gymnasts Scientific Abstract, Cong. ***Scientifque de Gymnastique***, Montreal, Canada 1985.

Ghosh, A. K., Khanna, G. L., Majumdar, P., Mathur, D. N. (1987b) : Sex differentiation in the physiological variables of Indian road cyclists at anaerobic threshold level. ***Pro. 74th Indian Science Congress***, Bangalore Abstract p. 34.

Ghosh, A. K., Ahuja, A., Khanna, G. L. (1987a) : Distance run as a predictor of aerobic endurance (VO_2 max) of sportsmen. ***Indian Journal of Medical Research*** 85 : 680-684.

Ghosh, A. K., Khanna, G. L., Ahuja, A., Mathur, D. N. (1986C) : Comparison of body composition, muscular strength and VO_2 max of mute Vs Indian national table tennis players. **XX III *FIMS World Congress on Sports Medicine***.

Ghosh, A. K., Goswami, A., Majumdar, P. and Mathur, D. N. (1991a) : Heart rate and blood lactate response in field hockey. ***Indian Journal of Medical Research*** 94[B], 10, 351-356.

Ghosh, A. K., Ahuja, A., Khanna, G. L. (1985a) : Body composition and maximal aerobic power of Indian national football players. Proc. 3rd ***International Congress of Sports Medicine Applied to Football***, 2-5 June 1985. Athens Greece.

Ghosh, A. K., Ahuja, A., Khanna, G. L., Kalley, S. (1985b) : Intergroup variation in characteristics of Indian national basketball players. Proc. ***FISU Conference***, Universiade, Kobe. pp. 345-346.

Ghosh, A. K., Ahuja, A., Khanna, G. L. (1986a) : Physiological status of Indian National Gymnasts., ***Congress Scientific de Gymnastique Universite de Montreal***, Canada.

Ghosh, A. K., Ahuja, A., Khanna, G. L. (1985c) : Pulmonary capacities of some group of sportsmen in India., ***British Journal of Sports Medicine*** 19 (4) : 85-88.

Gladder, B. Stainby, W. and Macintosh, B. (1982) : Norepinephrine increases canine muscle O_2 during recovery, ***Medicine and Science in Sports and Exercise*** 14 : 471-76.

Gledhill, N. (1985) : The influence of altered blood volume and oxygen transport capacity on aerobic performance. In (R.L. Terjung. ed.) ***Exercise and Sport Sciences Reviews*** Vol. 13 : 75-94. New York Macmillan Publishing Company.

Gleeson, M., Manghan, R. J., Greenhaft, P. L. (1986) : Comparison of the effects of pre-exercise feeding on glucose, glycerol and placebo on endurance and fuel homeostasis in man. ***Eur. Journal Applied Physiology*** 55 : 645-653.

Gollnic, P. D., Armstrong, R., Sanbert, C., Piew, K. and Saltin, B. (1972) : Enzyme activity and fiber composition in skeletal muscle of untrained and trained men. ***Journal of Applied Physiology*** 33 : 312-319.

Gollnick, P. et al (1973) Effect of training on enzyme activity and fibre composition of human skeletal muscle J. Appl. Physio 34, 107.

Gonyea, W. L., Sale, D. G., Gonyea, F, B and Mikesky A (1986) Exercise induced increases in muscle fiber number : European Journal of applied physiology 55. 137-147.

Gollnick, P. and Saltin, B. (1983) : Hypothesis significance of skeletal muscle oxidative capacity with endurance training, ***Clinical Physiology*** 2 : 1-12.

Gollnick, P. D. and Hodgson, D. R. (1986) : The identification of fibre types in skeletal muscle a continual dilema, ***Exercise and Sports Science Review*** 14 : 81-104.

Gore, C. and Withers (1990) : Effect of exercise intensity and duration on post exercise metabolism, ***Journal of Applid Physiology*** 68 : 2362-68.

Gorostiaga, E. M., Maurer, C. A., Eclache, J. P. (1989) : Decrease in respiratory quotient during exercise following L-carnitine supplementation. ***International Journal Sports Medicine*** 10 : 169-74.

Goswami, A., Mathur, D. N. and Ghosh, A. K. (1995) : Blood lactate removal pattern after submaximal and supramaximal exercises. ***NIS Scientific Journal*** 18, 2, 11-1.

Gracia-Sainz, J. (1991) : Cell responsiveness and protein Kinase C-receptor G Proteins and membrane effectors, ***News in Physiological Sciences*** 6 : 169-73.

Graham, T. E., Spriet, L. L. (1995) : Metabolic catecholamine, and exercise performance response to various dose of caffeine. ***Journal of Applied Physiology*** 78 : 867-74.

Graham, T. E., Spriet, L. L. (1991) : Performance and metabolic responses to a high caffeine dose during prolonged exercise. ***Journal of Applied Physiology*** 71 (6) : 2292-8.

Gtaham, T. E., Rush, J. W. E., Van soeren, M. H. (1994) : Caffeine and exercise metabolism and performance, ***Canadian Journal of Applied Physiology*** 19 : 111-38.

Green, J. and Sheldon, M. (1983) : Ventilatory changes associated with changes in pulmonary blood flow in dogs. ***Journal of Applied Physiology*** 54 : 997-1002.

Green, H. J., Sutton, J., Young, P., Cymerman, A. and Houston, C. S. (1989) : Operation Everest II. Muscle energetics during maximal exhaustive exercise. ***Journal of Applied Physiology*** 66 : 142-50.

Green H. (1986) : Muscle power: ***Fiber type recruitment, metabolism and fatigue***. In (N. Jones, N. Mccartney) and A Mccomas eds) Human Muscle power, 65-79. Champaign III. Human Kinetics Publishers.

Green, J. and Schmidt, N. (1984) : Mechanism of hyperpnea induced by changes in pulmonary blood flow. ***Journal of Applied Physiology*** 56 : 1418-1422.

Greenhaff, P. L., Casey, A., Shor,t A. H. et al, (1993) : Influence of oral creatine supplementation on muscle torque during repeated bouts of maximal voluntary exercise in man. ***Clinical Sciences*** 84 : 565-71.

Greenhaff, P. L. (1995) : Creatine and its application as an ergogenic aid. ***International Journal of Sports Nutrition*** 5 Suppl. : S100-S110.

Greenhaff, P. L., Bodin, K., Soderlund K. et al, (1994) : Effect of Oral creatine supplementation on skeletal muscle phosphocreatine resynthesis. ***American Journal of Physiology*** 266 : E725-30.

Greig, C., Finch, K. M., Jones, D. A. et al, (1987) : The effect of oral supplementation with L-carnitine on maximum and submaximum exercise capacity. ***European Journal of Applied Physiology*** 56 : 457-60.

Griffith, J., Humphreys, S., Clark, M. et al, (1994) : Forearm substrate utilization during exercise after a meal containing both fat and carbohydrate, ***Clinical Sciences*** 86 : 165-75.

Griffith, J., Humphreys, S., Clark, M. et al, (1994) : Immediate metabolic availability of dietary fat in combination with carbohydrate, ***American Journal of Clinical nutrition*** 59 : 53-59.

Harmansen, L. and Wachtlova, M. (1971) Capillary density of skeletal muscle in well trained and untrained men. ***Journal of Applied Physiology*** 30; 8670-863.

Grover, R. F., Reeves, J. T., Grover, E. B. and others (1979) : Muscular exercise in young men native to 3100m altitude. ***Journal of Applied Physiology*** 22 : 555, 1967. Frisancho.

Guezennec, C. Y., role of Lipid on endurance capacity in man, ***International Journal of Sports Medicine*** 1992 : 13 Suppl., 1 : S114-118j.

Gupta, S., Goswami, A., Sadhukhan, A. K. and Mathur, D. N. (1996) : Comparative study of lactate removal in short term massage of extremities, active recovery and a passive revovery period after supramaximal exercise session. ***International Journal of Sports Medicine***, (Germany) 17 : 106-110.

Guyton, A. C. (1986) : ***Test Book of Medical Physiology***, 7th eds, Philadelphia: WB Saunders.

Hagberg, J. et al, (1982) : Exercise hyperventilation in patients with McArdle's disease. ***Journal of Applied Physiology*** 52 : 991-994.

Hagberg, J., Mullin, J. and Nagle, N. (1978) : Oxygen consumption during constant load exercise, ***Journal of Applied Physiology*** 45 : 381-384.

Hagg, S. A., Morse, E. L. and Adibi, S. A. (1982) : Effect of exercise on rates of oxidation, turnover and plasma clearance of leucine in human subjects. ***American Journal of Physiology*** 242 : E407-E410.

Hammond, M. et al, (1986) : Pulmonary gas exchange in humans during exercise at sea level. ***Journal of Applied Physiology*** 60 : 1590-98.

Hargreaves, M., Costill, D. L., Fink, W. J., King, D. S., Fielding, R. A. (1987) : Effect of pre-exercise carbohydrate feeding on endurance cycling performance. ***Medicine & Science in Sports & Exercise*** 19 : 33-36.

Hargreaves, M. and Richter, E. A. (1988) : Regulation of skeletal muscle glycogenolysis during exercise. ***Canadian Journal of Sports Science*** 13 : 197-203.

Hargreaves, M. (1990) : Skeletal muscle Carbohydrate metabolism during exercise. ***Australian Journal of Science and Medicine in Sports*** 22 : 35-8.

Hargreaves, M., Kiens, B. and Richter, E. A. (1991) : Effect of increased plasma free fatty acid concentration on muscle metabolism in exercising man, ***Journal of Applied Physiology*** 70 : 194-201.

Harmansen, L. and Wachtlova, M. (1971) : Capillary density of skeletal muscle in well trained and untrained men. ***Journal of Applied Physiology*** 30 : 8670-863.

Harris, R. C., Soderlund, K., Hultman, E. (1992) : Elevation of creatine in resting and exercise muscle of normal subjects by creatine supplementation. ***Clinical Sciences*** 83 : 367-74.

Hawler, J. A., Dennis, S. C., Lindsay, F. H. et al, (1995) : Nutritional Practices of athletes: are they scale optimal? ***Journal of Sports Science*** 13 : 755-875.

Hermansen, I., Hultman, E., Saltin, B. (1967) : Muscle glycogen during prolonged severe exercise, ***Acta Physiologica Scandinavia*** 71 : 129-139.

Hermansen, L., Ekblom, B. and Saltin, B. (1970) : Cardiac output during submaximal and maximal treadmill and bicycle exercise, ***Journal of Applied Physiology*** 29 : 82-86.

Hickson, R., Bonze, M. and Hollaszy, J. (1978) : Faster adjustment of oxygen uptake to the energy requirement of exercise in the trained state, ***Journal of Applied Physiology*** 44 : 877-81.

Higginbotham, M. B., Marris, K. G. Willioms, R. S., McHale, P. A., Coleman, R. E. and Cobb, F. R. (1986) : Regulation of stroke volume during submaximal and naximal upright exercise in normal man. ***Circulation Research*** 85 : 281-291.

Hill, A. V. (1927) : "***Living Machinery***," Harcourt, Brace and World, Inc, New York.

Hill, R. and G, wyse (1989) : ***Animal Physiology***, New York Harper and Row.

Hill, A. V. (1923) : Muscular exercise lactic acid and the supply and utilization of oxygen,***Q. J Med*** 16 : 135-171.

Hill, A. V. (1914) : The oxidative removal of lactic acid, ***Journal of Physiology*** (London) 48: X-XI.

Hogberg, P. and O. Ljunggren (1947) : Uppvarmningens inverkan pa lopprestationerna, ***Svensk Idrott*** 40.

Hollmann, W., Frenkl, R., Bertean, P. & Rost, R. (1988) : The cardiovascular systems, ***The Olympic Book of Sports Medicine*** (ed) Dirix, A., Knuttgen, H. G. and Tittes, K Blackwell scientific publications pp 40-48.

Holloszy, J. O., Constable, S. H. and Young, D. A. (1986) : Activation of glucose transport in muscle by exercise. ***Diabetes/Metabolism Review*** 1 : 409-23.

Holloszy, J. O. and Coyle, E. F. (1984) : Adaptation of skeletal muscle to endurance exercise and their metabolic consequences. ***Journal of Applied Physiology*** 56 : 831-8.

Holloszy, J. (1982) : Muscle metabolism during exercise, ***Archives of Physical and Rehabilitation Medicine*** 63 : 231-34.

Hoppeler, H. (1986) : Exercise induced ultrastructure changes in skeletal muscle. ***International Journal of Sports Medicine*** 7 : 187-204.

Horstman, D. H., Weiskopf, R. and Robinson, S. (1979) : The nature of perception of effort at sea level and high altitude. ***Medicine and Science in Sports*** 11: 150.

Horswill, C. A. (1995) : Effects of bicarbonate, citrate, and phosphate loading on performance. ***International Journal of Sports Nutrition*** 5 Suppl. : S111-S119.

Houston, M. E., Morrin, D. A., Green, H. J. and Thomson, J. A. (1981) : The effect of rapid weight loss on physiological function in wrestlers, ***Physician and Sports Medicine*** 91 : 73-8.

Howley, E. T. (1976) : The effect of different intensities of exercise on the excretion of epinephrine and norepinephrine and epinephrine, ***Medicine and Science in Sports*** 8 : 219-22.

Huertas, R., Campos, Y., Diaz, E. et al, (1992) : Respiratory chain enzymes in muscle of endurance athletes: effect of L-carnitine. ***Biochemistry and Biophysics Research Commun*** 188 : 102-7.

Hultman, E. (1973) : Energy metabolism in human muscle, ***Journal of Physiology*** (London) 321 : 56.

Hurley, B. F., Nemeth, P. M., Martin, W. H., Hagberg, J., Dalsky, G. and Holloszy, J. O. (1986) : Muscle triglyceride utilisation during exercise. Effect of training, ***Journal of Applied Physiology*** 60 : 562-7.

Ikai, M. and Yabe, K. (1969) : Training effect of muscular endurance by means of voluntary and electrical stimulation. ***European Journal of Applied Physiology*** 28 : 55-60.

Ingler, F. (1979) : Capillary supply and mitochondrial content of different skeletal muscle fiber types in untrained and endurance trained men: A histological and ultrastructural study ***European Journal of Applied Physiology*** 40 : 197-209.

Ivy, J. L., Katz, A.L., Culle,r C. L., Sherman, W. M., Coyle, E. F. (1988) : Muscle glycogen synthesis after exercise; effect of time of carbohydrate ingestion. ***Journal of Applied Physiology*** 64 : 1480-1485.

Iyengar, S. (1984) : ***Computer Modelling of Complex Biological System*** Boca Raton Fl. CRC Press.

Jacobs, I., Romet, T. T. and Kerrigan-Brown, D. (1985) : Muscle glycogen depletion during exercise at 9°C and 21°C. ***European Journal of Applied Physiology*** 54 : 35-9.

James, D. E. (1995) : The mammalian facilitative glucose transporter family. International union of physiology sciences, ***American Physiology Society*** 10 : 67-71.

Janson, E. and Kaijser, L. (1987) : Substrate utilization and enzymes in skeletal muscle of extremely endurance trained men, ***Journal of Applied Physiology*** 62 : 999-1005.

Janssen, G. M. E., de Graef, C. J. J. and Saris, W. H. M. (1989) : Food intake and body composition in novice athletes during a training period to run a Marathon, ***International Journal of Sports Medicine*** 10 : S17-S21.

Johannessen, A., Hagen, C., Galbo, H. (1981) : Prolactin Growth hormone, thyrotrophin 3, 5, 3 triiodothyronine and thyroxine responses to exercise after fat and carbohydrate enriched diet. ***Journal Clinical Endocranial Metabolism*** 52 : 56-61.

Johnson, L. (1983) : ***Biology***: Dubuque, Ia : Wm C. Brown.

Jones, D. A. (1981) : Muscle fatigue due to changes beyond the neuromuscular junction. In ***Human Muscle Fatigue: Physiological Mechanisms*** 178-96. London: Pitman Medical.

Jones, N. L. et al, (1977) : Effect of pH on cardiorespiratory and metabolic responses to exercise. ***Journal of Applied Physiology*** 43 : 959-64.

Karlsson, J. and Saltin, B. (1970) : Lactate, ATP and C344 in working muscle during exhaustive exercise in man, ***Journal of Applied Physiology*** 29 : 598-602.

Karlsson, J. and Saltin, B. (1971) : Diet, Muscle glycogen and endurance performance, ***Journal of Applied Physiology*** 31 : 203-6.

Kartz, A. and Saltin, K. (1989) : Effect of hypoxia on glucose metabolism in human skeletal muscle during exercise. ***Acta Physiologica Scandinavica*** 136 : 377-82.

Kasper, C., Reeves, B., Flynn, M. et al, (1994) : L-carnitine supplementation and running performance. ***Medicine and Science in Sports and Exercise*** 26 (5) : S39.

Katz, A. et al, (1984) : Maximal exercise tolerance after induced alkalosis. ***International Journal of Sports Medicine*** 5 : 107-10.

Katz, A., Broberg, S., Saltin, K. and Wahren, J. (1986) : Leg glucose uptake during maximal dynamic exercise in human, ***American Journal of Physiology*** 251 : E65-E70.

Kaufmann, D. A. et al, (1974) : Pulmonary function of Marathon runners. ***Medicine and Science in Sports*** 6 : 114-118.

Keizer, H. A. and A. D. Rogal (1990) : Physical exercise and menstrual cycle alterations: what are the mechanism? ***Sports Medicine*** 10 (4) : 218-35.

Kenny, W. L. (1988) : Control of heat induced cutaneous vasodilatation in relation to age. ***European Journal of Applied Physiology*** 57 : 120-25.

Khanna, G. L. & Saha, M. (1991) : Effect of Six Months' training on Cardiorespiratory variables in talented children, ***Indian Journal of Sports Science & Physical Education*** Vol. 45 (4) : 31-32.

Khanna, G. L. (1991) : Physiological studies on effect of weight loss on Wrestling performance — a review. ***NIS Scientific Journal*** Vol. 14 (4) : 10-16.

Khanna, G. L., Ghosh, A. K., Ahuja, A. (1986a) : Body composition, muscular strength and cardiovascular efficiency of 252 sportsmen of various discipline ***SNIPES Journal***, 8 : 45-51.

Khanna, G. L., Ghosh, A. K., Majumdar, P. (1987b) : Assessment of aerobic anaerobic capacity and aerobic to anaerobic transition point of handball players. ***Proc. 74th Indian Science Congress, Bangalore*** Abstract p. 35.

Khanna, G. L., Ghosh, A. K., Ahuja, A., Mathur, D. N. (1986b) : Recovery oxygen debt analysis in graded maximal and supramaximal exercise. ***2nd National Conference on Physical Education and Sports Science*** Feb. 22-24, 1986. p. 4.

Khanna, G. L., Majumdar, P., Malik V., Mandal, M. (1995a) : Physiological demand of different positional players in women hockey. ***NIS Scientific Journal*** Vol. 18 (1) : 5-14.

khanna, G. L., Bhatnagar, D. P. (1993b) : A Cross-sectional analysis of submaximal and maximal oxygen consumption in Indian Boys. ***NIS Scientific Journal*** 16.

Khanna, G. L., Majumdar, P., Mandal, M. (1995c) : A secular trend in Maximum aerobic and anaerobic capacity in Indian National endurance sportsmen. ***NIS Scientific Journal*** 4 : 5-13.

Khanna, G. L., Ghosh, A. K., Sharma, J. G., Malhotra, M. S. (1983) : Physiological status of some judoists in India, ***SNIPES Journal*** 6 (2) ; 21-27.

Khanna, G. L., Majumdar, P., Mandal, M., Saha, M. (1994b) : Effects of six weeks conditioning training programe on submaximal and maximal cardiorespiratory variables in National badminton players. ***Indian Journal of Sports Science & Physical Education*** 6 (2) : 119-126.

Khanna, G. L., Saha, M., Majumdar, P. (1993a) : Physiological effects of three months training On Indian National volleyballers. ***Indian Journal of Sports Science & Physical Education*** 5 (2) : 1993.

Khanna, G. L., Majumdar, P., Malik, V., Vrinda, T., Mandal, M. (1996d) : A study of physiological responses during match on Indian National Kabaddi Players. ***British Journal of Sports Medicine*** Vol. 30 : 232-235.

Khanna, G. L., Majumdar, P., Saha, M., Mandal, M. (1998) : Cardiorespiratory fitness and body composition of Indian children of 10-16 yrs. ***Medicine and Sports Science*** 43 : 132-144.

Khanna, G. L., Majumdar, P., Vrinda, T., Mandal, M. (1996a) : Assessment of playing heart rate and fractional oxygen utilization in hockey as determining factor in game planning. Presented in the 1996, ***International Scientific Sports Congress and Exhibition*** held at Bangalore p. 67 (Abstract).

Khanna, G. L., Majumdar, P., Lal, P. R., Mandal, M. (1996b) : Comparative study of Iron status and lipid profile in elite endurance and strength trained athletes. Physical activity, sports and health, 1996 ***International Pre-Olympic Scientific Congress*** USA. p. 124 (Abstract).

Khanna, G. L., Saha, M. (1995b) : Effect of four weeks altitude training on cardiorespiratory variables in national cyclists. ***Indian Journal of Sports Science & Physical Education*** 7 (1) : 1-9.

Khanna, G. L., Bhatnagar, D. P. & Mathur, D. N. (1992b) : Prediction of aerobic and anaerobic capacity from maximal, submaximal and recovery cardiopulmonary responses in children. ***Indian Journal of Sports Science & Physical Education*** ED. 4 (1) : 1-7.

Khanna, G. L., Majumdar, P., Saha, M. (1994c) : A Comparative study of physiological profile of Indian National And Cuban Olympic boxers. ***Journal of Physical Education & Sports Sciences*** Vol. 94 : pp. 13-21.

Khanna, G. L., Saha, M. (1992c) : Physique and Physiological characteristics of Indian national Jr & Sr Swimmers with reference to age. ***NIS Scientific Journal*** 15 (3) : 87-94.

Khanna, G. L., Ghosh, A. K., Ahuja, A. and Bhatnagar, S. (1992a) : A Comparative study of Physiological variables in Senior and Junior National Cyclists. ***Indian Journal of Sports Science & Physical Education*** 4 (2) : 57-60.

Khanna, G. L., Majumdar, P., Ghosh, A. K., Mathur, D. N. (1986a) : Psycho-Physiological responses of Indian school footballers during graded ergometry. ***NIS Scientific Journal*** 11 (2), 1988. 8-12.

Khanna, G. L., & Bhatnagar, D. P. (1991) : Physiological profile of aerobic and anaerobic capacities and cardiopulmonary responses in 8-18 years children. ***Indian Journal of Sports Science & Physical Education*** 3 (2) : 68-76.

Khanna, G. L., Majumdar, P., Malik, V., Mandal, M. (1994a) : A study of physiological stress on different positional players in a hockey match. ***Proc. 81st Indian Science Congress*** Part-IV, p. 118 (Abstract).

Khanna, G. L., Ghosh, A. K., Ahuja, A., Mathur, D. N. (1987a) : Recovery oxygen debt analysis in graded maximal and supramaximal exercise. ***Sports Sciences*** 1987. 151-156.

Khanna, G. L., Ahuja, A., Ghosh, A. K. (1985) : Morpho-physiological characteristics of Indian basketball players. ***Hungarian Review of Sports Medicine*** 26 (4) : 243-249.

Kinderman, W., J. Keul and G. Huber, (1977) : Physical exercise after induced alkalosis (bicarbonate or Tris-buffer). ***European Journal of Applied Physiology*** 37 : 197-204.

Kingwell, B., McKenna, M. J., Sandstrom, E. R., Hargreaves, M. (1989) : Effect of glucose polymer ingestion on energy and fluid balance during exercise. ***Journal of Sports Sciences*** 7 : 3-8.

Kjellbergn, S., Rudhe, U. and Sjostrand, T. (1949) : Increase of the amount of haemoglobin and blood volume in connection with physical training, ***Acta Physiologica Scandinavia*** 19 : 146-151.

Klause, K., Dill, D. B., Phillips, E. E. and others (1967) : Metabolic reactions to work in the heat, ***Journal of Applied Physiology*** 22 : 292.

Klissoweas, V., Piray, F. and Petit, J. (1973) : Adaptation to maximal effort genetics and age, ***Journal of Applied Physiology*** 35 (2) : 288-293.

Kmuttgen, H. and Saltin, B. (1972) : Muscle metabolites and oxygen uptake in short-term submaximal exercise in man, ***Journal of Applied Physiology*** 32 : 690-94.

Knapic, J. J., Meredith, C. N., Jones, B. H., Suck, L., Young, V. R. and Evans, W. J. (1988) : Influence of fasting on carbohydrate and fat metabolism during rest and exercise in men, ***Journal of Applied Physiology*** 64 : 1923-9.

Kodama, T. (1985) : Thermodynamic analysis of muscle ATP mechanisms. ***Physiological Reviews*** 65 : 468-540.

Kozak-Collins, K., Burke, E., Schoene, R. B. (1994) : Sodium bicarbonate ingestion does not improve performance in women cyclists. ***Medicine Science in Sports and Exercise*** 26 : 1510-1515.

Kreider, R. B., Miller, G. W., Williams, M. H. et al, (1990) : Effects of phosphate loading on oxygen uptake, ventilatory anaerobic threshold, and run performance. ***Medicine Science in Sports Exercise*** 22 : 250-6.

La Grange, F. (1889) : ***Physiology of Bodily Exercise***, London : Kegan Paul International Ltd.

Lahiri, S. (1977) : Physiological responses and adaptations to high altitude. In Robertshow D., Ed. ***Environmental Physiology*** II, Baltimore, University Park Press.

Lambert, E. V., Speechly, D. P., Dennis, S. C. et al, (1994) : Enhanced endurance in trained cyclists during moderate intensity exercise following 2 weeks adaptation to a high fat diet. ***European Journal of Applied Physiology*** 69 : 287-93.

Larsson, L. (1982) : Physical training effect on muscle morphology in sedentary males at different ages. ***Medicine and Science in Sports Exercise*** 14 : 203.

Larsson, L. and Tasch, P. A. (1986) Motor unit, fiber density in extremely hypertrophied skeletal muscle in man: Electro physiological signs of muscle fiber hyperplasia — ***European Journal of Applied Physiology*** 55, 130-136.

Laycock, J. F. and Wise, P. H. (1983) : ***Essential Endocrinology***, New York, Oxford University Press.

Lemon, P. W. R., (1991b) : Protein and amino acid needs of the strength athlete. ***International Journal of Sports Nutrition*** 1 (in press).

Levine, L., Evans, W. J., Cararette, B. S., Fisher, E. C., Bullen, B. A. (1983) : Fructose and glucose ingestion and muscle glycogen during submaximal exercise. ***Journal of Applied Physiology*** 55 : 1776-1771.

Lewis, S. F. and Haller, R. G. (1986) : The pathophysiology of Mc Ardle's disease : Clues to regulation in exercise and fatigue, ***Journal of Applied Physiology*** 61 : 391-401.

Ljunghall, S. et al, (1988) : Increase in serum parathyroid hormone levels after prolonged exercise. ***Medicine and Science in Sports and Exercise*** 20 : 122-25.

Ljunghall, S. et al, (1986) : Prolonged low intensity exercise raises the serum parathyroid hormone levels, ***Clinical Endocrinology*** 25 : 535-42.

Lusk, G. (1928) : ***The Elements of the Science of Nutrition***, Philadelphia, WB Saunder.

Mac Dougall, J. D., Tuxen, D., Sale, D. B., Morz, J. R. and Sutton, J. R. (1985) : Arterial BP response to heavy resistance exercise, ***Journal of Appliad Physiology*** 58 : 785-790.

Mackintosh, B. R., Wrightm B. M. (1995) : Caffeine ingestion and performance of a 1,500 meter swim. Can ***Journal of Applied Physiology*** 20 : 168-77.

MacLean, D. A., Graham, T. E., Saltin, B. (1994) : Branched-chain amino acids augment ammonia metabolism while attenuating protein breakdown during exercise. ***American Journal of Physiology*** 267 : E1010-22.

Maitra, S. R., Chatterjee, S. and Das, S. (1968) : A quantitative information on normal values for respiratory functions in cat. ***Indian Journal of Physiology & Allied Sciences*** 22 : 28-33.

Maitra, S. R., Chatterjee, S. and Das, S. K. (1966) : Study on protein concentration in plasma and corpuscular changes of blood in man with minimal, submaximal and maximal work load. ***Proc. Symposium on Human Adaptability to Environments and Physical Fitness***. Ed. Malhotra M.S. : Defence Institute of Physiology and Allied Sciences, Madras, India pp. 130-140.

Maitra, S. R., Chatterjee, S., Chatterjee, P., Koyal, S. N. and Das Gupta, S. (1967) : Effect of heavy muscular work of five athletes on exchange of blood lactate, O_2 consumption, haemoglobin, RBC concentration and electrocardiogram. ***Indian Journal of Physiology & Allied Sciences*** 21 : 20.

Majumdar, P., Khanna, G. L., Mandal, M. (1998) : Anthropometric characteristics and Motor function of 8-12 years children in relation to auxological changes. ***Journal of Physical Education & Sports Sciences*** 3 : 32-39.

Majumdar, P., Khanna, G. L., Malik, V., Sachdeva, S., Arif, Md., Mandal, M. (1997) : Physiological analysis to quantify training load in Badminton, ***British Journal of Sports Medicine*** 31 : 342-345.

Majumdar, P., Khanna, G. L., Mandal, M., Ghosh, A. K. Analysis of training segment of National badminton players. (1994) : ***Proc. 81st Indian Science Congress*** Part-IV, p. 120.

Malhotra, M. S. (1971) : Physiological evaluation of Indian elite athletes. ***NIS Scientific Journal*** 5, 2 : 91-96.

Malhotra, M. S., Ramaswamy, S. S., Dua, G. L. and Sen Gupta (1966) : Physical work capacity as influenced by age. ***Ergonomics*** 9, 4 : 305-317.

Malhotra, M. S., Joseph, N. T. and Sen Gupta, J. (1973) : Physiological assessment of Indian Olympic hockey players. ***Indian Journal of Sports Medicine*** 2 : 5-10.

Mannix, E. T., Stager, J. M., Brechue, W. F. et al, (1988) : Phosphate Supplementation, cardiovascular function and exercise performance in humans. ***Journal of Applied Physiology*** 65 : 1821-6.

Marconi, C., Sassi, G., Carpinelli, A. et al, (1985) : Effects of L-Carnitine loading on the aerobic and anaerobic performance of endurance athletes. ***European Journal of Applied Physiology*** 54 : 131-5.

Maresh, C. M. (1981) : Influence of moderate altitude residents (2200 mts) on the acute mountain sickness and exercise response during early hypobaric hypoxia (4270 mt), Laramie, Wyoming, University of Wyoming ***Doctoral Dissertation***.

Martinean, L. and Jacobs, I. (1988) : Muscle glycogen utilization during shivering thermogenesis in humans, ***Journal of Applied Physiology*** 65 : 2046-50.

Mathur, D. N. (1970a) : Influence of interval training on blood sugar level. ***Track Technique*** 35 : 72-75.

Mathur, D. N. (1970b) : The physiological responses and requirements of participation in triple jump. In ***Encyclopaedia of Sports Sciences and Medicine***. Macmillan Press., New York, pp. 312-313.

Mathur, D. N. (1970b) : The physiological responses and requirements of participation in Hurdles. In ***Encyclopaedia of Sports Sciences and Medicine***. Macmillan Press, New Yorm., pp. 410-411.

Matson, L. G., Tran, Z. V. (1993) : Effects of sodium bicarbonate ingestion on anaerobic performance: a meta-analytic review. ***International Journal of Sports Nutrition*** 3 : 2-38.

Maughan, R. J. (1990) : Effect of diet composition on the performance of high intensity exercise. In ***Nutrition and Sports*** (Ed. H. Moncd) pp. 200-11 Masson, Paris.

Maughan, R. J. (1995) : Cratine supplementation and exercise performance. ***International Journal of Sports Nutrition*** 5 : 94-101.

McArdle, W. F. Katch and Katch, V. (1986) : ***Exercise Physiology***, Philadelphia, Lae & Febiger.

McNaughton, L. (1992) : Bicarbonate loading and its use in sports. ***International Clinical Nutrition Review*** 12 : 65-7.

McArdle, W. F. Katch and V. Katch (1986) : ***Exercise Physiology***, Energy, Nutrition and human performance, Philadelphia, Lae and Febiger.

McCully, K. et al, (1991) : Biochemical adaptation to training. Implications for resisting muscle fatigue. ***Canadian Journal of Physiology and Pharmacology*** 69 : 274-278.

Mckirnan, M. D., Gray, C. G. and White, F. C. (1991) : Effects of feeding on muscle blood flow during prolonged exercise in miniature swine. ***Journal of Applied Physiology*** 70 : 1097-1104.

Medbo, J. et al, (1988) : Anaerobic capacity determined maximal accumulated O_2 deficit, ***Journal of Applied Physiology*** 64 : 50-60.

Meijer, G. A. L., Janssen, GME., Westerterp, K. R., Verhoeven, F., Saris, WHM., Ten Hoor, F. (1991) : The effect of a 5 month endurance training program on Physical activity : evidence for a sex difference in the metabolic response to exercise. ***European Journal of Applied Physiology*** 62 : 11-17.

Meijer, G. A. L. (1990) : Physical activity, implications for human energy metabolism ***Thesis, University of Limburg***, Maastricht, The Netherlands.

Meredith, C. N., Frantera, W. R., Fisher, E. C., Hughes, V. A., Herland, J. C., Edward, J. and Evans, W. J. (1989) : Peripheral effects of endurance training in young and old subjects, ***Journal of Applied Physiology*** 66 : 2844-9.

Merton, P. A. (1954) : Voluntary strength and fatigue. ***Journal of Physiology*** 123 : 553-64.

Metzger, J. M., Fitts, R. H. (1986) : Fatigue from high and low frequency muscle stimulation role of sarcolemma action potentials. ***Experimental Neurology*** 43 : 320-333.

Mole, P. (1983) : "Exercise Metabolism" In ***Exercise Medicine : Physiological Principles and Clinical Application***, New York, Academic Press.

Morganroth, J., Maron, B., Henry, W. and Epstein, S. (1975) : Comparative left ventricular dimensions in trained athletes, ***Annals of International Medicine*** 82 : 521-524.

Muido, L. (1946) : The influence of Body Temperature on Performances in Swimming, ***Acta Physiologica Scandinavia*** 12 : 102.

Muoio, D. M., Leddy, J. J., Horvath, P. J. et al, (1994) : Effect of dietary fat on metabolic adjustments to maximal VO_2 and endurance in runners, ***Medicine and Science in Sports and Exercise*** 26 : 81-8.

Murray, R., Paul, G. L., Seifert, J. G., Eddy, D. E., Halaby, G. A. (1989) : The effect of glucose, fructose and sucrose ingestion during exercise. ***Medicine & Science in Sports and Exercise*** 21 : 275-282.

Mathur, D. N. (1969) : Influence of Interval training on blood sugar level. ***Track Technique*** 35 : 72-75.

Nair, C. S., Malhotra, M. S. and Gopinathan, P. M. (1971b) : Effect of altitude and cold acclimatization on the basal metabolism in man. ***Journal of Aerospace Medicine*** 42, 10 : 1056-1059.

Nair, C. S., Tiwari, O. P. and Malhotra, M. S. (1971a) : Effect of altitude acclimatization and cold on cold pressor response in man. ***Journal of Aerospace Medicine*** 42, 9 : 991-994.

Nakamura, Y. and S. Schwartz, (1972) : The influence of hydrogen ion concentration on calcium binding and release by skeletal muscle sarcoplasmic reticulum. ***Journal of General Physiology*** 59 : 22-32.

Natali, A., Santoro, D., Brandi, L. et al, (1993) : Effects of acute hypercarnitinemia during increased fatty substrate oxidation in man. ***Metabolism*** 42 : 594-600.

Newman, F. et al, (1961) : A comparison between body size and lung function of swimmers and normal school children. ***Journal of Physiology*** 156 : 9-16.

Nielsen, B., Savard, G., Richter, E. A., Hargreaves, M. and Saltin, B. (1990) : Muscle blood flow and muscle metabolism during exercise and heat stress. ***Journal of Applied Physiology*** 69 : 1040-6.

Norman, B., Sollevi, A., kaijser, L., Jansson, E. (1987) : ATP breakdown products in human skeletal muscle during prolonged exercise to exhaustion. ***Clinical Physiology*** 7 : 503-509.

Norman, B., Sollevi, A., Kaijser, L. and Jansson, E. (1987) : ATP breakdown products in human skeletal muscle during prolonged exercise to exhaustion. ***Clinical Physiology*** 7 : 503-9.

Nutter, D., Gilbert, C., Heymsfield, S., Perkins, J. and Schlant, R. (1975) : Cardiac hypertrophy in the endurance athletes, ***Physiologist*** 18 (3) : 336.

O' Reilly, K. P., Warhol, M. J., Fielding, R. A., Frontera, W., Meredith, C. N. et al, (1987) : Eccentric exercise induced muscle damage impairs muscle glycogen repletion. ***Journal of Applied Physiology*** 64 : 252-256.

Oscai, L., Williams, B. and Hertis, B. (1968) : Effect of exercise on blood volume, ***Journal of Applied Physiology*** 24 (5) : 622-624.

Owen, M. D., Kregel, K. C., Wall, P. T., Gislfi, C. V. (1986) : Effects of ingesting carbohydrate beverages during exercise in the heat. ***Medicine & Science in Sports and Exercise*** 18 : 568-575.

Oyono-Enguelle, S., Freund, H., Ott, C. et al, (1988) : Prolonged submaximal exercise and L-carnitine in humans. ***European Journal of Applied Physiology*** 58 : 53-61.

Parry-Billings, M. and D. M. MacLaren. (1986) : The effect of sodium bicarbonate and sodium citrate ingestion on anaerobic power during intermittent exercise. ***European Journal of Applied Physiology*** 55 : 524-29.

Pasman, W. J., Van Baak, M. A., Jeukendrup, A. E. et al, (1995) : The effect of different dosages of caffeine on endurance performance time. ***International Journal of Sports Medicine*** 16 : 225-30.

Pette, D. (1980) : ***Plasticity of muscle***, New York: Walter de Gruyter.

Pette, D. and Spamer, C. (1986) : Metabolic properties of muscle fibers, ***Federation Proceedings*** 45 : 2910-14.

Pette, D. (1987) : Activity induced fast to slow transition in mammalian muscle. ***Medicine and Science in Sports and Exercise*** 16 : 517-28.

Power, S. et al, (1987) : Oxygen deficit debt relationship in ponies during submaximal treadmill exercise. ***Respiratory Physiology*** 70 : 251-64.

Power, S. E., Howky and R. Cox. (1982) : Ventilatory and metabolic reactions to heat stress during prolonged exercise, ***Journal of Sports Medicine and Physical Fitness*** 22 : 32-36.

Power, S. et al, (1983) : Ventilatory threshold, running economy, and distance running performance. ***Research Quarterly*** 54 : 179-182.

Power, S., Dodd, S. and Beadle, R. (1985) : Oxygen uptake kinetics in trained athletes differing in O_2 max, ***European Journal of Applied Physiology*** 39 : 407-15.

Pugh, L. C. G. E. (1964) : Muscular exercise at great altitude. ***Journal of Applied Physiology*** 19 : 431.

Pugh, L. G. C. E. (1964) : Cardiac output in muscular exercise at 5,800 mt (19000 ft). ***Journal of Applied Physiology*** 19 : 441.

Railly, T. and Brooks, G. A. (1990) : Selective persistence of circadian rhythm in physiological responses to exercise. ***Chronobiology Internal*** 7 : 59-67.

Richter, D. (1982) : Generation and maintenance of the respiratory rhythm. ***Journal of Experimental Biology*** 100 : 93-107.

Richter, D., Ballantyne, D. and Remmers, J. (1986) : How is the respiratory rhythm generated? ***A Model News in Physiological Sciences*** 1 : 109-11.

Riley, W. S., Power, S. and Welch, H. (1981) : The effect of two levels of muscular work on urinary creatine excretion, ***Research Quarterly For Exercise and Sports*** 52 : 339-47.

Robertson, R. et al, (1982) : Effect of induced alkalosis on differentiated perceptions of exertion during arm and leg ergometry, ***Medicine and Science in Sports and Exercise*** 14 : 158.

Roggers, C. C. (1985) : Cyclists try caffeine suppositories, ***Physician and Sports Medicine*** 13 : 38-40.

Rowell, L. (1974) : ***Human Circulation Regulation During Physical Stress***, New York : Oxford press.

Rubin, S. (1987) : Core temparature regulation of heart rate during exercise in humans, ***Journal of Applied Physiology*** 62 : 1997-2002.

Saltion, K., Katz, A., Broberg, S. (1990) : Tricarboxylic acid cycle intermediates in human muscle during prolonged exercise. ***American Journal of Physiology*** 259 : C834-C841.

Sale, D. G. (1987) : Influence of exercise and training on motor unit activation. In (K.B. Pandolf. ed) ***Exercise and Sport Sciences Reviews***, Volume 15 : 95-151. New York : MacMillan Publishing Company.

Saltin, B. and Karlsson, J. (1971) : Muscle glycogen utilisation during work of different intensities. In ***Muscle Metabolism During Exercise***, (Eds B Pernon and B. Saltin) pp. 289-99, Plenum Press, New York.

Saltin, B., Blomqvist, G., Mitchell, J., Johnson, R. (1968) : Wildenthal, K. and Chapman, C. : Response to exercise after bedrest and after training. ***Circulation*** Suppl. 7.

Saltin, B., Grover, R. F., Blomquist, C. G. and others (1968) : Maximal oxygen uptake and cardiac output after 2 weeks at 4300 mt. ***Journal of Applied Physiology*** 25 : 400.

Saltin, B. and Karlsson, J. (1971) : Muscle glycogen utilization during work of different intensities, in pernow (ed) : ***Muscle Metabolism During Exercise***, pp. 289-299 (Pienum Press, New York).

Saltin, B. (1969) : Physiological effects of physical conditioning. ***Medicine Science Sports*** 1 : 50.

Saltin, B., Hartley, L., Kilbom, and Astrand, I. (1969) : Physical training sedentary middle aged and older men II, Oxygen uptake, heart rate and blood lactate concentrations at submaximal and maximal exercise, ***Scandinavian Journal of Clinical Lab Investigation*** 24 : 323-334.

Saltin, K., Katz, A. and Broberg, S. (1990) : Tricarboxylic acid cycle intermediates in human muscle during prolonged exercise. ***American Journal of Physiology*** 259 : C834-C841.

Saltin, B. et al, (1977) : Fiber types and metabolic potentials of skeletal muscles in sedentary man and endurance runners. ***Annal — New York Academy of Science*** 301-3.

Savabi, F., Geiger, P. J., Bessman, S. P. (1984) : Myofibrillar end of creatine phosphate energy shuttle. ***American Journal of Physiology*** 247 : C424-C432.

Schan, F. A., Hollmann, W., Liesen, H. and Waterloh, E. (1980) : Elektromen-mikroskopische Befunde am M. Vastur lat von Untrainlerten and Marathon Laufern Sowice iwea Beziehug zur relativen maximalen Sarerstoffanfnahme und laktat production. ***Dtsch. Z, Sportmed*** 31 (12) : 343.

Scheuer, J. et al, (1974) : Experimental observations on the effects of physical training upon intrinsic cardiac physiology and biochemistry. ***American Journal of Cardiology*** 33 : 744.

Schon, F. A., Hollmann, W., Leser, H & Sejersted, O. M., Vollestad, N. K. & Medbo, J. I. (1986) : Muscle fluid and electrolyte balance during and following exercise. ***Acta Physiologica Scandinavica*** 128 (Suppl. 5560 : 119-127).

Schön, F. A., Hollman, W., Liesen, H. and Waterioh, E. (1980) Elektronen — mikroskopische befunde an M. Vastus Lat. Von Untrainierten und Marathon laufern sowie ihre Beziehung zur relativen maximalev sauerstoffaufnane und laktatproducktion Disch z sportmed 31 (12) 343.

Scruggs, K. D., Martin, N. B., Broader, C. E., Hofman, Z., Thomas, E. L., Wambsgans, K. C. and Wilmore, J. H. (1991) : Stroke volume during submaximal exercise in endurance trained normotensive subject and in untrained hypertensive subject with β-blocked (Propranolo and Pindolol). ***American Journal of Cardiology*** 67 : 416 : 421.

Seals, D. R., Hagberg, J. M., Allen, W. K., Hurley, B. F., Dalsky, G. P., Ehsami, A. A. and Holloszy, J. O. (1984) : Glucose tolerance in young and older athletes and sedentary men, ***Journal of Applied Physiology*** 56 1521-5.

Sen, R. N. and Banerjee, S. (1958) : Determination of basal metabolic rate and blood concentration of protein bound iodine, cholesterol, and glucose in Indians. ***Indian Journal of Medical Research*** 46 : 759-765.

Sen, R. N., Chatterjee, S. K., Saha, P. N. and Subramanian A. (1964) : Assessment of work load and thermal stress in relation to physiological responses of workers in a cotton textile mill in Bombay. *Report no. 3*, ***Industrial Physiology Division, CLI, Bombay*** pp. 27.

Sen, R. N. (1954) : Studies on energy metabolism. ***Masters' Thesis***, Calcutta University, pp. 101.

Sen, Gupta, J., Malhotra, M. S. and Ramaswamy, S. S. (1972) : Exercise dyspnoea and work performance at sea level and at altitude. ***Indian Journal of Physiology and Pharmacology*** 16, 1 : 47-53.

Sen, R. N. (1955) : Fatigue and how to avoid it. Presidency College, ***Physiology Institute Journal*** 5 : 28-32.

Sen, R. N., Chatterjee, S. K., Saha, P. N. (1965) : Physiological stress and physiological strains on workers in a steel rolling mill in Bombay. Paper presented in the international seminar on ***Health Productivity*** Bombay.

Sharp, R. L., Costill, D. L., Fink, W. J. & Kind, D. S. (1986) : Effects of eight weeks of bicycle ergometer sprint training on human muscle buffer capacity, ***International Journal of Sports Medicine*** 7 : 3-17. Harmansen and Wachtlova 1971.

Sherman, W. M., Costill, D. L., Fink, W. J. and Miller, J. M. (1981) : The effect of exercise and diet manipulation on muscle glycogen and its subsequent utilization during performance. ***International Journal of Sports Medicine*** 2 : 114-18.

Sherman, W. M., Leenders, N. (1995) : Fat loading the next magic bullet? ***International Journal of Sports Nutrition*** 5 (Suppl.) S1-12.

Sherman, W. M., Brodowicz, G., Wright, D. A., Allen, W. K., Simonsen, J. et al, (1989) : Effect of 4th pre exercise carbohydrate feedings on cycling performance. ***Medicine and Science in Sports and Exercise*** 21 : 598-604.

Sherman, W. M., Costill, D. L., Fink, W. J., Hagerman, F. C., Armstrong, L. E. et al, (1983) : Effect of a 42.4 Km foot trace and subsequent rest or exercise on muscle glycogen and enzymes. ***Journal of Applied Physiology*** 55 : 1219-1224.

Simonson, E., N. Teslenko and M. Gorkin (1936) ; Einfluss von Vorubungen auf die Liestung beim 100 m. Lauf, ***Arbeitsphysiology*** 9 : 152.

Skinner, J. and Mclellal, T. (1980) : The transition from aerobic to anaerobic exercise. ***Research Quarterly*** 51 : 234-48.

Soderlund, K., Balsom, P. D., Ekblom, B. (1994) : Creatine supplementation and high intensity exercise: influence on performance and muscle metabolism. ***Clinical Science*** 87 : 120-1.

Sodhi, H. S. (1980b) : A study of morphology and body composition of Indian Basketball players, ***Journal of Sports Medicine and Physical Fitness*** 21 : 50.

Sodhi, H. S. (1980a) : Cardio-respiratory fitness and performance on cycle ergometer, ***Journal of Sports Medicine and Physical Fitness*** 20 : 100.

Soop, M., Bjorkman O., Cederblad G. et al, (1988) : Influence of carnitine supplementation on muscle substrate and carnitine metabolism during exercise. ***Journal of Applied Physiology*** 64 : 2394-9.

Spencer, M. K., Yan, Z., Katz, A. (1991) : Carbohydrate supplementation attenuate IMP accumulation in human muscle during prolonged exercise. ***American Journal of Physiology*** 261 : C71-C76.

Spriet, L. L., MacLean, Da., Dyck, D. J. et al, (1992) : Caffeine ingestion and muscle metabolism during prolonged exercise in humans. ***American Journal of Physiology*** 262 (Endocranial. Metab. 25) : E891-8.

Spriet, L. L. (1995) : Caffeine and performance, ***International Journal of Sports Nutrition*** 5 suppl. : S84-S99.

Stainsby, W. (1986) : Biochemical and physiological bases for lactate production, ***Medicine and Science in Sports and Exercise*** 18 : 341-43.

Steen, S. E., Opptiqer, R. A. and Brownell, K. D. (1988) : Metabolic effects of repeated weight loss and regain in adolescent wrestlers. ***Journal of American Medical Association*** 260 : 47-50.

Steak, M. J., Chopman, C., Stirling, J. L. and others (1978) : Effect of exercise, altitude and food on blood hormone and metabolites levels. ***Journal of Applied Physiology*** 45 : 350.

Stryer, L. (1981) : ***Biochemistry***, San Francisco, W. H. Freeman.

Stryer, L. (1988) : ***Biochemistry***, San Francisco, W. H. Freeman., Holloszy, J. (1982) : Muscle metabolism during exercise, ***Archieves of Physical and Rehabilitation Medicine*** 63 : 231-234.

Suttie, J. (1977) : ***Introduction to Biochemistry***, New York; Holt Rinehart & Winston.

Sutton, J. R. and Farrell, P. (1988) : ***Endocrine Responses to Prolonged Exercise***, Exercise science and sports medicine, Vol. 1, Edited by D. R. Lamb and Murray : Indianapolis, Benchmark Press 1.

Tarnapolsky, L. J., Mac Dougall, J. D., Atkinson, S. A., Tarnapolsky, M. A. and Sutton, J. R. (1990) : Gender differences in substrate for endurance exercise. ***Journal of Applied Physiology*** 61 : 2162-7.

Tarnopolshy, M. A. (1994) : Caffeine and endurance performance, ***Sports Medicine*** 18 : 109-25.

Tesch, P. et al, (1978) : Muscle fatigue and its relation to lactate accumulation and LDH activity in man. ***Acta Physiologica Scandinavia*** 103 : 413-420.

Tesch, P. A., Thorsson, and P. Kaiser (1984) : Muscle capillary supply and fibre type characteristics in weight and power fibers. ***Journal of Applied Physiology***, 56 : 35-38.

Tipton, C. (1965) : Training and bradycardia in rats. ***American Journal of Physiology*** 209 : 1089-1094.

Tipton, C., Barnard, R. and Tcheng, T. (1969) : Resting heart rate investigations with trained and non trained hypophysectomemed rats, ***Journal of Applied Physiology*** 26 (5) : 585-588.

Toates, F. (1975) : ***Control Theory in Biological and Experimental Physiology*** London, Hutchinson Education.

Tremblay, M. S., Galloway, S. D., Sexsmith, J. R. (1994) : Ergogenic effects of phosphate loading: Physiological fact and methodological fiction? ***Canadian Journal of Applied Physiology*** 9 : 1-11.

Trevidi, B. and W. H. Danforth, (1966) : Effect of pH on the kinetics of frog muscle phosphofructokinase. ***Journal of Biological Chemistry*** 241 : 4110-4112.

Turkevich D., Micco, A. and Reeves, J. T. (1988) : Non invasive measurement of the decrease in left ventricular filling time during maximal exercise in normal subjects. ***American Journal of Cardiology*** 62 : 650-652.

Van Handel, P. Caffeine. In: Williams, M. H., editor. (1983) : ***Ergogenic Aids in Sport***, Champaign: Human Kinetics Publishers, Inc. 128-63.

Vander, A. J., Sherman, J. H., Luciano, D. S. (1980) : Chapter 10 Muscle; in ***Human Physiology The Mechanism of Body Function*** 3rd ed. pp. 211-249 (McGraw-Hill, New York).

Vanier, M., Sarto, P., Martines, D. et al, (1994) : Effects of infusion branched chain amino acid during incremental exercise with reduced muscle glycogen content. ***European Journal of Applied Physiology*** 69 : 26-31.

Vecchiet, L., Di Lisa, F., Pieralisi, G. et al, (1990) : Influence of L-carnitine administration of maximal physical exercise. ***European Journal of Applied Physiology*** 61 : 486-90.

Vergara, J., Tsien, R. Y., Delay, M. (1985) : Inositoll, 4, 5 triphosphate, A possible chemical link in excitation contraction coupling in muscle. ***Proceeding of National Academy of Sciences*** USA. 82 : 6352-6356.

Voet, D. and Voet, J. G. (1990) : ***Biochemistry***, New York, John Wiley and Sons).

Vogel, J. A., Hartley, L. H., Cruz, J. C. and others (1974) : Cardiac output during exercise in sea level residents at sea level and altitude. ***Journal of Applied Physiology*** 36 : 169.

Vogel, J. A. and Hansen, J. E. (1966) : Cardio-vascular function during exercise at high altitude. In Goddard R. F. Ed. ***The Effect of Altitude on Physical Performance*** Chicago. The Athletic Institute.

Vollestad, N. and O. Sejersted (1988) : Biochemical correlates of fatigue, ***European Journal of Applied Physiology*** 57 : 336-37.

Vollestad, N. K., Vaage, O., Harmansen, L. (1984) : Muscle glycogen depletion pattern in type I and subgroups of type II fibers during prolonged severe exercise in man. ***Acta Physiologica Scandinavia*** 122 : 433-441.

Vollestad, N. K. and Blom, P. C. S. (1985) : Effect of varying exercise intensity on glycogen depletion in human muscle fibers. ***Acta Physiologica Scandinavica*** 125 : 395-405.

Vukovich, M. D., Costill, D. L., Hickey, M. S. et al, (1993) : Effect of fat emulsion infusion and fat feeding on muscle glycogen utilisation during cycle exercise. ***Journal of Applied Physiology*** 75 : 1513-8.

Vukovich, M., Costill, D., Fink, W. L. (1994) : Carnitine supplementation effect on muscle carnitine content and glycogen utilization during exercise. ***Medicine and Science in Sports and Exercise*** 26 : 1122-9.

Wahren, L., Fetig, P., Ahlborg, G. and Jorfeidt, L. (1971) : Glucose metabolism during leg exercise in man. ***Journal of Clinical Investigations*** 50 : 2715-25.

Wailer, B. A., Eriksen, M. and Jonbu, T. (1990) : The effect of a meal on cardiac output in man at rest and during moderate exercise, ***Acta Physiologica Scandinavica*** 140 : 167-173.

Wasserman, K. and M. Mclroy (1964) : Detecting the threshold on anerobic metabolism. ***American Journal of Cardiology*** 14 : 844-52.

Wasserman, K. et al, (1973) : Anaerobic threshold and respiratory gas exchange during exercise, ***Journal of Applied Physiology*** 35 : 236-43.

Waterloh, E. (1980) : Elektronen Nickroskopische Befunde asslafern sowie ihre Beziehug Zwe relative maximalen Sanerstoffanfanahme und Laktatproduktion, ***Dtsch Z, Sportmed*** 31 (12) : 343.

Weatherwax, R. S., Ahlberg, A., Deady, M. et al, (1986) : Effects of phosphate loading on bicycle time trial performance [abstract]. ***Medicine and Science in Sports and Exercise*** 18 : S11-S12.

Welch, H. G. (1987) : Effects of hypoxia and hyperoxia on human performance. In (K.B: Pandolf. ed.) ***Exercise and Sports Sciences Reviews***, Vol. 15 : 191-222. New York: Macmillan Publishing Company.

West, J. B., Boyer, S. J., Graber, D. J., Hackett, P. H., Maret, K. H., Milledge, J. S., Peters, Jr., R. M., Pizzo, C. J., Samaja, M., Sarnquist, F. H., Schoene, R. B. and Winslow, R. M. (1983) : Maximal exercise at extreme altitudes on Mount Everest. ***Journal of Applied Physiology*** 55 : 688-698.

Westerterp, K. R., Meijer, G. A. L., Janssen, G. M. E., Saris, W. H. M. and ten Hor, F. (1991) : Long term effect of physical activity on energy balance and body composition. ***British Journal of Nutrition*** (Submitted).

Westertrap, K. R., Saris, W. H. M., Van Es, M. and ten hoorf (1986) : Use of the doubly labelled water technique in humans during heavy sustained exercise. ***Journal of Applied Physiology*** 61 : 2162-7.

Wilcox, A. R., Caffeine and endurance performance (1990) : ***Sports Science Exchange*** May: 3 (26) : 1-4.

Wilkes, D. N., N. Gledhill, and R. Smyth. (1983) : Effect of acute induced metabolic alkalosis on 800-m racing time. ***Medicine and Science in Sports and Exercise*** 15 : 277-80.

Williams, M. H. (1995) : Nutritional ergogenics in athletics. ***Journal of Sports Science*** 13 : S63-74.

Williams, C. (1995) : Micronutrient and performance. ***Journal of Sports Science*** 13 : S1-10.

Williams, C. (1993) : Carbohydrate needs of elite athletes. In simpoulas AP, Pavion KN editors. ***Nutrition and Fitness for Athletes***, Vol. 70. 71. World Review of Nutrition and Dietetics. Basal Karger 34-60.

Wilmore, J. and Costill, D. (1988) Training for sports and activity Dubuque, La Wmc Brown.

Willmore, J. H. and Costill, D. L. (1994) : ***Physiology of Sports and Exercise*** Human Kinetics.

Wilmore, J. H. and Haskell, W. L. (1972) : Body composition and endurance capacity of professional football players. ***Journal of Applied Physiology*** 33 : 564-570.

Wolfe, R. R., Goodenough, R. D., Wolfe, M. H. et al, (1982) : Isotopic analysis of leucine and urea metabolism in exercising humans. ***Journal of Applied Physiology*** 52 : 458-66.

World Health Organization (1985) : Energy and protein requirements report of a joint ***FAO/WHO/UNU Expert Consultation.*** Technical Report Series, 724, Geneva.

Wyss, V., Ganzit, G. P., Rienzi, A. (1990) : Effects of L-carnitine administration on VO_2 max and the aerobic-anaerobic threshold in normoxia and acute hypoxia. ***European Journal of Applied Physiology*** 60 : 1-6.

Young, A. J., Sawaka, M. N., Levine, L., Cadarette, D. S. and Pandolf, K. B. (1985) : Skeletal muscle metabolism during exercise influenced by heat acclimatization, ***Journal of Applied Physiology*** 59 : 1929-35.

Young, A. J., Evans, W. J., Cymerman, A., Pandolf, K. B., Knapik, J. J. and Maher, J. T. (1982) : Sparing effect of chronic high altitude exposure on muscle glycogen utilisation, ***Journal of Applied Physiology*** 52 : 857-62.

